The alli™
Diet Plan

Your Essential Guide
to Success with alli™

Caroline Apovian, M.D.

Foreword by John P. Foreyt, Ph.D.

Produced by The Philip Lief Group, Inc.

Meredith® Books
Des Moines, Iowa

Meredith Books
1716 Locust Street
Des Moines, Iowa 50309–3023
www.meredithbooks.com

First Edition. Printed in the United States of America.
Library of Congress Control Number: 2006932660
ISBN: 978-0-696-23538-2

alli, alli Shuttle, and various design elements are trademarks of GlaxoSmithKline.

READ AND FOLLOW THE LABEL ON THE ALLI™ PRODUCT BEFORE TAKING.

This diet and fitness book is designed to provide helpful information on the subjects addressed. This book is sold with the understanding that the author, editors and consultants, producer, and publisher are not engaged in rendering medical, health, or any other kind of personal professional services. The suggestions for specific exercise routines, foods, medications, and lifestyle recommendations are not intended to replace medical advice or treatment by your physician. All questions and concerns regarding your health, metabolism, weight, nutrition, and physical activity or medication should be directed to your physician, particularly if you have any health problem or medical problems (including if you are pregnant or lactating). All reasonable attempts have been made to include the most recent and factual research and medical reports regarding exercise and nutrition. However, there is no guarantee that future research, particularly human studies, will not change the information presented here. Individual needs vary, and no nutrition or exercise program or medication will meet everyone's needs. Be sure to consult your physician prior to following any of the suggestions presented in this book and also before changing your diet or exercise routine or starting a new medication. You should rely on your physician's advice regarding whether the suggestions presented in this book are appropriate for you, and you should rely on your physician to establish your weight goal. The author, editors and consultants, producer, and publisher disclaim all liability associated with the recommendations and guidelines set forth in this book. The brands and restaurants listed are meant to give you an idea of the types of products and services being referred to. They are not being endorsed by the author, editors and consultants, producer, or publisher, nor have the products, companies who produce the products, or restaurants endorsed the diet or fitness plans in this book or the book.

To all those who have suffered emotionally
from their weight—may this book offer relief

contents

foreword

I was privileged to be one of the primary researchers charged with investigating the benefits of orlistat—the active ingredient of alli™—in one of the largest double-blind, placebo-controlled studies ever designed to evaluate a diet drug therapy for weight loss and prevention of weight gain. Researchers and scientists from renowned weight-loss and research centers around the world spent 22 years conducting more than 100 trials, all to ensure that alli™ would be the most effective and safest drug of its kind ever brought to market.

I can say with the utmost confidence that we succeeded. Studies have found that those who take alli™ and follow a reduced calorie, low-fat diet can lose 50 percent or more weight than through dieting alone.

For anyone who struggles with losing weight and keeping that weight off, alli™ offers help. It is the only over-the-counter weight-loss aid, clinically proven and approved by the Food and Drug Administration (FDA). And, unlike other medications, alli™ is absorbed minimally into the bloodstream. It is non-systemically acting, so it has no effect on the brain or heart. Rather, alli™ works directly in the intestine with the body's natural enzymes to prevent the digestive system from absorbing a portion of the fat you eat.

Alli™, however, is not a miracle drug. The power of alli™ comes from taking the alli™ capsule in combination with a reduced-calorie, low-fat diet and following a regular exercise plan. Dr. Caroline Apovian, Director of the Center for Nutrition and Weight Management at Boston University Medical Center, has developed the reduced-calorie, low-fat plan in this book complete with recipes, menus, and a fitness plan to help you gain the optimal effectiveness from alli™. This important book, *The alli™ Diet Plan*, is tailored to be a partner in helping you lose weight with alli™.

By committing to diet, fitness, taking the alli™ capsules, and following Dr. Apovian's plan, you can lose from 1 to 2 pounds a week, allowing you to reach and maintain your goal weight.

—John P. Foreyt, Ph.D.
Professor, Department of Medicine,
Director of the Behavioral Medicine Research Center
Baylor College of Medicine, Houston, Texas

the power of the alli™ diet plan

You are about to embark on a true revolution in dieting—an eating plan that works in tandem with alli™, the only FDA-approved, clinically tested, proven-to-work, over-the-counter weight loss aid. There is nothing else like it because the alli™ capsules, taken in combination with using *The alli™ Diet Plan*, can help accelerate the rate at which you lose weight by 50 percent or more.

As a physician, nutrition specialist, and Director of the Center for Nutrition and Weight Management at Boston University Medical Center, I've been helping women and men lose weight for over 20 years. I know how difficult it is to take off pounds and keep them off. I've seen thousands of intelligent, motivated people who are successful in other areas of their lives, except dieting. They've tried diets from Atkins to the Zone and everything in between. They come to me knowing the benefits of maintaining a healthy weight. Yet, in spite of their knowledge and determination, they still struggle to lose weight and keep it off permanently. That all changes, however, when I introduce them to *The alli™ Diet Plan*.

How alli™ Works

Alli™ is a weight loss aid that belongs to a class of drugs called lipase inhibitors. Lipase is a digestive enzyme that breaks down fat in the food you eat so that it can be absorbed, stored, and used by the body as needed. Alli™ works directly in the digestive tract by preventing the action of lipase, thus inhibiting your body's absorption of fat. Alli™ diverts about one-quarter of the fat you eat directly to your intestines and colon, where it gets flushed from your body.

Alli™ was designed to work most effectively when taken while eating a reduced-calorie, low-fat meal containing 30 percent of calories from fat. Thirty percent of fat on a limited number of calories is what will help you achieve the maximum benefit from alli™.

Alli™ is different from other diet aids on the market. Other weight loss products are appetite suppressants that work by altering brain chemistry and stimulating the central nervous system in ways that make you jittery, irritable, and restless. They may also have other negative side effects. Alli™, however, works directly within the digestive tract. It is only minimally systemic (meaning only a tiny amount is absorbed into your bloodstream), so it has no effect on brain chemistry or the central nervous system. In other words, it's not going to affect your mood, behavior, or body in any adverse way.

Safe and Steady Weight Loss

During the last 22 years, scientists have conducted more than 100 studies (in more than 30 countries) on the active ingredient in alli™, orlistat, and proven it to be safe and effective, even for long-term use. During the September 2006 International Congress on Obesity, researchers reported on 3 separate studies that followed more than 1,700 dieters for 6 to 12 months and found that more people taking alli™ lost a significantly larger amount of body weight than those who followed only a low-fat diet.

In addition to weight loss, alli™ can have other health benefits. The same studies found that the dieters who took alli™ also had greater decreases in cholesterol levels, blood pressure levels, and waist circumference.

Alli™ capsules are for overweight adults (18 years or older). Most people can take the alli™ capsules safely, but you should not take them, or you should get your doctor's advice first, if you have specific health conditions or take certain medications. Read the label on the alli™ product carefully.

With the assistance of alli™, this diet plan can help you attain the weight loss results that you've always wanted but have not yet been able to achieve. Alli™ is not a magic bullet, but if you take the alli™ capsules as directed and follow the menus and recipes according to this diet's three-phase plan, you should lose weight at a healthy and steady rate of 1 to 2 pounds a week.

Treatment Effects

The reduced-calorie, low-fat diet outlined in this book is designed to balance your fat intake throughout the day to help avoid any unwanted effects. Alli™ is tolerated well only if it is taken with a meal, that contains 30 percent or less fat calories. Eating more than 30 percent fat calories can cause treatment effects. They include more frequent bowel movements, an urgent need to go to the bathroom, and gas with an oily discharge. You may not experience treatment effects right after eating a high-fat meal, but you could within 24 to 72 hours after you've consumed the meal. The other time you could experience treatment effects is when you first begin taking the alli™ capsule. The important point to keep in mind in either case is that these effects are in no way harmful and should subside fairly quickly as you adjust to the new diet.

How the Plan Works

The alli™ diet consists of three phases. You will eat a specific number of calories and grams of fat each day. Your calories will remain the same, but the total amount of fat you are allowed to eat each day will increase as you advance to Phase 2 and Phase 3. In Phase 1, you will eat a diet in which 15 percent of your daily calories comes from fat. In Phase 2, 20 percent of your calories will come from fat. In Phase 3, you will eat meals that are 30-percent fat—the target for optimal weight loss. During all the phases, you will take one alli™ capsule with each main meal containing fat. Each phase is discussed in more detail later in the chapter.

This is not as hard as it might sound because all of the calorie and fat counting has already been done for you. *The alli™ Diet Plan* features more than 300 daily menus, specially developed and calibrated for each phase of the program at each calorie level. There are menus for those who love to cook and menus for those who hate to cook, menus for those with little time on their hands, and menus for those who enjoy being a weekend gourmet. There are meals without red meat, meals without fish, and even meals without any type of meat, fish, or poultry. There are no-cook menus for those days when you know you won't be able to cook. There is such a wide variety in menus, you should have no problem selecting meals that contain foods you love to eat. And you'll never go over your target fat and calorie intake or risk treatment effects.

More Food, Less Fat

On the alli™ diet, you'll be surprised by how much food you're able to eat. Because you'll be limiting the amount of fat in your diet, you'll end up with more room for protein and carbohydrate calories. This is because, ounce for ounce, fat contains more than twice the number of calories as the same amount of protein and carbohydrates—9 calories per gram of fat compared to 4 calories per gram of protein and carbohydrates.

Just because alli™ blocks your body's ability to absorb some fat doesn't mean that you can eat more fat than is recommended on the plan. Remember, alli™ blocks fat absorption relative to the amount of fat you eat. Therefore, the more fat you consume, the more fat alli™ will prevent from entering your system, which increases the risk of experiencing unwanted treatment effects.

A Vitamin a Day

Alli™ does not absorb all the fat you eat, and for good reason. Your body needs a certain amount of fat in order to maintain healthy cells. Fat is also the main transportation system for certain nutrients—specifically vitamins A, D, E, and K. Because some of the fat that would normally carry these essential nutrients and distribute them ultimately gets eliminated by taking alli™, you can help ensure that you are getting adequate amounts by taking a multivitamin every day that contains the daily value (DV) for each. Take your multivitamin at bedtime. It is a good health practice, just like brushing your teeth. In fact taking it at bedtime when you brush your teeth is a good way to remember. Just don't take your multivitamin within two hours, either before or after, of taking your alli™ capsule.

And Exercise Too

The alli™ Diet Plan also includes a fitness program that consists of easy-to-follow walking and toning exercises that will provide you with the blueprint you need to achieve good health for the rest of your life.

Before You Begin

1. **Be informed.** Read and follow all label instructions on the alli™ product.

2. **Set a realistic goal weight.** This means a weight that is healthy and appropriate to your size and build—not someone else's.

3. **Ease into the plan.** Start reducing the fat in your diet for a few days prior to beginning the program. Some high-fat foods to consider eating less of include mayonnaise, salad dressings, fried foods, baked goods, chips, and whole-dairy products. In their place try substituting mustard, flavored vinegars, grilled or broiled foods, fruit, and low-fat dairy products.

4. **Clean house—literally.** Go to your kitchen and remove those fatty foods that tempt you the most. If other people in your household still want to eat these foods, place them out of sight or on a hard-to-reach shelf. Or ask your family to support your efforts by eating these foods when you are not around.

5. **Go shopping.** Plan your meals before the start of each week, then go to the market and buy the ingredients you need for the entire week's menu. Make sure you get a variety of low-fat, low-calorie snacks as well.

6. **Prepare to get moving.** You may want to buy a comfortable pair of walking shoes and inexpensive hand weights to get you started on your fitness program. An inexpensive pedometer can also be very helpful; it will help you become aware of just how far you are walking.

7. **Set up a support system.** Having a diet buddy, or an encouraging friend, can make a difference. Recruit anyone you know who will help support your interest in losing weight and maintaining a healthy lifestyle.

8. **Keep a diet journal.** Studies have shown that the single biggest predictor of weight loss success is keeping a diet journal. Use it to record your weekly meal plans and what you eat each day, log your exercise, and keep track of your weekly weight loss. You can also use your journal to set your goals, follow their progress, and record your personal feelings about your dieting experience. You can even use your journal to help you identify meals that could be causing treatment effects, rate recipes, and note your new eating habits.

Pick Your Calorie Target

To find your calorie target, use the chart below as your guide. Find your current weight and your current activity level to determine the number of calories you will eat each day. This is the calorie level that should help you lose weight at a steady pace. And, because you are taking alli™, you should be able to lose at least 50 percent or more than you would if you followed the diet alone.

CURRENT WEIGHT	WOMEN		MEN	
	Low Activity	Moderate Activity	Low Activity	Moderate Activity
110–114	1,200 cals	1,200 cals	1,200 cals	1,500 cals
115–119				
120–124		1,500 cals		1,800 cals
125–129				
130–134			1,500 cals	
135–139				
140–144				
145–149			1,800 cals	
150–154	1,500 cals			
155–159				
160–164				
165–169		1,800 cals		
170–174				
175–179				
180–184				
185–189	1,800 cals			
190–194				
195 and up				

Low activity: Little or no walking, stair-climbing, doing yard work, or other physical activity.
Moderate activity: You burn at least 150 calories three or more days a week through physical activity such as walking approximately two miles, gardening for 30 to 45 minutes, or running 1.5 miles in 15 minutes.

Three Phases

Here's what you can expect during the three phases of the alli™ diet:

Phase 1

During this phase you will begin to get into the habit of taking one alli™ capsule with each main meal containing fat. As a reminder, set your bottle of capsules out where you can see it. Also keep some in the alli shuttle™ (the carrying case provided when you buy alli™) and put it in your purse or briefcase so you always have the capsules with you when you are at work or dining out.

You'll start out by reducing your total fat intake to 15 percent of the calories you eat per day. Stay on this phase for one week. Do not be discouraged if you do not lose weight during this week. It is designed primarily for you to adjust to the alli™ diet and minimize or eliminate treatment effects. If you feel comfortable and are adjusted to your new diet, you can move on to the next phase at any time during the first week.

The chart below shows how your calorie and fat allowance is spread throughout the day when you use the menus on pages 23 through 69. You'll be eating the same amount of fat at each main meal, but calories will vary to allow you a larger meal at lunch than at breakfast and a larger meal at dinner than at lunch.

PHASE 1 – 15% of Calories from Fat						
	1,200 Calories 20 Grams of Fat		1,500 Calories 25 Grams of Fat		1,800 Calories 30 Grams of Fat	
Meal	**Fat (g)**	**Calories**	**Fat (g)**	**Calories**	**Fat (g)**	**Calories**
Breakfast	6	250	7	350	8	400
Lunch	6	350	8	450	10	550
Dinner	6	400	8	500	10	650
Snacks	2	200	2	200	2	200

Phase 2

During this phase you will increase your total fat intake to 20 percent of calories per meal. Continue to take one alli™ capsule with each main meal containing fat, but no more than three a day. As with Phase 1, you will be in this phase for one week. You may experience minimal treatment effects during this phase. As long as you are comfortable with the diet, you can skip ahead to Phase 3 at any time during this week.

Notice that the percentage of fat you consume increases during this phase, even though your calories remain the same as in Phase 1. Below are the breakdowns used in the menus on pages 23 through 69.

PHASE 2 – 20% of Calories from Fat					
	1,200 Calories 26 Grams of Fat		1,500 Calories 33 Grams of Fat		1,800 Calories 40 Grams of Fat	
Meal	Fat (g)	Calories	Fat (g)	Calories	Fat (g)	Calories
Breakfast	8	250	10	350	12	400
Lunch	8	350	10	450	13	550
Dinner	8	400	11	500	13	650
Snacks	2	200	2	200	2	200

Phase 3

This is the phase when weight loss should shift into full gear. You'll increase your daily fat intake to 30 percent of calories per meal. This reduced-fat, low-calorie formula should get maximum benefit out of the alli™ capsule. Continue to take one alli™ capsule with each main meal containing fat, but still no more than three a day. In this final phase you should see a steady, moderate weight loss of 1 to 2 pounds a week as you have modified your diet to a healthy and realistic fat intake. You will stay with the 30 percent per meal fat level and one capsule with each meal until you reach your weight loss goal. The chart below shows how your fat and calorie intake is divided in the meal plans on pages 23 through 69.

PHASE 3 – 30% of Calories from Fat					
	1,200 Calories 40 Grams of Fat		1,500 Calories 50 Grams of Fat		1,800 Calories 60 Grams of Fat	
Meal	Fat (g)	Calories	Fat (g)	Calories	Fat (g)	Calories
Breakfast	9	250	13	350	14	400
Lunch	12	350	15	450	18	550
Dinner	13	400	16	500	22	650
Snacks	6	200	6	200	6	200

Notice that your fat intake increases even more in this phase, but your calories are still the same. This is the amount of fat and calories that will help you achieve your goal weight.

Make the Most of Every Meal

All the menus and recipes featured in this book are designed to provide you with the amount of fat and calories that work best with the alli™ capsules. A healthy diet needs a complement of the main nutrients. Carbohydrates, found in fruits, vegetables, and whole grains, are the body's main source of energy. Protein, found in meat, poultry, fish, eggs, dairy products, and beans, serves the primary role of keeping your cells healthy. Fats, found in oils, nuts, and animal products, provide energy and also perform essential functions that keep your organs and cells healthy. Any diet plan that eliminates one of these essential nutrients will not work in the long run and may actually be harmful.

I encourage you to take advantage of the menu plans in this book. The menus eliminate the need for daily food planning and counting fat grams and calories. The weekday meals are designed so that you can quickly get them on the table. The menu plans also include many already-prepared options. In fact, for your convenience, you'll find a no-cook alternative for every recipe in the book, starting on page 70.

I also encourage you to try the recipes. In addition to being delicious, the 200-plus recipes are quick and easy to make and provide fat and calorie counts for each serving. All the recipes use shortcut ingredients whenever possible, such as canned chicken broth instead of homemade stock and canned beans instead of dried. Most of the recipes can be on the table in 30 minutes or prepared ahead of time. Some, especially soups and casseroles, are easy to freeze.

Because you're likely to eat out sometime during the week, the book includes the best picks of more than 100 restaurants—even fast-food places—that will allow you to stay on the alli™ diet. Plus you'll find smart tips on how to spot fat in menu items in any restaurant.

The alli™ diet meal plans and recipes take the guesswork out of choosing what to eat and ensure that you never have to go it alone in terms of choosing the right foods, controlling fat, limiting calories, and managing portion sizes.

Planning Your Own Menus

If you prefer to plan your own meals rather than follow the meal plans, you need to figure out the amount of fat you should have each day. Take your calorie target level from page 12 and follow this simple two-step equation to find out your calories from fat and your total fat grams for each day.

Step 1: Multiply your calorie level by the percentage of fat (15, 20, or 30 percent) to get the total calories from fat each day.

Step 2: Divide the total calories from fat by 9 (the number of calories in a gram of fat) to get total grams of fat each day.

For example, let's say you are in Phase 3 of the 1,500-calorie-a-day plan, in which 30 percent of your calories should come from fat, and you are planning to eat a 500-calorie dinner.

500 calories × .30 (30% fat) = 150 calories from fat

150 calories ÷ 9 (calories per gram of fat) = 16.7 grams of fat

Make room for snacks. Make sure to plan snacks in your daily allotment. A good rule of thumb is to aim for a total of 200 calories and 2 to 6 grams of fat per day for snacks. (Thirty percent of a 100-calorie snack is 3 grams.) For suggestions, see the snack lists starting on page 80.

Consider your calories. The alli™ menus balance fat grams by providing 30 percent (or less) fat calories per meal. The meal plans in this book allow for more calories at lunch than at breakfast and more calories at dinner than at lunch. If you prefer your main meal at lunch, simply flip the meals. You can design your meals any way you want as long as you target and do not exceed 30 percent of calories from fat at any meal and stay within your daily calorie allowence.

Use the alli™ recipes. Planning menus using the alli™ recipes is easy because all the fat and calories in each dish are designed to fit within the alli™ diet. If you want to try other recipes, use only cookbooks that list calories and fat grams for each serving.

Watch your fats. Get familiar with the Nutrition Facts labels on packaged foods. Some foods that claim to be low-fat, reduced-fat, reduced-calorie, or light (or lite) can be misleading. For example, light olive oil suggests a lower fat content when, in fact, it refers to a lighter color (all oil is 100 percent fat). Also pay attention to the kinds of fat the food contains. Avoid trans fat, man-made fats that help extend the life of packaged foods, and saturated fat as much as possible. Saturated fats are found only in animal products. Opt for foods containing monounsaturated fat, such as olive oil and nuts, and omega-3 fatty acids, which are found in cold-water fish such as salmon.

Check the serving size. Note that product nutritional counts are given per serving, so make sure to check out how many servings are in the product or food you are buying.

Use this quick cheat sheet. Trying to keep tabs on your diet by the percentage of fat in your calories can get confusing. You can make sure you're getting no more than 30 percent of calories from fat in any food by using the formula on page 16 or the chart below when shopping:

If calories are:	15% of calories-fat grams should be less than:	20% of calories-fat grams should be less than:	30% of calories-fat grams should be less than:
50	1	1.1	2
100	1.6	2.2	3
150	2.5	3.3	5
200	3.3	4.4	7
250	4	5.5	8
300	5	6.6	10
350	6	8	12
400	6.6	9	13
450	7.5	10	15
500	8	11	17
550	9	12	18
600	10	13	20

You are embarking on a new, exciting chapter of your life—one that is steeped in good health and delicious meals—armed with the understanding that you can indeed lose and control your weight. The alli™ capsule and *The alli™ Diet Plan* are your partners in the journey.

Frequently Asked Questions

Q. Now that I have your book, do I need the booklets that came with my alli™ starter pack?

A. Yes. Use all the tools you can for the program—the capsules, the program education that comes with the starter pack, as well as the website myalliplan.com, which provides you with interactive tools and a community of individuals on the alli™ program.

Q. How do I best pick a starting date to begin taking alli™?

A. Pick the day you will begin taking alli™ capsules and start the diet before you begin taking the capsules. If possible, start taking alli™ capsules on a weekend when you are home, in case you experience treatment effects.

Q. What if I forget to take an alli™ capsule with a meal?

A. It simply means you won't get the fat-blocking benefits of alli™ for that meal. Alli™ works specifically on the meal you consume with the capsule, though you can take the forgotten capsule up to one hour after the meal. Never double up on the capsule at the next meal.

Q. I don't like to eat breakfast. Can I just pass on that meal?

A. Alli™ works best when you eat three healthy, low-fat meals a day. Also studies have shown that a healthy breakfast is an important forecaster of success when trying to lose weight and keep it off. People who skip breakfast tend to overeat later in the day. Eating a healthy breakfast also ignites your metabolism, which is key to losing weight. So consider why you don't like breakfast and write down the reason in your diet journal. Is it because you're too short on time, or is it just habit? Breakfast doesn't have to be an elaborate meal. There are plenty of quick, satisfying breakfast choices in the meal plans. Have breakfast when others would be having a morning snack. But don't skip it.

Q. A holiday is coming up. I know I'm going to eat more than 30 percent fat at dinner. Should I double up on my alli™?

A. No. You should not plan to eat high-fat meals when you are trying to lose weight—and that includes holidays. Plan a holiday meal using the recipes in this book instead. As you progress through the diet, you will discover new ways of eating that will lead you to automatically start making better choices! The menus and recipes in this book are planned to complement a normal lifestyle. That includes the holidays too.

Q. Can I have a glass of wine with dinner if I take alli™?

A. Drinking alcoholic beverages while taking alli™ capsules has no effect on the action of alli™ and alli™ has no effect on the action of alcohol. However, drinking alcohol can have an effect on your appetite. For many people alcohol whets the appetite. Also don't forget that alcoholic beverages contain calories—a glass of wine has about 120 calories. You need to adjust for it in your daily calorie allotment. Another reason to be cautious about alcohol is that it tends to weaken willpower. You might set out with good intentions, but after a couple of drinks, two servings of dessert seem quite irresistible.

Q. I'm on Phase 2 and I haven't lost any weight. What am I doing wrong?

A. Nothing. I designed Phases 1 and 2 in order for you to get accustomed to the diet and to help minimize or eliminate treatment effects. Although you may experience weight loss during these two phases, you should really start to notice steady, gradual weight loss during Phase 3.

Q. I started losing weight on the plan, but then stopped. What happened?

A. If you stop making progress after losing weight—especially if you have lost five percent or more of your body weight—you've probably reached a plateau. This means your body is at its new reduced weight and needs fewer calories to function than it did at your old weight. To continue losing weight, reset your calories and fat targets based on your new weight (see chart on page 12). If you are still not losing weight, you most likely are eating too many calories—probably more than you realize. This is another reason why keeping a diet journal is important. It is easy to forget a snack or extra serving you ate, especially if you're eating on the run or feeling stressed. In addition to tracking your food intake, use your journal to record events that may cause you to overeat.

Q. What should I do when I have a craving for chocolate or potato chips?

A. It's bound to happen! If you're craving sweets, eat some fruit. Grapes or cherries or any fruit you can eat one at a time will help keep you satisfied. Try the recipe for Frozen Grapes on page 304. Or try sugar-free hard candy. When salty snacks are on your mind, try some crunchy vegetables like celery or cucumber slices. Another tactic is to exercise or take a walk. It will distract you and boost your mood.

Q. I have high blood pressure and have been following the DASH (Dietary Approaches to Stop Hypertension) Diet. Is it okay to take alli™?

A. The alli™ diet complements the DASH Diet in that it is low in fat, concentrates on incorporating fruits and vegetables into your diet, and encourages a healthy eating style. However, some of the recipes do call for salt and canned ingredients, which tend to be higher in sodium than fresh foods. You can follow the alli™ recipes as long as you avoid salt, use low-sodium stocks, and rinse canned goods. That said, if you have high blood pressure, it means you are under a doctor's care and most likely take medication. As with anyone with a medical condition, you should not change your dietary habits without first consulting with your physician.

Q. Does it matter what kind of fat I eat?

A. For the sake of good health, the alli™ diet emphasizes good fats, mainly the monounsaturated variety found in such things as olive oil and nuts. Monos have the unique ability to lower bad LDL cholesterol and raise HDL cholesterol, among other healthy benefits. Plus the alli™ diet menus call for using artificial butter substitutes that contain no trans fats. Overall, the alli™ diet limits total fat intake to 30 percent or less calories per meal, so you can be confident you are following a healthy diet. As a general health rule, you should try to limit your intake of saturated fat, which is found only in animal products, and avoid trans fats, man-made fats that extend the shelf life of convenience foods and make french fries crispier and sweets smoother. Trans fats have been found to have negative health effects, including increasing the risk of heart disease and contributing to obesity. Manufacturers are making efforts to eliminate trans fats, but they are not totally off the market yet.

Q. I already walk 30 to 60 minutes every day, which is the goal time on the alli™ exercise program. What can I do to get more exercise?

A. Get in the 10,000 Steps Program. The program is sponsored by Shape Up America! and the only requirement to join is to buy an inexpensive pedometer. Clip it on in the morning and take it off at night. The goal is to cover 10,000 steps a day, about 5 miles. To find out more about the program go to the website at www.shapeup.org.

Q. Why do you put so much emphasis on keeping a diet journal?

A. Simply because weight loss research shows that those who keep a daily diet journal are more successful at weight loss than those who don't. You use a diet journal to keep a record of your calorie and fat intake, track your weight loss both in weight and inches, and log your exercise. You can even use it as a personal diary to write about your weight loss goals and your emotional ups and down while dieting. It can be a very effective tool.

Q. How long can I continue to take alli™?

A. You can continue taking alli™ until you reach your goal weight. Just remember that the maximum dosage is one capsule three times a day with each main meal containing fat.

meal plans

The essence of *The alli™ Diet Plan* is its menus. They are designed to guarantee that you'll get the correct amount of calories and fat—plus a good complement of nutrients—at every meal. These menus, which are designed around the 200-plus alli™ recipes in chapter six, will take you through each phase of the alli™ diet.

With almost 300 different menus, the plan provides a variety of meals, so finding ones that appeal to you should be easy. Created to accommodate today's busy lifestyle, these menus are divided into three categories: weekday menus, weekend menus, and no-cook menus. The majority should meet your weekday needs—simple to prepare and easy to get on the table in 30 minutes or less. Weekend menus are designed for when you have additional time to cook and experiment with the tasty alli™ recipes. However, the recipes are still easy to make and you won't spend the whole day in the kitchen. The no-cook menus are for those days when you simply don't have the time or the inclination to cook.

Like the menu, but you are less than enthusiastic about one or two of the recipe selections? That's covered too. Starting on page 70, you will find a list of convenience foods that can substitute for almost every recipe listed. The same goes for the snacks. All the recommended snacks in the menus can be substituted by any of the reduced-calorie, low-fat choices starting on page 80. Only choose a snack with more than 2 grams of fat if you are on the 1,800-calorie plan.

What menu you eat on any given day doesn't matter as long as you adhere to your calorie level and the phase of the diet that you are following. Rest assured, the menus were developed to promote weight loss *and* good health. All menus are:

- Designed to distribute fat intake throughout the day, which is key to getting the maximum effectiveness from taking alli™ capsules
- Nutritionally balanced
- Filled with a variety of foods to meet a variety of tastes

I recommend that you choose your menus at the beginning of each week so that you can do all your food shopping at one time. As you continue on the alli™ diet, you will grow accustomed to the alli™ style of eating. Eventually you may want to do your own menu planning. (To find out how to design your own menus, see page 16.) For now, though, leave it up to me.

A few words about using these menus:

- Recipes are for 1 serving unless otherwise indicated. Also choose medium fruits and vegetables unless indicated differently.
- "Margarine, reduced-fat" refers to any of the nonhydrogenated butter substitutes on the market. Buy the product of your preference; just make sure that it is free of trans fats.
- No-cook menus are included for those times when convenience foods are your only choice. Make them the exception rather than the rule. Eating natural foods is always your best choice.
- Whole grains help increase your fiber intake. So use whole grains whenever you can, even if it is not indicated in the menu.
- Brands are used in many places in order to keep calorie and fat counting accurate. They are in no way an endorsement for the product.

These menus and the wide variety of delicious foods they include will make your transition to the alli™ diet simple and successful. Good luck and enjoy!

Weekday Menu PHASE ① 15% Fat

1,200 CALORIES 20 GRAMS FAT	1,500 CALORIES 25 GRAMS FAT	1,800 CALORIES 30 GRAMS FAT
BREAKFAST Multi-Grain Cheerios, 1 c. Milk, 2%, 1 c. Strawberries, sliced, ½ c.	Multi-Grain Cheerios, 1½ c. Milk, 2%, 1 c. Blueberries, ½ c.	Multi-Grain Cheerios, 1½ c. Milk, 2%, 1¼ c. Banana, 1
LUNCH Roast beef, deli, 2 oz. Bread, whole wheat, 2 slices Mayonnaise, nonfat, 2 T. Horseradish, 1 tsp. Tomato, 3 thick slices Apple, 1	Roast beef, deli, 4 oz. Bread, whole wheat, 2 slices Mayonnaise, nonfat, 2 T. Horseradish, 1 tsp. Tomato, 3 thick slices Apple, 1	Roast beef, deli, 4 oz. Bread, whole wheat, 2 slices Mayonnaise, nonfat, 2 T. Horseradish, 1 tsp. Tomato, 3 thick slices Apple, 1
SNACK Health Valley Apple Granola Bar	Pretzels, 1 oz.	Pretzels, 1 oz.

DINNER
*Sizzlin' Shrimp w/Black-Eyed
  Peas* (p. 201)
Couscous, whole wheat, ½ c.
Steamed green beans, ½ c.
	*Sizzlin' Shrimp w/Black-Eyed
	  Peas,* (p. 201) 1½ srv.
	Couscous, whole wheat, ½ c.
	Steamed green beans, ½ c.
		*Sizzlin' Shrimp w/Black-Eyed
		  Peas,* (p. 201) 1½ srv.
		Couscous, whole wheat, ¾ c.
		Steamed green beans, 1 c.

SNACK Low-fat cake	Fat-free cake	Fat-free cake
20 grams fat 1,208 calories	**24 grams fat 1,502 calories**	**30 grams fat 1,817 calories**

Weekday Menu PHASE ① 15% Fat

1,200 CALORIES 20 GRAMS FAT	1,500 CALORIES 25 GRAMS FAT	1,800 CALORIES 30 GRAMS FAT
BREAKFAST *Cranberry Muffin* (p. 141), 1 Milk, 1%, 1 c.	*Cranberry Muffins* (p. 141), 2 Milk, fat-free, 1 c.	*Cranberry Muffins* (p. 141), 2 Milk, 1%, 1 c.; Grapefruit, ½

LUNCH
Campbell's Chunky Beef w/Country
  Vegetables Soup, 1½ c.
Sourdough roll, 1
	Campbell's Chunky Beef
	  w/Country Vegetables Soup,
	  2 c.
	Sourdough roll, 1
	Peach, 1
		Campbell's Select Three Cheese
		  Mushroom Ravioli w/Veg-
		  etables Soup, 2 c.
		Whole wheat dinner rolls, 2
		Plums, 2

SNACK Nabisco Ginger Snaps, 4	Nabisco Ginger Snaps, 4	Nabisco Ginger Snaps, 3

DINNER
Drunken Pork Chops (p. 247)
Baked potato
Steamed green beans, 1 c.
	Drunken Pork Chops (p. 247),
	  1½ srv.
	Baked potato
	Steamed green beans, 1 c.
		Drunken Pork Chops (p. 247),
		  1½ srv.
		Mashed Sweet Potatoes (p.
		  282), 2 srv.
		Peas, 1 c.

SNACK Dried figs, 2 pieces	Dried figs, 2 pieces	Dried apricots, 5 pieces
20.3 grams fat 1,213 calories	**25.2 grams fat 1,497 calories**	**29.4 grams fat 1,795 calories**

Weekday Menu PHASE ① 15% Fat

1,200 CALORIES 20 GRAMS FAT	1,500 CALORIES 25 GRAMS FAT	1,800 CALORIES 30 GRAMS FAT

BREAKFAST
Smart Ones English Muffin
  Sandwich, 1
Orange juice, 4 oz.
	Smart Ones English Muffin
	  Sandwich, 1
	Orange juice, 4 oz.
	Dannon Light 'n Fit yogurt,
	  4 oz.
		Smart Ones English Muffin
		  Sandwich, 1
		Orange juice, 8 oz.

LUNCH
*Warm Potato and Tuna
  Salad* (p. 174)
Whole wheat potato roll, 1
	Warm Potato and Tuna Salad
	  (p. 174), 1½ srv.
	Whole wheat potato roll, 1
		Warm Potato and Tuna Salad
		  (p. 174), 1¾ srv.
		Whole wheat dinner roll, 1

SNACK Dannon Light 'n Fit, 4 oz.	Dried apricots, 4 pieces	Plum, 1

DINNER
*Roast Chicken w/Winter
  Vegetables* (p. 230)
Mashed Potatoes (p. 284)
	*Roast Chicken w/Winter
	  Vegetables* (p. 230), 1½ srv.
	Mashed Potatoes (p. 284)
		*Roast Chicken w/Winter
		  Vegetables* (p. 230), 2 srv.
		Mashed Potatoes (p. 284), 1½ srv.

SNACK
*Mixed Fruit w/Strawberry-Ginger
  Sauce* (p. 298)
	*Mixed Fruit w/Strawberry-
	  Ginger Sauce* (p. 298)
		*Mixed Fruit / Strawberry-Ginger
		  Sauce* (p. 298)

19.6 grams fat **1,208 calories**	**24.3 grams fat** **1,522 calories**	**28.6 grams fat** **1,808 calories**

Weekday Menu PHASE ① 15% Fat

1,200 CALORIES 20 GRAMS FAT	1,500 CALORIES, 25 GRAMS FAT	1,800 CALORIES, 30 GRAMS FAT
BREAKFAST Grape-Nuts Flakes, ¾ c. Milk, 2 %, 1 c. Strawberries, sliced, ½ c.	Grape-Nuts Flakes, ¾ c. Milk, 2 %, 1 c. Banana, 1	Grape-Nuts Flakes, 1 c. Milk, 2 %, 1 c. Banana, 1

LUNCH
Amy's Whole Meals Chili &
  Cornbread
	Amy's Whole Meals Chili &
	  Cornbread
	Fig Newtons, 2
		Amy's Whole Meals Chili &
		  Cornbread
		Fig Newtons, 4

SNACK Plum, 1	Plum, 1	*Frozen Grapes* (p. 304), 1 c.

DINNER
*Sizzlin' Shrimp w/Black-Eyed
  Peas* (p. 201)
Polenta, ½ c.
Mixed greens w/ranch fat-free
  dressing, 2 T.
	*Sizzlin' Shrimp w/Black-Eyed
	  Peas* (p. 201), 1¼ srv.
	Polenta, ¾ c.
	Mixed greens w/ranch fat-
	  free dressing, 2 T.
		*Sizzlin' Shrimp w/Black-Eyed
		  Peas* (p. 201), 1¾ srv.
		Polenta, 1 c.
		Mixed greens w/ranch fat-free
		  dressing, 2 T.

SNACK *Baked Apples* (p. 294)	*Baked Apples* (p. 294)	*Baked Apples* (p. 294)
20.4 grams fat **1,202 calories**	**24.8 grams fat** **1,499 calories**	**29.7 grams fat** **1,812 calories**

Weekday Menu PHASE ① 15% Fat

1,200 CALORIES 20 GRAMS FAT	1,500 CALORIES 25 GRAMS FAT	1,800 CALORIES 30 GRAMS FAT
BREAKFAST		
Egg, boiled or poached, 1 Thomas' 100% Whole-Wheat English Muffin, 1 Grapefruit juice, 4 oz.	Egg, boiled or poached, 1 Thomas' 100% Whole-Wheat English Muffin, 1, w/margarine, reduced-fat, 1 tsp., and jam, 1 T. Grapefruit juice, 8 oz.	Egg, boiled or poached, 1 Thomas' 100% Whole-Wheat English Muffin, 1, w/margarine, reduced-fat, 2 tsp., and jam, 1 T. Grapefruit juice, 8 oz.
LUNCH		
Pineapple Chicken Sandwich (p. 232)	*Pineapple Chicken Sandwich* (p. 232) Potato chips, baked, 1 oz.	*Pineapple Chicken Sandwich* (p. 232) Potato chips, baked, 1 oz. Dannon Light 'n Fit yogurt, 4 oz.
SNACK		
Pear, 1	Pear, 1	Pear, 1
DINNER		
Greens w/*Balsamic Mustard Dressing* (p. 332) *Caribbean Fish Stew* (p. 195) Brown rice, ½ c.	Greens w/*Creamy Italian Dressing* (p. 336) *Caribbean Fish Stew* (p. 195) Brown rice, 1 c.	Greens w/*Balsamic Mustard Dressing* (p. 332) *Caribbean Fish Stew* (p. 195), 1½ srv. Brown rice, 1 c.
SNACK		
Apple, 1	Apple, 1	Apple, 1
19.7 grams fat 1,202 calories	**24.2 grams fat 1,542 calories**	**30.9 grams fat 1,789 calories**

Weekday Menu PHASE ① 15% Fat

1,200 CALORIES 20 GRAMS FAT	1,500 CALORIES 25 GRAMS FAT	1,800 CALORIES 30 GRAMS FAT
BREAKFAST		
Asparagus Omelet, (p. 144) Whole wheat toast, 1 slice	*Asparagus Omelet,* (p. 144) Whole wheat toast, 2 slices	*Asparagus Omelet,* (p. 144) Whole wheat toast, 2 slices, w/jam, 1 T.
LUNCH		
Turkey breast, deli, 4 oz., on a hard roll w/lettuce, tomato, and fat-free mayo, 2 T. *Creamy Coleslaw* (p. 286)	Turkey breast, deli, 4 oz., on a hard roll w/lettuce, tomato, and fat-free mayo, 2 T. Kraft Singles, Pepper Jack, 1 slice *Creamy Coleslaw* (p. 286), *1 c.*	Turkey breast, deli, 6 oz., on a hard roll w/lettuce, tomato, and fat-free mayo, 2 T. Kraft Singles, Pepper Jack, 1 slice *Creamy Coleslaw* (p. 286), 1 c.
SNACK		
Dried plums, 4 pieces	Dried plums, 6 pieces	Dried figs, 3 pieces
DINNER		
Spaghetti w/Fresh Mushrooms and Red Sauce (p. 259) Mixed greens w/mandarin oranges, ½ c., and *Orange Vinaigrette* (p. 342)	*Spaghetti w/Fresh Mushrooms and Red Sauce* (p. 259), 1¼ srv. Mixed greens w/mandarin oranges, ½ c., and *Orange Vinaigrette* (p. 342)	*Spaghetti w/Fresh Mushrooms and Red Sauce* (p. 259), 1¼ srv. Mixed greens w/mandarin oranges, ½ c., and *Orange Vinaigrette* (p. 342) Italian bread, 1½" piece
SNACK		
Spiced Apples (p. 295)	*Spiced Apples* (p. 295)	*Spiced Apples* (p. 295)
19.5 grams fat 1,205 calories	**25 grams fat 1,496 calories**	**30 grams fat 1,801 calories**

Weekday Menu PHASE 1 15% Fat

1,200 CALORIES 20 GRAMS FAT	1,500 CALORIES 25 GRAMS FAT	1,800 CALORIES 30 GRAMS FAT
BREAKFAST Swanson Low Fat Eggs w/Canadian Bacon	Swanson Low Fat Eggs w/Canadian Bacon Pillsbury Buttermilk Biscuits, lower-fat, 2	Swanson Low Fat Eggs w/Canadian Bacon Pillsbury Buttermilk Biscuits, lower- fat, 2; Grapefruit, ½
LUNCH *Little Caesar Salad* (p. 162), w/cooked shrimp, 8 large Club roll, 1	*Little Caesar Salad* (p. 162), 1¼ srv., w/cooked shrimp, 8 large Club roll, 1	*Little Caesar Salad* (p. 162), 2 srv., w/cooked shrimp, 8 large Whole wheat dinner roll, 1
SNACK Apple, 1	Stonyfield Farm Fat Free Yogurt, blueberry, 6 oz.	Stonyfield Farm Fat Free Yogurt, blueberry, 6 oz.
DINNER *Tomato-Corn Bisque* (p. 150) Lean Cuisine Grilled Chicken w/Teriyaki Glaze	*Tomato-Corn Bisque* (p. 150) Lean Cuisine Pork w/Cherry Sauce *Mixed Fruit w/Strawberry-Ginger Sauce* (p. 298)	*Tomato-Corn Bisque* (p. 150), 2 srv. Lean Cuisine Chicken a L'Orange *Mixed Fruit w/Strawberry-Ginger Sauce* (p. 298)
SNACK *Mixed Fruit w/Strawberry- Ginger Sauce* (p. 298)	Stella D'oro Anisette Sponge Cookies, 2	Stella D'oro Sponge Anisette Cookies, 2
19.4 grams fat **1,201 calories**	**24.5 grams fat** **1,490 calories**	**29.8 grams fat** **1,807 calories**

Weekday Menu (Meatless) PHASE 1 15% Fat

1,200 CALORIES 20 GRAMS FAT	1,500 CALORIES 25 GRAMS FAT	1,800 CALORIES 30 GRAMS FAT
BREAKFAST Thomas' 100% Whole- Wheat English Muffin w/peanut butter, reduced- fat, 2 tsp., and Smucker's Low Sugar Fruit Preserves, 1 T. Milk, 1%, ½ c.	Thomas' 100% Whole-Wheat English Muffin w/peanut butter, reduced-fat, 2 tsp., and Smucker's Low Sugar Fruit Preserves, 1 T. Milk, 1%, 1 c.	Thomas' 100% Whole-Wheat English Muffin w/peanut butter, reduced-fat, 2 tsp., and Smucker's Low Sugar Fruit Preserves, 1 T. Milk, 1%, 1 c.; Orange, 1
LUNCH Amy's Fat Free Split Pea Soup, 1 c. Greens w/3 oz. tuna, hard- boiled egg, 1, and ranch dressing, fat-free, 2 T.	Amy's Fat Free Split Pea Soup, 1½ c. Greens w/3 oz. tuna, hard-boiled egg, 1, Kraft Shredded Cheddar, 2%, 2 T., and ranch dressing, fat-free, 2 T.	Amy's Fat Free Split Pea Soup, 1½ c. Greens w/3 oz. tuna, hard-cooked egg, 1, Kraft Shredded Cheddar, 2%, 2 T., and ranch dressing, fat-free, 2 T. Whole wheat potato roll, 1
SNACK Pear, 1	Pear, 1	Pear, 1
DINNER *Spinach Risotto* (p. 266)	*Spinach Risotto* (p. 266), 1¼ srv.	*Spinach Risotto* (p. 266), 1¾ srv.
SNACK Tangerine, 1	Dried figs, 2 pieces	Dried figs, 2 pieces
19.8 grams fat **1,221 calories**	**24.7 grams fat** **1,497 calories**	**29.4 grams fat** **1,820 calories**

Weekday Menu PHASE 1 · 15% Fat

1,200 CALORIES 20 GRAMS FAT	1,500 CALORIES 25 GRAMS FAT	1,800 CALORIES 30 GRAMS FAT
BREAKFAST Aunt Jemima Cinnamon French Toast, 2 slices, w/Smucker's Sugar Free Pancake Syrup, 2 T. Milk, 1%, ½ c. Orange juice, 4 oz.	Aunt Jemima Cinnamon French Toast, 3 slices, w/Smucker's Sugar Free Pancake Syrup, 3 T. Milk, 1%, ½ c. Orange juice, 4 oz.	Aunt Jemima Cinnamon French Toast, 3 slices, w/Smucker's Sugar Free Pancake Syrup, 3 T. Milk, 1%, 1 c. Orange juice, 4 oz.
LUNCH *Asparagus Soup* (p. 149), ¾ srv. *Shrimp Salad Sandwich* (p. 202) Plum, 1	*Asparagus Soup* (p. 149) *Shrimp Salad Sandwich* (p. 202) Fresh cherries, 20	*Asparagus Soup* (p. 149), 1¼ srv. *Shrimp Salad Sandwiches* (p. 202), 1½; Fresh cherries, 20
SNACK Dried apricots, 2 pieces	Dried apricots, 4 pieces	Dried apricots, 3 pieces
DINNER *Vegetable Risotto* (p. 276) Grilled chicken breast, skinless and boneless, 4 oz.	*Vegetable Risotto* (p. 276) Grilled chicken breast, skinless and boneless, 6 oz.	*Vegetable Risotto* (p. 276), 1½ srv. Grilled chicken breast, skinless and boneless, 6 oz.
SNACK *Mixed Fruit* (p. 298)	*Mixed Fruit* (p. 298)	*Mixed Fruit* (p. 298)
19.2 grams fat 1,205 calories	**24.5 grams fat 1,513 calories**	**29 grams fat 1,793 calories**

Weekday Menu PHASE 1 · 15% Fat

1,200 CALORIES 20 GRAMS FAT	1,500 CALORIES 25 GRAMS FAT	1,800 CALORIES 30 GRAMS FAT
BREAKFAST Fruit plate of ⅛ cantaloupe and berries, ½ c. Cottage cheese, 2%, ½ c. *Cranberry Muffin*, (p. 141) 1	Fruit plate of ⅛ cantaloupe and berries, 1 c. Cottage cheese, 2%, ¾ c. *Cranberry Muffin*, (p. 141) 1	Fruit plate of ⅛ cantaloupe and berries, 1 c. Cottage cheese, 2%, 1 c. *Cranberry Muffin*, (p. 141) 1
LUNCH Lean Pockets Ultra Meatballs & Mozzarella, 1 Mixed lettuce salad w/Italian dressing, fat-free, 2 T. Health Valley Low-Fat Double Chocolate Cookies, 3	Lean Pockets Ultra Meatballs & Mozzarella, 1 Mixed lettuce salad w/Kraft Roasted Red Pepper Dressing, 2 T. Pretzels, 1 oz. Apple, 1	Hot Pockets Steak Fajita, 1 Mixed lettuce salad w/Italian dressing, fat-free, 2 T. Health Valley Low-Fat Double Chocolate Cookies, 4 Fresh cherries, 20
SNACK *Frozen Grapes* (p. 304), 1 c.	*Frozen Grapes* (p. 304), 1 c.	Pretzels, 1 oz.
DINNER *Tuna Noodle Casserole* (p. 203), 1½ srv. Steamed green beans, 1 c.	*Tuna Noodle Casserole* (p. 203), 1½ srv. Steamed green beans, 1 c. Buttermilk biscuits, 2	*Tuna Noodle Casserole* (p. 203), 2 srv. Steamed green beans, 1 c. Buttermilk biscuits, 2
SNACK *Spiced Apples* (p. 295)	*Spiced Apples* (p. 295)	*Spiced Apples* (p. 295)
20.3 grams fat 1,209 calories	**25.3 grams fat 1,481 calories**	**30.7 grams fat 1,807 calories**

Weekend Menu (Meatless) PHASE ① 15% Fat

1,200 CALORIES 20 GRAMS FAT	1,500 CALORIES 25 GRAMS FAT	1,800 CALORIES 30 GRAMS FAT
BREAKFAST *Sweet Potato Jacks* (p. 136), 1 Cottage cheese, ½ c. Pineapple chunks, ¼ c.	*Sweet Potato Jacks* (p. 136), 1 Cottage cheese, ½ c. Pineapple chunks, ¼ c. Banana, 1	*Sweet Potato Jacks* (p. 136), 2 Cottage cheese, ½ c. Pineapple chunks, ¼ c.
LUNCH *Texas Black Bean Soup* (p. 157) *Classic Spinach Salad* (p. 161)	*Texas Black Bean Soup* (p. 157), w/sour cream, light, 1 T. *Classic Spinach Salad* (p. 161) Soft breadstick, 1	*Texas Black Bean Soup* (p. 157), w/sour cream, light, 2 T. *Classic Spinach Salad* (p. 161) Soft breadsticks, 2
SNACK Peach, 1	Orange, 1	Banana, 1
DINNER *Sweet and Spicy Shrimp* (p. 200) *Tropical Rice* (p. 274) *Glazed Carrots* (p. 279)	*Sweet and Spicy Shrimp* (p. 200) *Tropical Rice* (p. 274) *Creamed Spinach* (p. 277)	*Caribbean Fish Stew* (p. 195) *Tropical Rice* (p. 274) *Glazed Carrots* (p. 279), 2 srv.
SNACK *Carrot Cake* (p. 293)	*Carrot Cake* (p. 293)	*Carrot Cake* (p. 293)
19 grams fat 1,205 calories	**25.3 grams fat 1,499 calories**	**30 grams fat 1,779 calories**

Weekend Menu PHASE ① 15% Fat

1,200 CALORIES 20 GRAMS FAT	1,500 CALORIES 25 GRAMS FAT	1,800 CALORIES 30 GRAMS FAT
BREAKFAST *Cranberry Muffin* (p. 141), 1 Fruit plate of ⅛ cantaloupe, blueberries, ¼ c., and strawberries, sliced, ¼ c. Ricotta cheese, light, ¼ c.	*Cranberry Muffin* (p. 141), 1 Fruit plate of ⅛ cantaloupe, blueberries, ¼ c., and strawberries, sliced, ¼ c. Ricotta cheese, light, ¼ c. Banana, 1	*Cranberry Muffin* (p. 141), 1 Fruit plate of ⅛ cantaloupe, blueberries, ¼ c., and strawberries, sliced, ¼ c. Ricotta cheese, light, 6 T. Banana, 1
LUNCH *Pasta w/Tomatoes* (p. 257) Italian bread, 1" piece Mixed lettuce salad, 1½ c. Kraft Roasted Red Pepper Dressing, 2 T.	*Pasta w/Tomatoes* (p. 257) Italian bread, 2" piece Mixed lettuce salad, 1½ c. Kraft Roasted Red Pepper Dressing, 2 T.	*Spaghetti w/Fresh Mushrooms* (p. 259) Italian bread, 1" piece Mixed lettuce salad, 1½ c. Kraft Roasted Red Pepper Dressing, 2 T. Crumbled blue cheese, 1 T.
SNACK *Pineapple-Mango Topping w/Frozen Yogurt* (p. 297)	Ice cream, Edy's or Breyers, light, ½ c.	*Pineapple-Mango Topping w/Frozen Yogurt* (p. 297)
DINNER *Tomato-Corn Bisque* (p. 150) *Shrimp Salad Sandwich* (p. 202)	*French Onion Soup* (p.152) *Shrimp Salad Sandwich* (p. 202)	*French Onion Soup* (p. 152) *Grilled Pineapple Chicken Sandwich* (p. 232); *Creamy Coleslaw* (p. 286), ½ c.
SNACK Sara Lee Free & Light Pound Cake, ⅛ cake	Archway Fat Free Oatmeal Raisin Cookie, 1	Sara Lee Free & Light Pound Cake, ⅛ cake
20 grams fat 1,207 calories	**24.7 grams fat 1,512 calories**	**30.5 grams fat 1,787 calories**

Weekend Menu PHASE (1) 15% Fat

1,200 CALORIES 20 GRAMS FAT	1,500 CALORIES 25 GRAMS FAT	1,800 CALORIES 30 GRAMS FAT

BREAKFAST
Blueberry Muffin (p. 140), 1
Dannon Natural Flavors
   Yogurt, 6 oz.
	Blueberry Muffins (p. 140), 2
	Dannon Natural Flavors
	   Yogurt, ½ c.
		Blueberry Muffins (p. 140), 2
		Dannon Natural Flavors
		   Yogurt, 6 oz.

LUNCH
Buttery Squash Soup (p. 151)
Tuna Noodle Casserole (p. 203)
	Buttery Squash Soup (p. 151),
	   1½ srv.
	Tuna Noodle Casserole (p. 203)
		Buttery Squash Soup (p. 151),
		   1½ srv.
		Tuna Noodle Casserole (p. 203),
		   1½ srv.

SNACK Peach, 1	Dried plums, 5 pieces	Dried plums, 5 pieces

DINNER
Drunken Pork Chops (p. 247)
Mashed Sweet Potatoes
   (p. 282), 1½ srv.
Steamed green beans, 1 c.
	Drunken Pork Chops (p. 247), 1½
	   srv.
	Mashed Sweet Potatoes (p. 282),
	   1½ srv.
	Steamed green beans, 1 c.
		Drunken Pork Chops (p. 247),
		   2 srv.
		Mashed Sweet Potatoes (p. 282),
		   2 srv.
		Steamed green beans, 1 c.

SNACK *Spiced Apples* (p. 295)	*Spiced Apples* (p. 295)	*Spiced Apples* (p. 295)
19.1 grams fat **1,201 calories**	**25 grams fat** **1,515 calories**	**30.4 grams fat** **1,800 calories**

Weekend Menu PHASE (1) 15% Fat

1,200 CALORIES 20 GRAMS FAT	1,500 CALORIES 25 GRAMS FAT	1,800 CALORIES 30 GRAMS FAT

BREAKFAST
Raisin Bran Muffin
w/Orange Glaze (p. 143)
Dannon Light 'n Fit Smoothie
   yogurt, 7 oz.
	Raisin Bran Muffin w/
	Orange Glaze (p. 143)
	Breyers Light Yogurt, 8 oz.
		Raisin Bran Muffin w/Orange
		Glaze (p. 143)
		Dannon Creamy Fruit Blends
		   Yogurt, 6 oz.

LUNCH *Linguine w/Clam Sauce* (p. 263)	*Linguine w/Clam Sauce* (p. 263) Italian bread, 1" piece	*Linguine w/Clam Sauce* (p. 263), 1¼ srv. Italian bread, 1" piece
SNACK Dried figs, 2 pieces	Dried figs, 2 pieces	Dried figs, 3 pieces

DINNER
Two-Potato Bisque (p. 159)
Grilled Chicken Caesar Salad
   (p. 170) w/grated Parmesan
   cheese, 1 T.
	Two-Potato Bisque (p. 159)
	Grilled Chicken Caesar Salad
	   (p. 170), 1½ srv., w/grated
	   Parmesan cheese, 2 T.
		Two-Potato Bisque (p. 159), 2 srv.
		Grilled Chicken Caesar Salad
		   (p. 170), 1½ srv., w/grated
		   Parmesan cheese, 2 T.

SNACK Pear, 1	Pear, 1	Pear, 1
19.8 grams fat **1,224 calories**	**25.4 grams fat** **1,503 calories**	**29.9 grams fat** **1,794 calories**

No-Cook Menu PHASE ① (Meatless) 15% Fat

1,200 CALORIES 20 GRAMS FAT	1,500 CALORIES 25 GRAMS FAT	1,800 CALORIES 30 GRAMS FAT
BREAKFAST Cheerios, 1 c., Milk, 2%, 1 c. Blueberries, ½ c.	Cheerios, 1 c., Milk, 2%, 1 c. Banana, 1	Raisin Bran, 1 c., Milk, 2%, 1 c. Banana, 1
LUNCH Lean Cuisine Salmon w/Basil Mixed greens, 2 c. Ranch dressing, fat-free, 2 T.	Lean Cuisine Salmon w/Basil Mixed greens, 2 c. Wish-Bone Light! Parmesan Peppercorn Ranch Dressing, 2 T. Whole wheat toast, 2 slices	Lean Cuisine Salmon w/Basil Mixed greens, 2 c. Wish-Bone Light! Parmesan Pep- percorn Ranch Dressing, 2 T. Whole wheat toast, 2 slices Fat-free oatmeal raisin cookie, 1
SNACK Pretzels, 1 oz.	Ice cream, fat-free, 1 c.	Orange, 1 large
DINNER Health Valley Potato Leek Soup 1 c. Amy's Shepherd's Pie Club roll, 1	Progresso Macaroni and Bean Soup, 1 c. Amy's Shepherd's Pie Club roll, 1	Progresso Macaroni and Bean Soup, 1 c. Amy's Whole Meals Chili & Corn- bread w/sour cream, fat-free, 2 T. Club roll, 1
SNACK Dried figs, 2 pieces	Fresh cherries, 20	Health Valley Apple Granola Bar, 1
20.5 grams fat **1,201 calories**	**25.5 grams fat** **1,519 calories**	**29 grams fat** **1,815 calories**

No-Cook Menu PHASE ① 15% Fat

1,200 CALORIES 20 GRAMS FAT	1,500 CALORIES 25 GRAMS FAT	1,800 CALORIES 30 GRAMS FAT
BREAKFAST Lean Pockets Bacon, Egg & Cheese Orange	Swanson Low-Fat Eggs w/Pancakes and syrup, 1 T. Orange	Swanson Low-Fat Eggs w/Canadian Bacon Whole-wheat toast, 2 slices
LUNCH Salad bar greens/vegetables, 2 c., w/Italian dressing, light, 2 T. Tuna (in water), 3 oz. Whole wheat bread, 2 slices Peach	Salad bar greens/vegetables, 2 c., w/Italian dressing, light, 2 T. Tuna (in water), 3 oz. Whole wheat bread, 2 slices Pear	Vegetable soup, 1 c. Salad bar greens/vegetables, 2 c., w/Italian dressing, light, 2 T. Tuna (in water), 3 oz. Whole wheat bread, 2 slices Pear
SNACK Kashi GoLean Crunch Bar, 1	Ice cream, fat-free, ½ c.	Ice cream, fat-free, ½ c.
DINNER Amy's Whole Meals Chili & Cornbread Sour cream, fat-free, 2 T. Pie, 6 oz.	Amy's Whole Meals Enchilada w/Spanish Rice and Beans Sour cream, fat-free, 2 T. Salsa, fat-free, ¼ c. YoPlait Light Custard Style Yogurt, 6 oz.	Amy's Whole Meals Enchilada w/Spanish Rice and Beans Sour cream, fat-free, 2 T. Salsa, fat-free, ¼ c. Guiltless Gour. Tortilla Chips, 1 oz. YoPlait Light Custard Style Yogurt, 6 oz.
SNACK YoPlait Light Yogurt, 6 oz.	Pretzels, 1 oz.	Kashi GoLean Crunch Bar, 1
19 grams fat **1,200 calories**	**25 grams fat** **1,480 calories**	**31 grams fat** **1,765 calories**

No-Cook Menu PHASE ① 15% Fat

1,200 CALORIES 20 GRAMS FAT	1,500 CALORIES 25 GRAMS FAT	1,800 CALORIES 30 GRAMS FAT
BREAKFAST Kellogg's Nutri-Grain Muffin Bar, 1 Dannon Light 'n Fit Yogurt, 6 oz. Strawberries, sliced, ½ c.	Nutri-Grain Muffin Bar, 1 Dannon Yogurt, 6 oz Strawberries, sliced, ½ c.	Quaker Oatmeal to Go Square, 1 Dannon Yogurt, 6 oz. Strawberries, sliced, ½ c.

LUNCH
Lean Pockets Ultra Ham &
  Cheese, 1
Campbell's Select Bean Soup, 1 c.
	Lean Pockets Turkey, Broccoli &
	  Cheese, 1
	Campbell's Select Bean Soup,
	  1 c.
		Lean Pockets Turkey, Broccoli &
		  Cheese, 1
		Campbell's Select Bean Soup, 1½ c.

SNACK Orange, 1 large	Orange, 1 large	Orange, 1

DINNER
Mixed greens, 2 c., w/ranch dress-
  ing, fat-free, 2 T.
Smart Ones Fajita Chicken
  Supreme, Corn, ¼ c.
	Mixed greens, 2 c., w/ranch
	  dressing, fat-free, 2 T.
	Smart Ones Chicken Enchilada
	  Suiza, Corn, ½ c.
	Sour cream, fat-free, 2 T.
		Mixed greens, 2 c. w/ranch dressing,
		  fat-free, 2 T.
		Smart Ones Chicken Enchilada Suiza
		  Corn, ½ c., Sour cream, fat-free, 2 T.,
		  Ready Rice, Spanish Style, ¾ c.

SNACK Pretzels, 1 oz.	Pretzels, 1 oz.	Vitalicious VitaBrownie, 1
19.5 grams fat **1,218 calories**	**24.5 grams fat** **1,503 calories**	**29 grams fat** **1,816 calories**

No-Cook Menu PHASE ① 15% Fat

1,200 CALORIES 20 GRAMS FAT	1,500 CALORIES 25 GRAMS FAT	1,800 CALORIES 30 GRAMS FAT

BREAKFAST
Cantaloupe, ¼
Yoplait Whips! Yogurt, 4 oz.
Oatmeal Raisin Cookie, 1
	Eggo Homestyle Waffles, 2,
	  w/Smucker's Strawberry
	  Topping, 2 T.
	Milk, 1%, ¾ cup
		Cantaloupe, ¼
		Eggo Homestyle Waffles, 2, w/
		  Smucker's Strawberry Topping, 2 T.
		Milk, 1%, 1 c.

LUNCH Turkey, deli, 4 oz. Mayonnaise, fat-free, 2 T. Whole wheat bread, 2 slices Fruit Roll-Ups, 1	Turkey, deli, 4 oz. Mayonnaise, fat-free, 2 T. Whole wheat bread, 2 slices Dried figs, 2 pieces	Turkey, deli, 6 oz. Mayonnaise, fat-free, 2 T. Whole wheat bread, 2 slices Laughing Cow Light Cheese Wedge, 2 Apple, 1

SNACK
Baby carrots, 1 c., w/Wish-Bone
  Light! Dressing, 2 T.
	Baby carrots, 1 c., w/Wish-Bone
	  Light! Dressing, 2 T.
		Baby carrots, 1 c., w/Wish-Bone
		  Light! Dressing, 2 T.

DINNER
Smart Ones Chicken Carbonara
Mixed greens, 2 c., w/Kraft Free
  Italian Dressing, 2 T.
Apple, 1
	Campbell's Select Clam
	  Chowder, 2 c.
	Smart Ones Chicken Carbonara
	Mixed greens, 2 c., w/Kraft Free
	  Italian Dressing, 2 T.
		Campbell's Select Clam Chowder, 2 c.
		Amy's Whole Meals Chili & Cornbread
		Mixed greens, 2 c., w/Kraft Free
		  Italian Dressing, 2 T.
		Healthy Choice Fudge Bar

SNACK Nabisco Gingersnaps, 4	Nabisco Gingersnaps, 4	Nabisco Gingersnaps, 3
20 grams fat **1,212 calories**	**24.7 grams fat** **1,497 calories**	**30.7 grams fat** **1,805 calories**

Weekday Menu PHASE 2 20% Fat

1,200 CALORIES 26 GRAMS FAT	1,500 CALORIES 33 GRAMS FAT	1,800 CALORIES 40 GRAMS FAT
BREAKFAST		
Clif Bar, Caramel Apple Cobbler, 1, Milk, 2%, ½ c.	Clif Bar, Caramel Apple Cobbler, 1, Milk, 2%, 1 c.	Odwalla Bar! Peanut Crunch, 1, Milk, 2%, 1 c.
LUNCH		
Aloha Fruit Salad w/Macadamia Crunch (p. 167) Campbell's Select Savory Lentil Soup, 1 c.	*Aloha Fruit Salad /w Macadamia Crunch* (p. 167), 1½ srv. Campbell's Select Savory Lentil Soup, 1 c.	*Aloha Fruit Salad w/Macadamia Crunch* (p. 167), 2 srv. Campbell's Select Savory Lentil Soup, 1 c.
SNACK		
Dannon La Crème Mousse Yogurt, 4 oz.	Dried apricots, 5 pieces	Kashi GoLean Crunchy! Bar, Chocolate Caramel, 1
DINNER		
Mixed lettuce salad, 1½ c. Ranch dressing, fat-free, 2 T. *Chicken Pot Pie* (p. 228)	Mixed lettuce salad, 1½ c. Kraft Light Done Right! Ranch Dressing, 2 T. *Chicken Pot Pie* (p. 228)	Mixed lettuce salad, 1½ c. Wish-Bone Light! Parmesan Peppercorn Ranch Dressing, 2 T. *Chicken Pot Pie* (p. 228), 1½ srv.
SNACK		
Mango chunks, ½ c.	Chocolate cake, fat-free	Chocolate cake, fat-ree
25 grams fat **1,231 calories**	**33 grams fat** **1,468 calories**	**39 grams fat** **1,803 calories**

Weekday Menu PHASE 2 20% Fat

1,200 CALORIES 26 GRAMS FAT	1,500 CALORIES 33 GRAMS FAT	1,800 CALORIES 40 GRAMS FAT
BREAKFAST		
Raisin Bran Muffin w/Orange Glaze (p. 143) Milk, 2%, ½ c.	*Raisin Bran Muffin w/Orange Glaze* (p. 143) Milk, 2%, 1 c.	*Raisin Bran Muffin w/Orange Glaze* (p. 143), Milk, 2%, 1 c. Orange and grapefruit sections, 1 c.
LUNCH		
Progresso Traditional Chickarina Soup, 1½ c. Whole wheat roll, 1 Orange, 1	Progresso Vegetable Classics Macaroni and Bean Soup, 2 c. Whole wheat potato roll, 1 Peach, 1	Campbell's Chunky Baked Potato w/Cheddar and Bacon Bits, 2 c. Whole wheat potato rolls, 2 Plums, 2
SNACK		
Healthy Choice Ice Cream Vanilla Bar w/Fudge Coating, 1	Fudgsicle, 1	Healthy Choice Caramel Swirl Ice Cream Sandwich, 1
DINNER		
Stir-Fried Pork w/Apples and Figs (p. 248) Polenta, ½ c. *Creamed Spinach* (p. 277)	*Stir-Fried Pork w/Apples and Figs* (p. 248) Polenta, ½ c. *Creamed Spinach,* (p. 277), 1½ srv.	*Stir-Fried Pork w/Apples and Figs* (p. 248), 1½ srv. Polenta, ½ c. *Creamed Spinach* (p. 277), 1½ srv.
SNACK		
Grapes, 1 c.	Stella D'oro Anisette Cookies, 2 Watermelon chunks, 1 c.	Reduced-Fat Nilla Wafers, 4
25.6 grams fat **1,180 calories**	**32.7 grams fat** **1,506 calories**	**39.8 grams fat** **1,835 calories**

Weekday Menu PHASE 2 20% Fat

1,200 CALORIES 26 GRAMS FAT	1,500 CALORIES 33 GRAMS FAT	1,800 CALORIES 40 GRAMS FAT
BREAKFAST Eggo Nutrigrain Waffles, 2, w/2T. sugar-free syrup Orange juice, 6 oz.	Eggo Nutrigrain Waffles, 2, w/2T. sugar-free syrup Orange juice, 6 oz. Dannon Light 'n Fit Yogurt, 4 oz.	Eggo Nutrigrain Waffles, 2, w/2T. sugar-free syrup Orange juice, 8 oz. Dannon La Crème Yogurt, 4 oz.
LUNCH *Grilled Shrimp w/Corn-and-Tomato Salad* (p. 173) Whole wheat roll, 1 Cantaloupe, ¼	*Grilled Shrimp w/Corn-and-Tomato Salad* (p. 173) 1½ srv. Whole wheat roll, 1 Cantaloupe, ¼	*Grilled Shrimp w/Corn-and-Tomato Salad* (p. 173), 2 srv. Whole wheat roll, 1 Honeydew melon, ¼
SNACK Jell-O Pudding Snack, 1	Jell-O Fat Free Pudding Snack, 1	Jell-O Fat Free Pudding Snack, 1
DINNER *Chicken Paprikash* (p. 223) Egg noodles, ½ c. Peas, ½ c.	*Chicken Paprikash* (p. 223), 1½ srv. Egg noodles, ½ c. Peas, ½ c.	*Chicken Paprikash* (p. 223) 2 srv. Egg noodles, ½ c. Peas, ½ c.
SNACK Stella D'oro Anisette Sponge Cookies, 2	Stella D'oro Almond Toast Cookies, 2	Stella D'oro Anisette Sponge Cookies, 2
26.3 grams fat **1,219 calories**	**32.4 grams fat** **1,502 calories**	**39.4 grams fat** **1,783 calories**

Weekday Menu PHASE 2 20% Fat

1,200 CALORIES 26 GRAMS FAT	1,500 CALORIES 33 GRAMS FAT	1,800 CALORIES 40 GRAMS FAT
BREAKFAST Oatmeal, 1 c. Milk, 2%, 1 c.	Oatmeal, 1¼ c. Milk, 2%, 1¼ c.	Oatmeal, 1½ c. Milk, 2%, 1½ c.
LUNCH Mixed lettuce salad w/Italian dressing, fat-free, 2 T. Lean Cuisine Creamy Basil Chicken Crisp breadstick, 1	Mixed lettuce salad w/Italian dressing, low-fat, 2 T. Lean Cuisine Creamy Basil Chicken Soft breadstick, 1	Mixed lettuce salad w/Italian dressing, low-fat, 2 T. Lean Cuisine Orange Peel Chicken Soft breadsticks, 2
SNACK Pear, 1	Pear, 1	Keebler Country Style Oatmeal Cookie, 1
DINNER *Veal Marsala* (p. 251) *Lean and Mean Mashed Potatoes* (p. 284), ¾ srv. Steamed broccoli florets, 1 c.	*Veal Marsala* (p. 251) 1½ srv. *Lean and Mean Mashed Potatoes* (p. 284) Steamed broccoli florets, 1 c.	*Veal Marsala* (p. 251), 1½ srv. *Lean and Mean Mashed Potatoes* (p. 284), 1½ srv. Steamed broccoli florets, 1 c.
SNACK *Mixed Fruit w/Strawberry-Ginger Sauce* (p. 298)	*Mixed Fruit w/Strawberry-Ginger Sauce* (p. 298)	*Mixed Fruit w/Strawberry-Ginger Sauce* (p. 298)
25.2 grams fat **1,239 calories**	**33 grams fat** **1,508 calories**	**40.7 grams fat** **1,812 calories**

Weekday Menu PHASE ② 20% Fat

1,200 CALORIES 26 GRAMS FAT	1,500 CALORIES 33 GRAMS FAT	1,800 CALORIES 40 GRAMS FAT
BREAKFAST Egg, boiled or scrambled dry, 1 Whole wheat toast, 1 slice Sharp Cheddar, 2%, 1 slice Grapefruit, ½	Egg, boiled or scrambled dry, 1 Whole wheat toast, 2 slices Sharp Cheddar, 1 slice Grapefruit, ½	Eggs, boiled or scrambled dry, 2 Whole wheat toast, 2 slices, w/jam or preserves, 1 T. Grapefruit, ½
LUNCH *Tuna Salad Sandwich* (p. 218) Apple, 1	*Tuna Salad Sandwich* (p. 218) Nabisco Ginger Snaps, 5	*Tuna Salad Sandwich* (p. 218) Reduced-Fat Nilla Wafers, 4 Apple, 1
SNACK Country Style Oatmeal Cookie, 1	*Sesame Cheese Balls* (p. 304)	*Sesame Cheese Balls* (p. 304)

DINNER
Beef and Vegetable Stew
  (p. 246)
Uncle Ben's Ready Rice, ¾ c.
	Beef and Vegetable Stew
	  (p. 246), 1¼ srv.
	Uncle Ben's Ready Rice, 1 c.
		Beef and Vegetable Stew (p. 246),
		  1½ srv.
		Uncle Ben's Ready Rice, 1¼ c.

SNACK
Pineapple-Mango Topping
  w/Frozen Yogurt (p. 297)
	Red, White, and Blue Parfaits
	  (p. 292)
		Red, White, and Blue Parfaits
		  (p. 292)

26.6 grams fat **1,235 calories**	**33.5 grams fat** **1,493 calories**	**39 grams fat** **1,814 calories**

Weekday Menu PHASE ② 20% Fat

1,200 CALORIES 26 GRAMS FAT	1,500 CALORIES 33 GRAMS FAT	1,800 CALORIES 40 GRAMS FAT
BREAKFAST *Eggs-and-Potato Hash* (p. 146) Whole wheat toast, 1 slice	*Eggs-and-Potato Hash* (p. 146) Whole wheat toast, 2 slices	*Eggs-and-Potato Hash* (p. 146) Whole wheat toast, 2 slices, w/ margarine, reduced-fat, 2 tsp. Orange juice, 4 oz.

LUNCH
Pita Bread, 6", w/ham, 3 oz.,
  Swiss cheese, low-fat, 1 slice,
  lettuce, tomato, and mayo,
  fat-free, 2 T.
	Pita bread, 6", w/ham, 4 oz.,
	  Swiss cheese, low-fat, 1 slice,
	  lettuce, tomato, and reduced-
	  fat mayo, 1 T.
	Plum, 1
		Pita bread, 6", w/ham, 4 oz., Swiss
		  cheese, low-fat, 1 slice, lettuce,
		  tomato, and reduced-fat mayo,
		  2 T.
		Apple, 1

SNACK Apple, 1	Apple, 1	Dried figs, 2 pieces

DINNER
Spaghetti w/Summer Tomatoes,
  Basil, and Garlic (p. 256)
Mixed greens w/Kraft Thousand
  Island Dressing, 2 T.
Crisp breadstick, 1
	Spaghetti w/Summer Tomatoes,
	  Basil, and Garlic (p. 256),
	  1¼ srv.
	Mixed greens w/Kraft Thousand
	  Island Dressing, 2 T.
	Crisp breadsticks, 2
		Spaghetti w/Summer Tomatoes,
		  Basil, and Garlic (p. 256),
		  1½ srv.
		Mixed greens w/Kraft Thousand
		  Island Dressing, 2 T.
		Crisp breadsticks, 3.

SNACK
Fresh Raspberry Sauce (p. 300)
  over 1 sliced pear
	Fresh Raspberry Sauce (p. 300)
	  over 1 sliced pear
		Fresh Raspberry Sauce (p. 300) over
		  1 sliced pear

24.3 grams fat **1,223 calories**	**32.7 grams fat** **1,500 calories**	**39.3 grams fat** **1,782 calories**

Weekday Menu PHASE 2 20% Fat

1,200 CALORIES 26 GRAMS FAT	1,500 CALORIES 33 GRAMS FAT	1,800 CALORIES 40 GRAMS FAT
BREAKFAST Pepperidge Farm Homestyle French Toast, 1 slice, w/margarine, reduced-fat, 1 tsp., and Smucker's Sugar Free Pancake Syrup, 2 T. Milk, 1%, ½ c.	Pepperidge Farm Homestyle French Toast, 1 slice, w/margarine, reduced-fat, 1 tsp., and Smucker's Sugar Free Pancake Syrup, 2 T. Milk, 1%, 1 c.; Orange juice, 4 oz.	Pepperidge Farm Homestyle French Toast, 1 slice, w/margarine, reduced-fat, 1 tsp., and Smucker's Sugar Free Pancake Syrup, 2 T. Milk, 1%, 1 c.
LUNCH *Grilled Cheese/Bacon* (p. 250) Apple, 1	*Grilled Cheese/Bacon* (p. 250) *Creamy Coleslaw* (p. 286), 1 c. Plums, 2	*Grilled Cheese/Bacon* (p. 250), 1½ srv. *Creamy Coleslaw* (p. 286), ½ c. Plums, 2
SNACK Archway Home Style Fat Free Oatmeal Raisin Cookie, 1	Health Valley Moist n' Chewy Dutch Apple Granola Bar, 1	Fat Free Banana Crunch Cake, ⅛ cake
DINNER *Grilled Vegetables w/Garlic Vinaigrette* (p. 179) Grilled chicken breast, skinless and boneless, 4 oz.	*Grilled Vegetables w/Garlic Vinaigrette* (p. 179) Grilled chicken breast, skinless and boneless, 4 oz.	*Grilled Vegetables w/Garlic Vinaigrette* (p. 179), 1½ srv. Grilled chicken breast, skinless and boneless, 6 oz.
SNACK Pear w/*Raspberry Sauce* (p. 300)	Pear w/*Raspberry Sauce* (p. 300)	Pear w/*Raspberry Sauce* (p. 300)
26.4 grams fat **1,223 calories**	**32.6 grams fat** **1,505 calories**	**39 grams fat** **1,783 calories**

Weekday Menu PHASE 2 20% Fat

1,200 CALORIES 26 GRAMS FAT	1,500 CALORIES 33 GRAMS FAT	1,800 CALORIES 40 GRAMS FAT
BREAKFAST Melon, ⅛, w/berries, ½ c. Cottage cheese, whole-milk, ½ c. *Cranberry Muffin* (p. 141)	Melon, ⅛, w/berries, ½ c. Cottage cheese, whole-milk, ¾ c. *Carrot-Raisin Bran Muffin* (p. 142)	Melon, ⅛, w/berries, ½ c. Cottage cheese, whole-milk, ¾ c. *Carrot-Raisin Bran Muffin* (p. 142), 1
LUNCH Lean Pockets Cheeseburger, 1 Mixed lettuce salad w/ranch dressing, fat-free, 2 T.	Lean Pockets Cheeseburger, 1 Mixed lettuce salad w/Wish-Bone Light! Parmesan Peppercorn Ranch Dressing, 2 T. Snackwell's Fat Free Cookie, 1	Hot Pockets Jalapeño Steak and Cheese, 1 Mixed lettuce salad w/ranch dressing, fat-free, 2 T. Health Valley Low-Fat Cookies, 3
SNACK Health Valley Low-Fat Cookies, 2	Pear, 1	Apples, 2
DINNER *Stir-Fried Pork w/Apples and Figs* (p. 248) *Sweet Potato Jack* (p. 136) *Cheesy Broccoli* (p. 264)	*Stir-Fried Pork w/Apples and Figs* (p. 248), 1½ srv. *Sweet Potato Jack* (p. 136) *Cheesy Broccoli* (p. 264), 1½ srv.	*Stir-Fried Pork w/Apples and Figs* (p. 248), 2 srv. *Sweet Potato Jack* (p. 136) *Cheesy Broccoli* (p. 264), 1½ srv.
SNACK *Grilled Peaches* (p. 299)	*Grilled Peaches* (p. 299)	*Grilled Peaches* (p. 299), 1½ srv.
26.3 grams fat **1,209 calories**	**33 grams fat** **1,507 calories**	**41 grams fat** **1,806 calories**

Weekday Menu PHASE ② 20% Fat

1,200 CALORIES 26 GRAMS FAT	1,500 CALORIES 33 GRAMS FAT	1,800 CALORIES 40 GRAMS FAT
BREAKFAST Eggs-and-Potato Hash (p. 146) Whole wheat toast, 1 slice	Eggs-and-Potato Hash (p. 146), 1½ srv. Whole wheat toast, 1 slice	Eggs-and-Potato Hash (p. 146), 1½ srv. Whole wheat toast, 2 slices
LUNCH Mixed lettuce salad w/Italian dressing, fat-free, 2 T. Healthy Choice Meat Loaf	Mixed lettuce salad w/Italian dressing, fat-free, 2 T. Healthy Choice Meat Loaf Sourdough roll, 1	Mixed lettuce salad w/Italian dress- ing, fat-free, 2 T. Healthy Choice Meat Loaf Sourdough roll, 1 Pear, 1
SNACK Plums, 2	Plums, 2	Dried fig, 1 piece
DINNER Vegetarian Chili (p. 182) Baked potato, ½ Shredded cheddar, 2%, 1 T.	Vegetarian Chili (p. 182) Baked potato Shredded cheddar, 2%, 2 T.	Vegetarian Chili (p. 182), 1½ srv. Baked potato Shredded cheddar, 2%, 2 T.
SNACK Fresh Raspberry Sauce (p. 300) over ice cream, fat-free, ½ c.	Fresh Raspberry Sauce (p. 300) over ice cream, fat-free, ½ c.	Fresh Raspberry Sauce (p. 300) over ice cream, fat-free, ½ c.
25.8 grams fat 1,198 calories	**32 grams fat 1,514 calories**	**38.4 grams fat 1,822 calories**

Weekday Menu PHASE ② 20% Fat

1,200 CALORIES 26 GRAMS FAT	1,500 CALORIES 33 GRAMS FAT	1,800 CALORIES 40 GRAMS FAT
BREAKFAST Raisin bran, ¾ c. Milk, whole, ¾ c. Strawberries, sliced, ½ c.	Raisin bran, 1 c. Milk, whole, 1 c. Strawberries, sliced, ½ c.	Raisin bran, 1 c. Milk, whole, 1¼ c. Strawberries, sliced, ½ c.
LUNCH Tuna Salad Sandwich (p. 218) Grapes, 1 c.	Tuna Salad Sandwich (p. 218) Plums, 2 Health Valley Low-Fat Healthy Chips Double Chocolate Cookies, 2	Tuna Salad Sandwich (p. 218), 1½ srv. Apple, 1 small Health Valley Low-Fat Healthy Chips Double Chocolate Cookies, 2
SNACK Keebler Oatmeal Cookie, 1	Orange, 1	Dried figs, 2 pieces
DINNER Green Giant Chicken Cheesy Pasta Skillet Meal, 2 c. Lettuce and tomato salad w/Basil-Cream Dressing (p. 334)	Green Giant Chicken Cheesy Pasta Skillet Meal, 2½ c. Lettuce and tomato salad w/ Poppy Seed Dressing (p. 340)	Green Giant Chicken Cheesy Pasta Skillet Meal, 2½ c. Lettuce and tomato salad w/Poppy Seed Dressing (p. 340) Soft breadsticks, 2
SNACK Plums, 2	Keebler Oatmeal Cookies, 2	Chips Ahoy Thin Crisps, 1 pack
25.6 grams fat 1,191 calories	**33.3 grams fat 1,486 calories**	**39 grams fat 1,820 calories**

Weekend Menu (Meatless) PHASE **2** 20% Fat

1,200 CALORIES 26 GRAMS FAT	1,500 CALORIES 33 GRAMS FAT	1,800 CALORIES 40 GRAMS FAT
BREAKFAST *Asparagus Omelet w/Summer* *Herbs* (p. 144) Whole wheat toast, 1 slice Tomato, 3 thick slices	*Asparagus Omelet w/Summer* *Herbs* (p. 144) Whole wheat toast, 1 slice, w/melted low-fat Swiss cheese, 1 oz. Tomato, 3 thick slices	*Asparagus Omelet w/Summer* *Herbs* (p. 144) Whole wheat toast, 1 slice, w/melted Swiss cheese, 1 oz. Tomato, 3 thick slices, w/*Basil-* *Cream Dressing* (p. 334), 2 T.
LUNCH *Autumn Bean and Squash Stew* (p. 177) Egg noodles, ½ c.	*Autumn Bean and Squash* *Stew* (p. 177) Egg noodles, 1 c.	*Autumn Bean and Squash* *Stew* (p. 177) Egg noodles, 1 c. Buttermilk biscuit, 1
SNACK *Stuffed Celery* (p. 305), 2 stalks	Health Valley Apple Granola Bar, 1	Health Valley Apple Granola Bar, 1
DINNER *Fish Sticks* (p. 198), 3, w/cocktail sauce, 2 T. *Creamy Coleslaw* (p. 286), 1 c.	*Fish Sticks* (p. 198), 4, w/cocktail sauce, 2 T. *Creamy Coleslaw* (p. 286), 1 c.	*Fish Sticks* (p. 198), 5, w/cocktail sauce, ¼ c. *Creamy Coleslaw* (p. 286), 1 c.
SNACK *Baked Apple* (p. 294)	*Baked Apple* (p. 294)	*Baked Apple* (p. 294)
24.4 grams fat **1,206 calories**	**32 grams fat** **1,530 calories**	**40 grams fat** **1,813 calories**

Weekend Menu PHASE **2** 20% Fat

1,200 CALORIES 26 GRAMS FAT	1,500 CALORIES 33 GRAMS FAT	1,800 CALORIES 40 GRAMS FAT
BREAKFAST Egg, boiled or fried in nonstick pan, 1 Whole wheat toast, 1 slice Orange sections, 1 c.	*Eggs-and-Potato Hash* (p. 146) Whole wheat toast, 1 slice Orange sections, 1 c.	*Eggs-and-Potato Hash* (p. 146) Whole wheat toast, 2 slices Orange sections, 1 c.
LUNCH *Buttery Squash Soup* (p. 151) *Roasted Chicken Salad* *w/Raspberry Vinaigrette* (p. 172)	*Asparagus Soup* (p. 149) *Roasted Chicken Salad* *w/Raspberry Vinaigrette* (p. 172) Soft breadstick, 1	*Asparagus Soup* (p. 149) *Roasted Chicken Salad w/* *Raspberry Vinaigrette* (p. 172) Soft breadsticks, 2
SNACK Dannon Light 'n Fit Creamy Nonfat Yogurt, 6 oz.	Dannon La Crème Yogurt, 4 oz.	Dannon La Crème Mousse Yogurt, 4 oz.
DINNER *Stir-Fried Pork and Greens* (p. 249) Brown rice, ½ c. *Glazed Carrots* (p. 279)	*Stir-Fried Pork and Greens* (p. 249) Brown rice, ¾ c. *Glazed Carrots* (p. 279)	*Stir-Fried Pork and Greens* (p. 249), 1½ srv Brown rice, 1 c. *Glazed Carrots* (p. 279)
SNACK Pear, 1	Pear, 1	Archway Home Style Cookie, 1
25 grams fat **1,240 calories**	**32.8 grams fat** **1,516 calories**	**40.9 grams fat** **1,819 calories**

Weekend Menu PHASE 2 — 20% Fat

1,200 CALORIES 26 GRAMS FAT	1,500 CALORIES 33 GRAMS FAT	1,800 CALORIES 40 GRAMS FAT
BREAKFAST *Banana-Nut Hotcakes* (p. 137), 1 Dannon La Crème Mousse Yogurt, 4 oz.	*Banana-Nut Hotcakes* (p. 137) Dannon La Crème Mousse Yogurt, 4 oz.	*Banana-Nut Hotcakes* (p. 137) Dannon La Crème Yogurt, 4 oz.
LUNCH *Veal Scallops w/Fennel and Grapes* (p. 252) Egg noodles, ½ c.	*Veal Scallops w/Fennel and Grapes* (p. 252) Egg noodles, ¾ c.	*Veal Scallops w/Fennel and Grapes* (p. 252), 1½ srv. Egg noodles, 1 c.
SNACK *Mixed Fruit w/Strawberry-Ginger Sauce* (p. 298)	*Mixed Fruit w/Strawberry- Ginger Sauce* (p. 298)	*Mixed Fruit w/Strawberry-Ginger Sauce* (p. 298)
DINNER *Mini Pizzas Two Ways w/ Vegetable Topping* (p. 192) Mixed lettuce salad w/fat-free ranch dressing, 2 T.	*Green Olive Tapenade* (p. 306) w/Rosemary & Olive Oil Triscuits, 2 *Mini Pizzas Two Ways w/Veg- etable Topping* (p. 192) Salad w/fat-free dressing, 2 T.	*Green Olive Tapenade* (p. 306), 2 srv., w/Rosemary & Olive Oil Triscuits, 4 *Mini Pizzas Two Ways w/ Vegetable Topping* (p. 192) Salad w/fat-free dressing, 2 T.
SNACK Stella D'oro Anisette Cookies, 2	Stella D'oro Anisette Cookies, 2	Stella D'oro Anisette Cookies, 2
25.8 grams fat **1,232 calories**	**31.8 grams fat** **1,513 calories**	**38.7 grams fat** **1,810 calories**

Weekend Menu PHASE 2 — 20% Fat

1,200 CALORIES 26 GRAMS FAT	1,500 CALORIES 33 GRAMS FAT	1,800 CALORIES 40 GRAMS FAT
BREAKFAST *Asparagus Omelet w/Summer Herbs* (p. 144) *Grilled Portobello Mushrooms* (p. 271), ½ srv. Whole wheat toast, 1 slice	*Asparagus Omelet w/Summer Herbs* (p. 144) *Grilled Portobello Mushrooms* (p. 271), ½ srv. Whole wheat toast, 2 slices	*Asparagus Omelet w/Summer Herbs* (p. 144) *Grilled Portobello Mushrooms* (p. 271) Whole wheat toast, 2 slices
LUNCH *Tomato-Corn Bisque* (p. 150) *Warm Potato and Tuna Salad* (p. 174)	*Tomato-Corn Bisque* (p. 150) *Warm Potato and Tuna Salad* (p. 174) Sourdough roll, 1	*Two-Potato Bisque* (p. 159), 1½ srv. *Warm Potato and Tuna Salad* (p. 174) Sourdough roll, 1, w/margarine, reduced-fat, 1 T.
SNACK Newton Caramel Apple Bars, 1	Keebler Oatmeal Cookie, 1	Newton Caramel Apple Bars, 2
DINNER *Chicken Paprikash* (p. 223) Egg noodles, ½ c. Peas, ½ c.	*Chicken Paprikash* (p. 223), 1½ srv. Egg noodles, ½ c. Peas, ½ c.	*Chicken Paprikash* (p. 223), 2 srv. Egg noodles, ½ c. Peas, ½ c.
SNACK *Spiced Apples* (p. 295)	*Spiced Apples* (p. 295)	*Spiced Apples* (p. 295)
25.8 grams fat **1,235 calories**	**32.4 grams fat** **1,530 calories**	**39 grams fat** **1,823 calories**

No-Cook Menu PHASE 2 20% Fat

1,200 CALORIES 26 GRAMS FAT	1,500 CALORIES 33 GRAMS FAT	1,800 CALORIES 40 GRAMS FAT

BREAKFAST
Hot Pockets Ham, Egg, &
  Cheese, 1
Orange, 1 large
	Hot Pockets Bacon, Egg, &
	  Cheese, 1
	Orange, 1 large
	Dannon Smoothie, 7 oz.
		Hot Pockets Biscuits Bacon Egg
		  & Cheese, 1
		Orange, 1 large

LUNCH
Smart Ones Four Cheese Pizza
	Smart Ones Four Cheese Pizza
	Campbell's Soup at Hand Chicken
	  and Stars
		Smart Ones Four Cheese Pizza
		Campbell's Chunky Microwav-
		  able Bowls Beef w/Country
		  Vegetables

SNACK Peach, 1	Pear, 1	Apple, 1 large

DINNER
Lean Cuisine Lemon Garlic
  Shrimp
Tomato, 3 thick slices, w/
  Italian dressing, fat-free, 2 T.
	Lean Cuisine Lemon Garlic Shrimp
	Tomato, 3 thick slices, w/ Italian
	  Dressing, low-fat, 2 T.
	Crisp breadsticks, 2
		Lean Cuisine Lemon Garlic
		  Shrimp w/cooked shrimp,
		  8 extra-large
		Tomato, 3 thick slices, w/ Italian
		  dressing, low-fat, 2 T.
		Soft breadsticks, 2

SNACK Pear, 1	Low-fat granola	Low-fat granola
25 grams fat **1,201 calories**	**32.5 grams fat** **1,470 calories**	**39.5 grams fat** **1,785 calories**

No-Cook Menu PHASE 2 20% Fat

1,200 CALORIES 26 GRAMS FAT	1,500 CALORIES 33 GRAMS FAT	1,800 CALORIES 40 GRAMS FAT

BREAKFAST
Aunt Jemima Cinnamon French
  Toast, 2 slices
Margarine, reduced-fat, 2 tsp.
Maple syrup, 2 tsp.
Blueberries, ½ cup
	Aunt Jemima Cinnamon French
	  Toast, 3 slices
	Margarine, reduced-fat, 1 T.
	Maple syrup, 1 T.
	Blueberries, ½ cup
		Aunt Jemima Cinnamon French
		  Toast, 3 slices
		Margarine, reduced-fat, 1 T.
		Maple syrup, 2 T.
		Blueberries, ½ cup

LUNCH Turkey breast, deli, 3 oz. Swiss cheese, low-fat, 1 oz. Lettuce and tomato Mayonnaise, reduced-fat, 2 T. Whole wheat bread, 2 slices	Turkey breast, deli, 3 oz. Swiss cheese, low-fat, 1 oz. Lettuce and tomato Mayonnaise, reduced-fat, 2 T. Whole wheat bread, 2 slices Potato chips, baked, 1 oz.	Turkey breast, deli, 4 oz. Swiss cheese, low-fat, 2 oz. Lettuce and tomato Mayonnaise, reduced-fat, 2 T. Whole wheat bread, 2 slices Potato chips, baked, 1 oz.
SNACK Dried Apricots, 5 pieces	Apple, 1	Dried Figs, 3 pieces
DINNER Lean Cuisine Spaghetti Mixed lettuce salad, 1½ c. Italian dressing, low-fat, 2 T. Crisp breadsticks, 2	Lean Cuisine Jumbo Rigatoni Mixed lettuce salad, 1½ c. Italian dressing, low-fat, 2 T. Crisp breadsticks, 2	Lean Cuisine Jumbo Rigatoni Mixed lettuce salad, 1½ c. Italian dressing, light, 2 T. Soft breadsticks, 2
SNACK Pear, 1	Pear, 1	Pear, 1
25 grams fat **1,190 calories**	**33 grams fat** **1,511 calories**	**40 grams fat** **1,816 calories**

No-Cook Menu PHASE 2 20% Fat

1,200 CALORIES 26 GRAMS FAT	1,500 CALORIES 33 GRAMS FAT	1,800 CALORIES 40 GRAMS FAT
BREAKFAST Wheaties, 1 c. Milk, 2%, 1 c. Strawberries, sliced, ½ cup	Raisin bran, 1 c. Milk, whole, 1 c. Strawberries, sliced, ½ cup	Raisin bran, 1 c. Milk, whole, 1 c. Strawberries, sliced, ½ cup Walnuts, chopped, 2 tsp.
LUNCH Spinach tortilla, 1 Roast beef, deli, 2 oz. Kraft Singles, 1 slice Lettuce and tomato Mayonnaise, fat-free, 2 T.	Spinach tortilla, 1 Roast beef, deli, 4 oz. Kraft Singles, 1 slice Lettuce and tomato Mayonnaise, fat-free, 2 T.	Spinach tortilla, 1 Roast beef, deli, 4 oz. Kraft Singles, 2 slices Lettuce and tomato Mayonnaise, fat-free, 2 T. Apple, 1
SNACK Low-fat cake, 1 slice	Low-fat granola bar, 1	Low-fat granola bar, 1
DINNER Progresso Garden Vegetable Soup, 1 c. Lean Cuisine Steak Tips Dijon	Progresso Traditional Beef Barley Soup, 1 c. Lean Cuisine Chicken Fettuccini	Progresso Split Pea Soup, 1 c. Lean Cuisine Orange Peel Chicken Crisp breadsticks, 2
SNACK Pear, 1	Pear, 1	Pear, 1
25.5 grams fat 1,230 calories	**32.5 grams fat 1,525 calories**	**40.3 grams fat 1,797 calories**

No-Cook Menu PHASE 2 20% Fat

1,200 CALORIES 26 GRAMS FAT	1,500 CALORIES 33 GRAMS FAT	1,800 CALORIES 40 GRAMS FAT
BREAKFAST Egg, hard-cooked, 1 Wheat toast, 1 slice, w/ margarine, reduced-fat, 1 tsp. Grapefruit, ½	Nutri-Grain Blueberry Cereal Bars, 2 Dannon La Crème Mousse Yogurt, 4 oz.	Aunt Jemima French Toast, 3 slices, w/maple syrup, 1 T. Silk Soymilk, Very Vanilla, 8 oz.
LUNCH Lean Cuisine Three Bean Chili Pear, 1	Lean Cuisine Fiesta Grilled Chicken Whole wheat bread, 1 slice Pear, 1	Cheeseburger Lean Pockets, 1 Mixed greens, 2 c., w/olives, 3, and fat-free Dressing, 2 T. Guiltless Gourmet Corn Chips, 1 oz. Orange, 1
SNACK Jell-O Fat Free Pudding, 1	Dole Individual Fruit Bowl, 1	Health Valley Granola Bar, 1
DINNER Lean Cuisine Baked Lemon Pepper Fish Stonyfield Farm Lowfat Luscious Lemon Yogurt, 6 oz., w/blueberries, ½ c.	V8 100% Vegetable Juice, 8 oz. Healthy Choice Herb Baked Fish w/Kraft Tartar Sauce, 1 T.	Campbell's Select Minestrone Soup, 1½ c. Green Giant Garlic Chicken Pasta Skillet Meal, 1½ c. Soft Breadsticks, 2
SNACK Vitalicious VitaBrownie, 1	Vitalicious VitaBrownie, 1 Ice cream, fat-free, ½ c.	Dannon La Crème Yogurt, 4 oz. Strawberries, sliced, ½ c.
25.6 grams fat 1,212 calories	**33.5 grams fat 1,505 calories**	**40.3 grams fat 1,807 calories**

Weekday Menu PHASE (3) 30% Fat

1,200 CALORIES 40 GRAMS FAT	1,500 CALORIES 50 GRAMS FAT	1,800 CALORIES 60 GRAMS FAT
BREAKFAST		
Nutri-Grain Bar, 1 Milk, whole, ½ c.	Nutri-Grain Bar, 1 Milk, whole, 1 c. Blueberries, ½ c.	Quaker Breakfast Bar, 1 Milk, whole, 1 c. Blueberries, ½ c.
LUNCH		
Watercress/Strawberry Salad (p. 168), w/turkey, 4 oz. Whole wheat roll, 1	*Watercress/Strawberry Salad* (p. 168), w/turkey, 6 oz. Whole wheat roll, 1, w/reduced fat marg., 1 tsp.	*Watercress/Strawberry Salad* (p. 168), 1½ srv. w/turkey, 6 oz. Soft breadsticks, 2
SNACK		
Newton Caramel Apple Bar, 1	*Stuffed Celery* (p. 305), 3	Archway Oatmeal Raisin Cookie, 1
DINNER		
Pumpkin Soup (p. 153) Amy's Shepherd Pie Whole wheat roll, 1, w/reduced-fat margarine, 2 tsp.	*Pumpkin Soup* (p. 153) Amy's Shepherd Pie Soft breadsticks, 2, w/reduced-fat marg., 2 tsp. Grapes, ½ c.	*French Onion Soup* (p. 152) Amy's Cheese Enchilada Meal
SNACK		
Jell-O Pudding Snack Cup, 1	Jell-O Pudding Snack Cup, 1	Jell-O Pudding Snack Cup, 1
38 grams fat 1,201 calories	**46 grams fat 1,498 calories**	**56 grams fat 1,795 calories**

Weekday Menu PHASE (3) 30% Fat

1,200 CALORIES 40 GRAMS FAT	1,500 CALORIES 50 GRAMS FAT	1,800 CALORIES 60 GRAMS FAT
BREAKFAST		
Blueberry Banana Split for Breakfast (p. 291) w/strawberries, ½ c.	*Blueberry Banana Split for Breakfast* (p. 291), 1½ srv., w/berries, ½ c.	*Blueberry Banana Split for Breakfast* (p. 291) *Carrot-Raisin Bran Muffin* w/reduced-fat marg., 1 tsp. (p. 142)
LUNCH		
Tortilla wrap w/roast beef, 2 oz., reduced-fat mayo., 2 T., lettuce, tomato Peach, 1	Tortilla wrap w/roast beef, 4 oz., reduced-fat mayo, tomato, lettuce Peach, 1	Tortilla wrap w/roast beef, 3 oz., 2% cheddar, 1 oz., reduced-fat mayo., 2 T., tomato, lettuce Grapes, 1 c.
SNACK		
Ginger snaps, 3	Ginger snaps, 3	Ginger snaps, 6
DINNER		
Baked Halibut w/Pepper & Parsley Crust (p. 213), *Creamed Spinach* (p. 277), 1½ srv.	*Baked Halibut w/Pepper & Parsley Crust* (p. 213) *Creamed Spinach* (p. 277), 1½ srv. Uncle Ben's Ready Rice, 1 c.	*Baked Halibut w/Pepper & Parsley Crust* (p. 213) *Creamed Spinach* (p. 277), 2 srv. Uncle Ben's Ready Rice, 1 c.
SNACK		
Light ice cream, ½ c.	Light ice cream, ½ c.	Light ice cream, ½ c.
35 grams fat 1,192 calories	**43 grams fat 1,509 calories**	**53 grams fat 1,794 calories**

Weekday Menu PHASE 3 30% Fat

1,200 CALORIES 40 GRAMS FAT	1,500 CALORIES 50 GRAMS FAT	1,800 CALORIES 60 GRAMS FAT
BREAKFAST		
Oatmeal, 1 c. w/chopped walnuts, 1 tsp., raisins, 1 T. Milk, whole, ½ c.	Oatmeal, 1¼ c. w/chopped walnuts, 1 tsp., raisins, 1 T. Milk, whole, ¾ c.	Oatmeal, 1½ c. Milk, whole, 1 c. Blueberries, ½ c.
LUNCH		
Pita Sandwich to Go (p. 189) w/provolone, 1 oz. extra	*Pita Sandwich to Go* (p. 189) w/provolone, 1½ oz., & turkey, 2 oz. (extra)	*Pita Sandwich to Go* (p. 189) w/provolone, 1½ oz., & turkey, 4 oz. (extra)
SNACK		
Laughing Cow Light Cheese Wedge, 1 Low-fat wheat crackers, 4	Laughing Cow Light Cheese Wedge, 1 Low-fat wheat crackers, 4	Laughing Cow Light Cheese Wedge, 1 Low-fat wheat crackers, 5
DINNER		
Lettuce/tomato salad w/ *Raspberry-Walnut Dressing*, (p. 333) Lean Cuisine Salmon w/Basil Sourdough roll, 1	Lettuce/tomato salad w/ *Raspberry-Walnut Dressing*, (p. 333) Lean Cuisine Dinnertime Chicken Florentine	Lettuce/tomato salad w/*Raspberry-Walnut Dressing* (p. 333) Lean Cuisine Chicken Fettuccini Soft breadsticks, 2, w/reduced-fat marg., 2 tsp.
SNACK		
Chips Ahoy Thin Crisps, 1 pack	Healthy Choice Ice Cream Sandwich, 1	Healthy Choice Ice Cream Sandwich, 1
38 grams fat **1,210 calories**	**47 grams fat** **1,484 calories**	**56 grams fat** **1,796 calories**

Weekday Menu PHASE 3 30% Fat

1,200 CALORIES 40 GRAMS FAT	1,500 CALORIES 50 GRAMS FAT	1,800 CALORIES 60 GRAMS FAT
BREAKFAST		
Corn Chex, 1 c. Milk, whole, 1 c. Strawberries, ½ c.	Cracklin' Oat Bran, ½ c. Milk, whole, ¾ c. Banana	Cracklin' Oat Bran, ¾ c. Milk, whole, ¾ c. Banana
LUNCH		
Lettuce/Tomato Salad w/Kraft Red Pepper Dressing, 2 T. Lean Cuisine Deluxe French Bread Pizza	Lettuce/Tomato salad w/*Garlic Vinaigrette* (p. 341) Lean Cuisine Spinach & Mushroom Pizza Grapes, ½ c.	Lettuce/Tomato salad w/*Garlic Vinaigrette* (p. 341) Lean Cuisine Four Cheese Pizza Grapes, ½ c.
SNACK		
Stuffed Celery (p. 305), 2	Jell-O Pudding Snack Cup, 1	Healthy Choice Ice Cream Sandwich, 1
DINNER		
Poached Salmon w/Balsamic Tomato Sauce (p. 209) *Tropical Rice* (p. 274) Peas, ½ c.	*Poached Salmon w/Balsamic Tomato Sauce* (p. 209) *Tropical Rice* (p. 274) Peas, ¾ c.	*Poached Salmon w/Balsamic Tomato Sauce* (p. 209) 1½ srv. *Tropical Rice* (p. 274), 1½ srv. Peas, ¾ c.
SNACK		
Planters Peanut Butter Cookie Crisps, 1 pack	Chips Ahoy Thin Crisps, 1 pack	Chips Ahoy Thin Crisps, 1 pack
38 grams fat **1,227 calories**	**46 grams fat** **1,493 calories**	**56 grams fat** **1,834 calories**

Weekday Menu PHASE ③ 30% Fat

1,200 CALORIES 40 GRAMS FAT	1,500 CALORIES 50 GRAMS FAT	1,800 CALORIES 60 GRAMS FAT

BREAKFAST
Aunt Jemima Pancakes, 3,
  w/reduced-fat marg., 1T.,
  sugar-free syrup, 1 T.
	Banana Nut-Hotcakes (p. 137)
	  w/reduced-fat marg., 1 T.,
	  sugar-free syrup, 1 T.
		Banana-Nut Hotcakes (p. 137),
		  w/reduced-fat marg. 1 T.,
		  sugar-free syrup, 1 T.
		Milk, whole, ½ c.

LUNCH
Greens w/mandarin oranges,
  ½ c., *Honey-Lime Dressing*
  (p. 338)
Smart Ones Meatloaf w/Mashed
  Potatoes
	Greens w/sliced pear, *Honey-Lime*
	  Dressing (p. 338)
	Smart Ones Meatloaf w/Mashed
	  Potatoes
		Greens salad w/*Garlic Vinaigrette*
		  (p. 341)
		Italian bread, 2" piece
		Lean Cuisine Meatloaf with/
		  Whipped Potato

SNACK *Stuffed Celery* (p. 305), 1	*Stuffed Celery* (p. 305), 3	*Stuffed Celery* (p. 305), 3

DINNER
Chicken Fajitas (p. 222)
	Super-Quick Pumpkin Soup
	  (p. 153)
	Chicken Fajitas (p. 222)
		Super-Quick Pumpkin Soup
		  (p. 153), 1½ srv.
		Chicken Fajitas (p. 222), w/light
		  sour cream, 1 T.

SNACK Archway Oatmeal Raisin Cookie, 1	Low-fat ice cream sandwich, 1	Low-fat ice cream sandwich, 1
36 grams fat **1,212 calories**	**44 grams fat** **1,498 calories**	**57 grams fat** **1,794 calories**

Weekday Menu PHASE ③ 30% Fat

1,200 CALORIES 40 GRAMS FAT	1,500 CALORIES 50 GRAMS FAT	1,800 CALORIES 60 GRAMS FAT
BREAKFAST Grape-Nuts Flakes, ¾ c. Milk, whole, ¾ c. Blueberries, ¼ c.	Grape-Nuts Flakes, 1¼ c. Milk, whole, 1¼ c. Blueberries, ½ c.	Grape-Nuts Flakes, 1½ c. Milk, whole, 1¼ c. Blueberries, ½ c.
LUNCH *Turkey Burger* (p. 234) Low-fat Swiss, 1 oz.	*Turkey Burger* (p. 234) Low-fat Swiss, 1½ oz. Grapes, ½ c.	*Turkey Burger* (p. 234) Low-fat Swiss, 2 oz. Baked Tostitos, 1 oz.

SNACK
Planters Peanut Butter Crisps,
  1 pack
	Planters Peanut Butter Crisps,
	  1 pack
		Gingersnaps, 4

DINNER
Greens w/*Creamy Italian*
  Dressing (p. 336)
Bird's Eye Skillet Garlic Shrimp,
  1¼ c.
Soft breadstick, 1, w/reduced-
  fat marg., 1 tsp
	Greens w/*Creamy Italian Dressing*
	  (p. 336)
	Bird's Eye Skillet Garlic Shrimp,
	  1½ c.
	Soft breadstick, 2, w/reduced-fat
	  marg., 1 tsp
		Greens w/*Creamy Italian Dressing*
		  (p. 336)
		Bird's Eye Skillet Garlic Shrimp,
		  1¾ c.
		Italian bread, 2" piece w/reduced-
		  fat marg., 2 tsp.

SNACK Vitalicious Brownie, 1	Vitalicious Brownie, 1	Vitalicious Brownie, 1
37 grams fat **1,203 calories**	**47 grams fat** **1,521 calories**	**54 grams fat** **1,799 calories**

Weekday Menu PHASE 3 30% Fat

1,200 CALORIES 40 GRAMS FAT	1,500 CALORIES 50 GRAMS FAT	1,800 CALORIES 60 GRAMS FAT

BREAKFAST
Hot Pockets Ham, Egg &
  Cheese, 1
Citrus sections, 1 c.
	Hot Pockets Bacon, Egg &
	  Cheese, 1
	Citrus sections, 1 c.
	Milk, 1%, 1 c.
		Hot Pockets Biscuit w/Bacon, Egg &
		  Cheese, 1
		Citrus sections, 1½ c.

LUNCH
Spinach wrap w/ham, 2oz., low
  fat Swiss, 1 oz., light mayo,
  1 tsp., lettuce & tomato
	Spinach wrap w/ham, 4oz., low
	  fat Swiss, 1 oz., light mayo,
	  1 T., lettuce & tomato
		Spinach wrap w/roast beef, 4 oz.,
		  low fat Swiss, 1 oz., light mayo,
		  1 T., lettuce and tomato
		Apple, 1

SNACK *Stuffed Celery* (p. 305), 2	*Stuffed Celery* (p. 305), 1	*Stuffed Celery* (p. 305), 2
DINNER *Fish Sticks* (p. 198), 4 *Tartar Sauce* (p. 330) *Creamy Coleslaw* (p. 286)	*Fish Sticks* (p. 198), 5 *Tartar Sauce* (p. 330) *Creamy Coleslaw* (p. 286)	*Fish Sticks* (p. 198), 6 *Tartar Sauce* (p. 330), 2 srv. *Creamy Coleslaw* (p. 286), 2 srv.

SNACK
Raspberry Sauce (p. 300) over
  light ice cream, ½ c.
	Raspberry Sauce (p. 300) over
	  light ice cream, ½ c.
		Raspberry Sauce (p. 300) over light
		  ice cream, ½ c.

36 grams fat **1,223 calories**	**48 grams fat** **1,511 calories**	**57 grams fat** **1,796 calories**

Weekday Menu PHASE 3 30% Fat

1,200 CALORIES 40 GRAMS FAT	1,500 CALORIES 50 GRAMS FAT	1,800 CALORIES 60 GRAMS FAT

BREAKFAST
English muffin
Cranberry-Walnut Spread
  (p. 324)
Milk, whole, ¾ c.
	English muffin
	Cranberry-Walnut Spread
	  (p. 324)
	Milk, whole, 1 c.
		English muffin
		Cranberry-Walnut Spread (p. 324),
		  2 srv.
		Milk, whole, 1 c.

LUNCH
Hero's Hoagie (p. 236)
	Hero's Hoagie (p. 236), w/turkey
	  breast, 2 oz. extra
		Hero's Hoagie (p. 236), w/turkey
		  breast, 2 oz. extra
		Archway Oatmeal Raisin Cookie, 1

SNACK Plum, 1	Fudgsicle, 1	Plum, 1

DINNER
Birds Eye Skillet Beefsteak &
  Potatoes, 1½ c.
Peas, ½ c.
Dinner roll, 1
	Birds Eye Skillet Beefsteak &
	  Potatoes, 2 c.
	Peas, ½ c.
	Dinner roll, 1
		Birds Eye Skillet Beefsteak &
		  Potatoes, 2 c.
		Peas, 1 c.
		Dinner roll, 1, w/reduced-fat
		  margarine, 2 tsp.

SNACK *Grilled Peaches* (p. 299)	*Grilled Peaches* (p. 299) Stella D'Oro Anisette Cookie, 1	*Mixed Fruit w/Strawberry-Ginger Sauce* (p. 298) Light ice cream, ½ c.
37 grams fat **1,209 calories**	**46 grams fat** **1,507 calories**	**55 grams fat** **1,821 calories**

Weekday Menu PHASE ③ 30% Fat

1,200 CALORIES 40 GRAMS FAT	1,500 CALORIES 50 GRAMS FAT	1,800 CALORIES 60 GRAMS FAT
BREAKFAST Egg, scrambled dry, 1, w/lean ham, 1 oz. Whole wheat toast, 1 slice, w/ reduced-fat margarine, 1 tsp. Grapefruit, ½	Egg, scrambled dry, 1, w/lean ham, 2 oz. Whole wheat toast, 2 slices, w/ reduced fat margarine, 2 tsp. Citrus sections, ½ c.	Egg, scrambled dry, 2 Whole wheat toast, 2 slices Citrus sections, 1 c.
LUNCH Progresso Macaroni and Bean Soup, ½ c. *Grilled Cheese and Bacon* (p. 250)	Progresso Macaroni and Bean Soup, 1 c., w/ Parmesan, 2 tsp. *Grilled Cheese and Bacon* (p. 250)	Progresso Macaroni and Bean Soup, ¾ c., w/ Parmesan, 1 T. *Grilled Cheese and Bacon* (p. 250), 1½ srv.
SNACK Plum, 1	Plum, 1	Plum, 1
DINNER Baked tilapia fillet, 6 oz. *Tomato Chutney* (p. 322) Uncle Ben's Ready Rice, ½ c. *Cheesy Broccoli* (p. 264)	Baked tilapia fillet, 6 oz. *Tomato Chutney* (p. 322) Uncle Ben's Ready Rice, 1 c. *Cheesy Broccoli* (p. 264)	Baked tilapia fillet, 6 oz. *Tomato Chutney* (p. 322), 2 srv. Uncle Ben's Ready Rice, 1½ c. *Cheesy Broccoli* (p. 264), 1½ srv.
SNACK *Fresh Raspberry Sauce* (p. 300), over light ice cream, ½ c.	*Fresh Raspberry Sauce* (p. 300), over light ice cream, ½ c.	*Fresh Raspberry Sauce* (p. 300), over light ice cream, ½ c.
36 grams fat **1,211 calories**	**45 grams fat** **1,520 calories**	**54 grams fat** **1,797 calories**

Weekday Menu PHASE ③ 20% Fat

1,200 CALORIES 40 GRAMS FAT	1,500 CALORIES 50 GRAMS FAT	1,800 CALORIES 60 GRAMS FAT
BREAKFAST *Aloha Fruit Salad* (p. 167), no lettuce Cottage cheese, whole milk, ½ c.	*Aloha Fruit Salad* (p. 167), no lettuce Cottage cheese, whole milk, ¾ c.	*Aloha Fruit Salad* (p. 167), no lettuce, 1¼ srv. Cottage cheese, whole milk, ¾ c.
LUNCH Mixed greens w/low-fat Italian dressing, 2 T. Birds Eye Voila Garlic Shrimp Skillet, ¾ c. Uncle Ben's Ready Rice, ½ c.	Mixed greens w/low-fat Italian dressing, 2 T. Birds Eye Voila Garlic Shrimp Skillet, 1¼ c. Uncle Ben's Ready Rice, ½ c.	Mixed greens w/low-fat Italian dressing, 2 T. Birds Eye Voila Garlic Shrimp Skillet, 1½ c. Uncle Ben's Ready Rice, ¾ c.
SNACK Laughing Cow Light Cheese Wedge, 1 Low-fat wheat crackers, 4	Laughing Cow Light Cheese Wedge, 1 Low-fat wheat crackers, 4	Laughing Cow Light Cheese Wedge, 1 Low-fat wheat crackers, 5
DINNER *Brook Trout w/Tomato Relish* (p. 212) *Creamed Spinach* (p. 277) Steamed carrots, ¾ c.	*Brook Trout w/Tomato Relish* (p. 212) *Creamed Spinach* (p. 277) *Glazed Carrots* (p. 279), 1½ srv.	*Brook Trout w/Tomato Relish* (p. 212), 1½ srv. *Creamed Spinach* (p. 277) *Glazed Carrots* (p. 279), 2 srv.
SNACK *Carrot Cake* (p. 293)	*Carrot Cake* (p. 293)	*Carrot Cake* (p. 293)
38 grams fat **1,215 calories**	**47 grams fat** **1,488 calories**	**57 grams fat** **1,804 calories**

Weekday Menu PHASE ③ 30% Fat

1,200 CALORIES 40 GRAMS FAT	1,500 CALORIES 50 GRAMS FAT	1,800 CALORIES 60 GRAMS FAT
BREAKFAST Toasted French bread, 1 slice Goat cheese, ¾ oz. Apple, 1	Toasted French bread, 2 slices Goat cheese, 1¼ oz. Apple, 1	Toasted French bread, 2 slices Goat cheese, 1¼ oz. Apple, 1

LUNCH
Tuna Salad Sandwich (p. 218)
Campbell's Select Creamy Potato/
  Garlic Soup, ½ c.
	Tuna Salad Sandwich (p. 218)
	Kraft Singles 2 % sharp Cheddar,
	  1 slice
	Campbell's Cream of Potato
	  Soup, ½ c.
		Tuna Salad Sandwich (p. 218),
		  1½ srv.
		Campbell's Cream of Potato
		  Soup, 1 c.

SNACK Gingersnaps, 4	Gingersnaps, 3	Kashi Go Lean Crunch Bar, Chocolate Caramel, 1

DINNER
Grilled Tofu Burger (p. 188),
  w/roll
Creamy Coleslaw (p. 286)
	Grilled Tofu Burger (p. 188),
	  w/roll
	Creamy Coleslaw (p. 286), 2 srv.
	Baked potato chips, 1 oz.
		Grilled Tofu Burger (p. 188), w/roll
		Creamy Coleslaw (p. 286), 2 srv.
		Baked Tostitos, 1 oz.
		Guacamole (p. 323)

SNACK
Healthy Choice Ice Cream
  Sandwich, 1
	Healthy Choice Ice Cream
	  Sandwich, 1
		Healthy Choice Ice Cream
		  Sandwich, 1

36 grams fat **1,209 calories**	**45 grams fat** **1,501 calories**	**55 grams fat** **1,804 calories**

Weekday Menu PHASE ③ 30% Fat

1,200 CALORIES 40 GRAMS FAT	1,500 CALORIES 50 GRAMS FAT	1,800 CALORIES 60 GRAMS FAT

BREAKFAST
Kashi Go Lean cereal, ¾ c.,
  w/milk, whole, 1 c.
Strawberries, ½ c.
	Kashi Go Lean cereal, 1 c.,
	  w/milk, whole, 1 c.
	Strawberries, ½ c.
		Kashi Go Lean Crunch cereal, 1 c.,
		  w/milk, whole, 1 c., & walnuts,
		  chopped, 1 tsp.
		Blueberries, ½ c.

LUNCH
Chicken Soup with Soba Noodles
  (p. 155)
Lettuce and tomato salad w/lean
  ham, 2 oz., 2% shredded
  cheddar, 1 T., Wish-Bone Light!
  Ranch Dressing, 2 T.
	Chicken Soup with Soba Noodles
	  (p. 155)
	Lettuce and tomato salad w/lean.
	  ham, 4 oz., 2% shredded
	  cheddar, 2 T., Wish-Bone
	  Light! Ranch Dressing, 2 T.
		Chicken Soup with Soba Noodles
		  (p. 155)
		Lettuce and tomato salad w/lean
		  ham, 4 oz., low fat Swiss
		  cheese, 2 oz., Wish-Bone Light!
		  Ranch Dressing, 2 T.

SNACK Stella D'Oro Breakfast Treat, 1	Stella D'Oro Breakfast Treat, 1	Pear, 1

DINNER
Pork tenderloin, 3 oz.
Braised Cabbage w/Apples
  (p. 270)
Egg noodles, ½ c.
	Pork tenderloin, 5 oz.
	Braised Cabbage w/Apples
	  (p. 270)
	Egg noodles, ½ c.
		Pork tenderloin, 6 oz.
		Braised Cabbage w/Apples,
		  (p. 270), 1½ srv.
		Egg noodles, ¾ c.

SNACK *Grilled Peaches* (p. 299)	*Grilled Peaches* (p. 299)	*Grilled Peaches* (p. 299)
38 grams fat **1,217 calories**	**47 grams fat** **1,494 calories**	**57 grams fat** **1,832 calories**

Weekday Menu PHASE ③ 30% Fat

1,200 CALORIES 40 GRAMS FAT	1,500 CALORIES 50 GRAMS FAT	1,800 CALORIES 60 GRAMS FAT
BREAKFAST Cantaloupe, ½ Cottage cheese, whole milk, ½ c., w/slivered almonds, 2 tsp	Cantaloupe, ½ Cottage cheese, whole milk, ¾ c., w/blackberries, ½ c., slivered almonds, 2 tsp.	Cantaloupe, ½ Cottage cheese, whole milk, ¾ c., w/mixed berries, 1 c., slivered almonds, 1 T.
LUNCH Mixed greens w/1 chopped apple, *Raspberry-Walnut Dressing* (p. 333) *Arizona Jerk Turkey* (p. 233), 1¼ srv.	Mixed greens w/1 chopped apple, chopped walnuts, 1 tsp., *Raspberry-Walnut Dressing* (p. 333) *Arizona Jerk Turkey* (p. 233), 1½ srv.	Mixed greens w/1 chopped apple, chopped walnuts, 3 tsp., *Raspberry-Walnut Dressing* (p. 333) *Arizona Jerk Turkey* (p. 233), 2 srv.
SNACK Laughing Cow Light Cheese Wedge, 1 Low-at wheat crackers, 4	Chips Ahoy Thin Crisps, 1 pack	Laughing Cow Light Cheese Wedge, 1 Low-fat wheat crackers, 7
DINNER *Spaghetti and Meatballs* (p. 267), w/1 T. Parmesan	*Spaghetti and Meatballs* (p. 267), w/2 T. Parmesan Soft breadstick, 1	*Spaghetti and Meatballs* (p. 267), 1½ srv., w/2 T. Parmesan
SNACK Jell-O Pudding Snack Cup, 1	Jell-O Pudding Snack Cup, 1	Jell-O Pudding Snack Cup, 1
38 grams fat **1,334 calories**	**47 grams fat** **1,521 calories**	**56 grams fat** **1,803 calories**

Weekday Menu PHASE ③ 30% Fat

1,200 CALORIES 40 GRAMS FAT	1,500 CALORIES 50 GRAMS FAT	1,800 CALORIES 60 GRAMS FAT
BREAKFAST Wheaties, 1 c. w/milk, whole, ¾ c. Strawberries, ½ c.	Wheaties, 1¼ c. w/ milk, whole, 1¼ c. Blueberries, ½ cup	Wheaties, 1½ c. w/ milk, whole, 1¼ c. Blueberries, ½ cup
LUNCH Whole wheat bread, 2 slices, w/ lean ham, 2 oz., low-fat Swiss, 1½ oz., lettuce, tomato, and reduced-fat mayo, 1 T.	Whole wheat bread, 2 slices, w/lean ham, 4 oz., low-fat Swiss, 2 oz., lettuce, tomato, and reduced-fat mayo, 1 T.	Whole wheat bread, 2 slices, w/lean ham, 4 oz., low-fat Swiss, 2 oz., lettuce, tomato, and reduced-fat mayo, 1 T. Plums, 2
SNACK Plum, 1	Plum, 1	Graham cracker, 1
DINNER Mixed greens with *Garlic Vinaigrette* (p. 341) *Jambalaya* (p. 216)	Mixed greens with *Garlic Vinaigrette* (p. 341) *Jambalaya* (p. 216), 1¼ srv.	Mixed greens w/*Garlic Vinaigrette* (p. 341) and crumbled blue cheese, 1 T. *Jambalaya* (p. 216), 1½ srv.
SNACK *Spiced Apples* (p. 295) Keebler Country Oatmeal Cookie, 1	*Spiced Apples* (p. 295) Keebler Country Oatmeal Cookie, 1	*Spiced Apples* (p. 295) Keebler Country Oatmeal Cookie, 2
37 grams fat **1,220 calories**	**47 grams fat** **1,521 calories**	**56 grams fat** **1,819 calories**

Weekday Menu PHASE ③ 30% Fat

1,200 CALORIES 40 GRAMS FAT	1,500 CALORIES 50 GRAMS FAT	1,800 CALORIES 60 GRAMS FAT
BREAKFAST Pumpernickel bread, 2 slices Monterey Jack cheese, 1¼ oz. Grapes, 1 c.	Pumpernickel bread, 2 slices Monterey Jack cheese, 1½ oz. Grapes, ½ c.; Pear, 1	Pumpernickel bread, 2 slices Monterey Jack cheese, 1¼ oz. Pear, 1; Milk, 1%, 1 c.
LUNCH Chicken breast, no skin, 6 oz. Mixed greens with light Italian dressing, 2 T.	Chicken breast, no skin, 5 oz. Mixed greens w/light Italian dressing, 2 T. Whole wheat roll w/ margarine, reduced fat, 2 tsp.	Chicken breast, no skin, 6 oz. Mixed greens w/ light Italian dressing, 2 T., and crumbled feta, 2 T. Club roll w/margarine, reduced-fat, 2 tsp.
SNACK Plum, 1	Plum, 1	Plum, 1
DINNER *Baby Greens with Avocado/ Strawberries* (p. 169) *Mussels Marinière* (p. 196) Italian bread, 1½" piece	*Baby Greens with Avocado/ Strawberries* (p. 169) *Mussels Marinière* (p. 196) *Orzo with Cherry Tomatoes, Capers, and Pine Nuts* (p. 260)	*Baby Greens with Avocado/ Strawberries* (p. 169) *Mussels Marinière* (p. 196) w/ Parmesan cheesse, 1 T. *Orzo with Cherry Tomatoes, Capers, and Pine Nuts* (p. 260), 1½ srv.
SNACK Breyers Light Ice Cream, ½ c.	Breyers Light Ice Cream, ½ c.	Breyers Light Ice Cream, ½ c.
40 grams fat 1,233 calories	**48 grams fat 1,517 calories**	**58 grams fat 1,820 calories**

Weekday Menu PHASE ③ 30% Fat

1,200 CALORIES 40 GRAMS FAT	1,500 CALORIES 50 GRAMS FAT	1,800 CALORIES 60 GRAMS FAT
BREAKFAST *Cranberry Muffin* (p. 141) Milk, 2%, 1 c. Sliced strawberries, ½ c.	*Cranberry Muffin* (p. 141) Milk, whole, 1 c. Mixed berries, ½ c.	*Cranberry Muffins* (p. 141), 2 Milk, whole, 1 c. Blueberries, ½ c.
LUNCH *Penne w/Broccoli* (p. 264) Plum, 1	*Penne w/Broccoli* (p. 264), 1¼ srv. Plum, 1	*Penne w/Broccoli* (p. 264), 1½ srv. Plum, 1
SNACK Archway Oatmeal Raisin Cookie, 1	Archway Oatmeal Raisin Cookie, 1	Archway Oatmeal Raisin Cookie, 1
DINNER Mixed greens w/*Creamy Italian Dressing* (p. 336) Birds Eye Voila Beefsteak and Garlic Potatoes, 1½ c. Buttermilk biscuit, 1	Mixed greens w/*Creamy Italian Dressing* (p. 336) Birds Eye Voila Beefsteak and Garlic Potatoes, 1½ c. Club roll w/margarine, reduced-fat, 2 tsp.	Mixed greens w/*Poppy Seed Dressing* (p. 340) Birds Eye Voila Beefsteak and Garlic Potatoes, 2 c. Soft breadsticks, 2, w/margarine, reduced-fat, 1 tsp.
SNACK *Chocolate-Covered Strawberries* (p. 289) Stella D'Oro Anisette Cookie, 1	*Chocolate-Covered Strawberries* (p. 289) Stella D'Oro Anisette Cookie, 1	*Chocolate-Covered Strawberries* (p. 289) Stella D'Oro Anisette Cookie, 1
38 grams fat 1,236 calories	**48 grams fat 1,502 calories**	**58 grams fat 1,799 calories**

Weekday Menu PHASE ③ 30% Fat

1,200 CALORIES 40 GRAMS FAT	1,500 CALORIES 50 GRAMS FAT	1,800 CALORIES 60 GRAMS FAT

BREAKFAST
Almond-Pumpkin Breakfast
  Bread (p. 139)
Milk, 1%, 1 c.
	Almond-Pumpkin Breakfast
	  Bread (p. 139), 1½ srv.
	Milk, 1%, 1 c.
		Almond-Pumpkin Breakfast
		  Bread (p. 139), 2 srv.
		Milk, 1%, 1 c.

LUNCH
Lean Pockets Ultra Meatballs &
  Mozzarella, 1
Lettuce and tomato salad w/
  Italian dressing, light, 2 T.
Grapes, 1 cup
	Lean Pockets Jalapeno Steak, 1
	Lettuce and tomato salad w/
	  Italian dressing, low-fat, 2 T.
	Peach, 1
		Lean Pockets Jalapeno Steak, 1
		Lettuce and tomato salad
		  w/Italian dressing, light, 2 T.,
		  and blue cheese, crumbled,
		  1 T.
		Cherries, 30

SNACK
Archway Oatmeal Raisin
  Cookie, 1
	Archway Oatmeal Raisin
	  Cookie, 1
		Archway Oatmeal Raisin
		  Cookie, 1

DINNER
Pasta Primavera (p. 261)
	Pasta Primavera (p. 261) w/
	  steamed shrimp, 8 large
		Pasta Primavera (p. 261)
		  w/steamed shrimp, 8 large
		Italian bread, 1" piece, w/mar-
		  garine, reduced-fat, 1 T.

SNACK Pear, 1	Jell-O Pudding Snack Cup, 1	Plum, 1
37.2 grams fat **1,241 calories**	**48 grams fat** **1,549 calories**	**57 grams fat** **1,783 calories**

Weekday Menu PHASE ③ 30% Fat

1,200 CALORIES 40 GRAMS FAT	1,500 CALORIES 50 GRAMS FAT	1,800 CALORIES 60 GRAMS FAT

BREAKFAST
Almond-Pumpkin Breakfast
  Bread (p. 139)
Milk, 1%, 1 c.
	Almond-Pumpkin Breakfast Bread
	  (p. 139)
	Milk, 2%, ½ c.
	Blueberries, ½ c.
		Almond-Pumpkin Breakfast
		  Bread (p. 139)
		Cream cheese, 1 T.
		Milk, 1%, 1 c.
		Orange, 1

LUNCH
Campbell's Chunky Turkey Pot
  Pie Soup, 1¼ c.
Buttermilk biscuit, lower-fat, 1
Plum, 2
	Campbell's Chunky Chicken &
	  Dumplings Soup, 1½ c.
	7-grain french roll, 1
	Peach, 1
		Campbell's Chunky Chicken &
		  Dumplings Soup, 1½ c.
		Whole wheat roll, 1
		Oatmeal raisin cookie, 1
		Apple, 1

SNACK Fat-free popcorn, 1 bag	Fat-free popcorn, 1 bag	Jell-O Pudding Snack Cup, 1

DINNER
Greek Lamb Kabobs (p. 253)
Uncle Ben's Ready Rice, 1 c.
	Greek Lamb Kabobs (p. 253),
	  1½ srv.
	Uncle Ben's Ready Rice, 1 c.
		Greek Lamb Kabobs (p. 253),
		  2 srv.
		Uncle Ben's Ready Rice, 1½ c.

SNACK Snackwell Fat-Free Cookie, 1	Ice cream, light, ½ c.	Peach, 1
36 grams fat **1,211 calories**	**47 grams fat** **1,501 calories**	**56 grams fat** **1,813 calories**

Weekday Menu PHASE (3) 30% Fat

1,200 CALORIES 40 GRAMS FAT	1,500 CALORIES 50 GRAMS FAT	1,800 CALORIES 60 GRAMS FAT
BREAKFAST Amy's Breakfast Burrito, 1	Amy's Breakfast Burrito, 1 Milk, 1%, 1 c.	Amy's Breakfast Burrito, 1 Milk, 2%, 1 c.
LUNCH *Warm Eggplant, Tomato, and Mozzarella Salad* (p. 165), Steamed shrimp, 8 large Crisp breadsticks, 2 Margarine, reduced-fat, 1t.	*Warm Eggplant, Tomato, and Mozzarella Salad* (p. 165), 1½ srv., w/steamed shrimp, 8 large Club roll, 1	*Warm Eggplant, Tomato, and Mozzarella Salad* (p. 165), 1½ srv., w/steamed shrimp, 12 large Whole wheat roll, 1 Apple, 1
SNACK Jell-O Pudding Snack Cup, 1	Jell-O Sugar Free Pudding, 1	Jell-O Pudding Snack, 1
DINNER *Chicken Fajitas* (p. 222)	*Chicken Fajitas* (p. 222) Sour cream, 2T.	Campbell's Chunky Potato w/Bacon, 1c. *Chicken Fajitas* (p. 222) Sour cream, 2T
SNACK *Fresh Raspberry Sauce* (p. 300) over 1 sliced peach	*Fresh Raspberry Sauce* (p. 300) over 1 sliced pear	Planters Peanut Butter Cookie Crisps, 1 packet
36 grams fat **1,228 calories**	**48 grams fat** **1,509 calories**	**57 grams fat** **1,808 calories**

Weekday Menu PHASE (3) 30% Fat

1,200 CALORIES 40 GRAMS FAT	1,500 CALORIES 50 GRAMS FAT	1,800 CALORIES 60 GRAMS FAT
BREAKFAST Dannon La Crème Mousse Yogurt, 4 oz. Granola, ½ c. Strawberries, sliced, ¼ c.	Dannon La Crème Mousse Yogurt, 4 oz. Granola, ½ c. Strawberries, sliced, ½ c.	Dannon La Crème Mousse Yogurt, 4 oz. Granola, ½ c. Strawberries, sliced, ½ c. Walnuts, chopped, 2 t.
LUNCH Stouffer's Chicken à la King	Stouffer's Chicken à la King Buttermilk biscuit, 1, w/margarine, reduced-fat, 1 tsp.	Stouffer's Chicken à la King Buttermilk biscuits, 2, w/ margarine, reduced-fat, 2t.
SNACK Planters Peanut Butter Cookie Crisps, 1 packet	Chips Ahoy Thin Crisps, 1packet	Chips Ahoy Thin Crisps, 1packet
DINNER Mixed lettuce salad, 1½ c., w/ranch dressing, fat-free, 2 T. *Brook Trout w/Tomato and Red Onion Relish* (p. 212) *Garden Peas* (p. 269)	Mixed lettuce salad, 1½ c., w/ranch dressing, fat-free, 2 T. *Brook Trout w/Tomato and Red Onion Relish* (p. 212) *Garden Peas* (p. 269), 2 srv.	Mixed lettuce salad, 1½ c., w/ranch dressing, fat-free, 2 T. *Brook Trout w/Tomato and Red Onion Relish* (p. 212) *Garden Peas* (p. 269), 1½ srv. Uncle Ben's Ready Rice, 1 c.
SNACK *Strawberry Sauce* (p. 300) over 1 sliced peach	*Strawberry Sauce* (p. 300) over 1 sliced peach	*Strawberry Sauce* (p. 300) over 1 sliced peach
38 grams fat **1,226 calories**	**48 grams fat** **1,514 calories**	**55 grams fat** **1,825 calories**

Weekday Menu PHASE ③ 30% Fat

1,200 CALORIES 40 GRAMS FAT	1,500 CALORIES 50 GRAMS FAT	1,800 CALORIES 60 GRAMS FAT
BREAKFAST Eggs, scrambled dry, 1 Cantaloupe, ¼ Wheat toast, 2 slices, w/margarine, reduced-fat, 1 tsp.	Eggs, scrambled dry, 2 Cantaloupe, ¼ Wheat toast, 2 slices	Eggs, scrambled dry, 2 Cantaloupe, ½ Wheat toast, 2 slices, w/margarine, reduced-fat, 1 T.
LUNCH *Portobello Burger* (p. 189) w/fresh mozzarella, ½ oz. Greens w/*Poppy Seed Dressing* (p. 340), 2 T.	*Portobello Burger* (p. 189) w/fresh mozzarella, 1 oz., and roasted red pepper, 1 oz. Greens w/*Poppy Seed Dressing* (p. 340), 2 T.	*Portobello Burger* (p. 189) w/fresh mozzarella, 1 oz., and roasted red pepper, 2 oz. Greens w/*Poppy Seed Dressing* (p. 340), 2 T.
SNACK Honey Maid Cinnamon Thin Crisps, 1 pack	Planters Peanut Butter Cookie Crisps, 1 pack	Archway Oatmeal Raisin Cookie, 1
DINNER *Pan-Seared Red Snapper* (p. 211) *Baked Asparagus* (p. 281)	*Pan-Seared Red Snapper* (p. 211) *Baked Asparagus* (p. 281) Uncle Ben's Ready Rice, ½ c.	*Pan-Seared Red Snapper* (p. 211) *Baked Asparagus* (p. 281) Uncle Ben's Ready Rice, 1¼ c.
SNACK Raspberries and blueberries, 1 c. *Yogurt Cheese* (p. 305), 2T. Walnuts, chopped, 1 T.	Raspberries and blueberries, 1 c. *Yogurt Cheese* (p. 305), ¼ c. Walnuts, chopped, 1 T.	Raspberries and blueberries, 1 c. *Yogurt Cheese* (p. 305), ¼ c. Walnuts, chopped, 1 T.
39 grams fat **1,211 calories**	**48 grams fat** **1,488 calories**	**57 grams fat** **1,830 calories**

Weekday Menu PHASE ③ 30% Fat

1,200 CALORIES 40 GRAMS FAT	1,500 CALORIES 50 GRAMS FAT	1,800 CALORIES 60 GRAMS FAT
BREAKFAST *Ratatouille Omelet* (p. 145) Cantaloupe, ½	*Ratatouille Omelet* (p. 145) Cantaloupe, ½	*Ratatouille Omelet* (p. 145), Cantaloupe, ¼ Whole wheat toast, 1 slice, w/margarine, reduced-fat, 1t.
LUNCH Spinach tortilla wrap, w/roast beef, 4 oz., lettuce, tomato, and reduced-fat mayo, 1 T.	Spinach tortilla wrap, w/roast beef, 6 oz., Kraft Singles, 1 slice, lettuce, tomato, and reduced-fat mayo, 1 T.	Spinach tortilla wrap, w/roast beef, 6 oz., Kraft Singles, 1 slice, lettuce, tomato, and reduced-fat mayo, 1 T. *Creamy Coleslaw* (p. 286)
SNACK Plum, 1	Archway Oatmeal Raisin Cookie, 1	Pear, 1
DINNER *Spaghetti w/Summer Squash* (p. 258) Lettuce and tomato salad w/ *Poppy Seed Dressing* (p. 340)	*Spaghetti w/Summer Squash* (p. 258), 1¼ srv. Lettuce and tomato salad w/ *Poppy Seed Dressing* (p. 340)	*Spaghetti w/Summer Squash* (p. 258), 1½ srv. Lettuce and tomato salad w/ *Poppy Seed Dressing* (p. 340)
SNACK Chips Ahoy Thin Crisps, 1 pack	Low-fat ice cream, ½ c.	Low-fat ice cream, ½ c.
37 grams fat **1,236 calories**	**48 grams fat** **1,523 calories**	**57 grams fat** **1,808 calories**

Weekday Menu PHASE 3 30% Fat

1,200 CALORIES 40 GRAMS FAT	1,500 CALORIES 50 GRAMS FAT	1,800 CALORIES 60 GRAMS FAT
BREAKFAST Amy's Breakfast Burrito, 1 Sour cream, 1T.	Amy's Breakfast Burrito, 1 Sour cream, 2T. Grapefruit, ½	Hot Pockets Biscuits Bacon Egg & Cheese, 1 Milk, fat-free, 1c. Strawberries, ½ c.
LUNCH *Watercress and Strawberry Salad* (p. 168), 1½ srv., w/steamed shrimp, 8 large Watermelon chunks, 1 c.	*Watercress and Strawberry Salad* (p. 168), 2 srv., w/steamed shrimp, 8 large Watermelon chunks, 1 c.	*Watercress and Strawberry Salad* (p. 168), 2 srv., shrimp, 12 Watermelon chunks, 1 c. Crisp breadsticks, 2
SNACK *Stuffed Celery* (p. 305), 2 srv.	*Stuffed Celery* (p. 305), 2 srv.	*Stuffed Celery* (p. 305), 2 srv.
DINNER *Chicken Soup* (p. 155) Lean Cuisine Stuffed Cabbage w/ Whipped Potatoes	*Chicken Soup* (p. 155) Lean Cuisine Steak Tips Dijon	*Chicken Soup* (p. 155), 2 srv. Stouffer's Beef Pot Roast w/ Browned Potatoes
SNACK *Fresh Raspberry Sauce* (p. 300) Breyers Light Ice Cream, ½ c.	*Fresh Raspberry Sauce* (p. 300) Breyers Light Ice Cream, ½ c.	*Fresh Raspberry Sauce* (p. 300) Breyers Light Ice Cream, ½ c.
38.5 grams fat **1,238 calories**	**48 grams fat** **1,525 calories**	**57 grams fat** **1,818 calories**

Weekday Menu (Meatless) PHASE 3 30% Fat

1,200 CALORIES 40 GRAMS FAT	1,500 CALORIES 50 GRAMS FAT	1,800 CALORIES 60 GRAMS FAT
BREAKFAST English Muffin w/cream cheese, 1½ T., and Smucker's Low Sugar Fruit Preserves, 1 T. Orange, 1	English Muffin w/cream cheese, 2 T., and Smucker's Low Sugar Fruit Preserves, 2 T. Dannon Light 'n Fit Yogurt, 6 oz.	English Muffin w/cream cheese, 2 T., and Smucker's Low Sugar Fruit Preserves, 1 T. Dannon Natural Flavors Yogurt, 4 oz., over blueberries, ½ c.
LUNCH Campbell's Potato Soup, 1 c. Lettuce and tomato salad w/tuna (in water), 3 oz., and Italian dressing, fat-free, 2 T.	Campbell's Potato Soup, 1 c. Lettuce and tomato salad w/tuna (in water), 3 oz., and Italian dressing, light, 2 T Cherries, 20	Campbell's Potato Soup, 1½ c. Lettuce and tomato salad w/tuna (in water), 3 oz., Swiss cheese, low-fat, 1 oz., and Italian dressing, light, 2 T Cherries, 20
SNACK Edy's Light Ice Cream, ½ c.	Edy's Light Ice Cream, ½ c.	Low-fat popcorn, 1 bag
DINNER *Grilled Tofu Burger* (p. 188) Kraft 2% Sharp Cheddar, 1 slice *Creamy Coleslaw* (p. 286)	*Sesame Cheese Balls* (p. 304), 2 srv. *Grilled Tofu Burger* (p. 188) *Baked Beans* (p. 273), ½ srv.	*Grilled Tofu Burger* (p. 188) Kraft 2% Sharp Cheddar, 1 slice Potato chips, baked, 1 oz. *Chocolate-Covered Strawberries* (p. 289) Sara Lee Light Pound Cake, 1 slice
SNACK Low-fat popcorn, 1 bag	Low-fat popcorn, 1 bag	Health Valley Granola Bar, 1
39 grams fat **1,232 calories**	**47 grams fat** **1,508 calories**	**59.9 grams fat** **1,840 calories**

Weekday Menu PHASE ③ 30% Fat

1,200 CALORIES 40 GRAMS FAT	1,500 CALORIES 50 GRAMS FAT	1,800 CALORIES 60 GRAMS FAT
BREAKFAST Pepperidge Farm Homestyle French Toast, 1 slice, w/Smucker's Sugar Free Pancake Syrup, 2 T. Milk, 1%, ¾ c.	Pepperidge Farm Homestyle French Toast, 1 slice, w/ Smucker's Sugar Free Pancake Syrup, 2 T. Dannon La Crème Yogurt, 4 oz. Blueberries, ½ c.	Eggo Blueberry Waffles, 2, w/ Smucker's Sugar Free Pancake Syrup, 2 T. Dannon La Crème Yogurt, 4 oz. Blueberries, ½ c.
LUNCH *Hero's Hoagie* (p. 236)	*Hero's Hoagie* (p. 236) w/turkey breast, deli, 1 oz. Plum, 1	*Hero's Hoagie* (p. 236) plus turkey breast, deli, 2 oz. Progresso Healthy Minestrone, 1c.
SNACK Plums, 1	Breyers Light Ice Cream, ½ c.	Plums, 2
DINNER Roasted chicken breast, skinless and boneless, 4 oz. *Rosemary Roasted New Potatoes* (p. 280), 1½ srv. *Baked Asparagus* (p. 281)	Roasted chicken breast, skinless and boneless, 6 oz. *Rosemary Roasted New Potatoes* (p. 280) *Cheesy Broccoli* (p. 264)	Roasted chicken breast, skinless and boneless, 6 oz. *Rosemary Roasted New Potatoes* (p. 280), 1½ srv. *Cheesy Broccoli* (p. 264), 2 srv.
SNACK Breyers Light Ice Cream, ½ c.	Planters Peanut Butter Cookie Crisps, 1 pack	Edy's Light Ice Cream, ½ c. Stella D'Oro Anisette Cookies, 2
37 grams fat 1,229 calories	**48 grams fat 1,489 calories**	**54.3 grams fat 1,835 calories**

Weekday Menu PHASE ③ 30% Fat

1,200 CALORIES 40 GRAMS FAT	1,500 CALORIES 50 GRAMS FAT	1,800 CALORIES 60 GRAMS FAT
BREAKFAST *Aloha Fruit Salad w/Macadamia Crunch* (p. 167) (no lettuce) Cottage cheese, 2%, ½ c.	*Aloha Fruit Salad w/Macadamia Crunch* (p. 167) (no lettuce) Cottage cheese, 2%, ¾ c.	*Aloha Fruit Salad w/Macadamia Crunch* (p. 167) (no lettuce) Cottage cheese, 2%, 1 c.
LUNCH Hot Pockets Steak Fajita, 1 Mixed lettuce salad w/Wish-Bone Light! Peppercorn Ranch Dressing, 2 T. Plum, 1	Hot Pockets Jalapeño Steak and Cheese, 1 Mixed lettuce salad w/fat-free ranch dressing, 2 T.	Hot Pockets Four Cheese Pizza, 1 Mixed lettuce salad w/fat-free ranch dressing, 2 T. Snackwell's Fat Free Cookie Cakes, 2
SNACK Snackwell Fat-Free Cookie, 1	Healthy Choice Ice Cream Sandwich, 1	Wise Popcorn, butter flavor, ½ oz.
DINNER *Chilean Sea Bass* (p. 217) *Tropical Rice* (p. 274), ¾ srv. Tomato, 3 thick slices, w/*Basil-Cream Dressing* (p. 334)	*Chilean Sea Bass* (p. 217) *Tropical Rice* (p. 274), 1¼ srv. Tomato, 3 thick slices, w/*Basil-Cream Dressing* (p. 334)	*Chilean Sea Bass* (p. 217) *Tropical Rice* (p. 274), 1½ srv. *Creamed Spinach* (p. 277)
SNACK *Mixed Fruit w/Strawberry-Ginger Sauce* (p. 298)	Jell-O Pudding Snack Cup, 1	Planters Peanut Butter Cookie Crisps, 1 pack
36 grams fat 1,234 calories	**45 grams fat 1,519 calories**	**55 grams fat 1,800 calories**

Weekday Menu PHASE ③ 30% Fat

1,200 CALORIES 40 GRAMS FAT	1,500 CALORIES 50 GRAMS FAT	1,800 CALORIES 60 GRAMS FAT
BREAKFAST Quaker Oatmeal to Go Bar, 1 Milk, whole, ½ c.	Quaker Oatmeal to Go Bar, 1 Milk, whole, ¾ c.	Quaker Oatmeal to Go Bar, 1 Milk, whole, 1 c.
LUNCH *Watercress and Strawberry Salad* (p. 168), 1¼ srv., w/steamed shrimp, 8 large Whole wheat potato roll, 1	*Watercress and Strawberry Salad* (p. 168), 1¾ srv., w/shrimp, 8 large Whole wheat potato roll, 1	*Watercress and Strawberry Salad* (p. 168), 2 srv., w/shrimp, 12 large Whole wheat potato roll, 1
SNACK Peach, 1	Planters Peanut Butter Cookie Crisps, 1 pack	Nabisco Gingersnap Cookies, 4
DINNER Campbell's Chunky Roadhouse Chili, 1 c., w/Kraft Shredded Cheddar, 2%, 2 T. *Red, White, and Blue Parfait* (p. 292)	Campbell's Chunky Roadhouse Chili, 1 c., w/Kraft Shredded Cheddar, 2%, ¼ c. Uncle Ben's Flavorful Rice, Four Cheese, 1 c.	Campbell's Chunky Roadhouse Chili, 1½ c., w/Kraft Shredded Cheddar, 2%, ¼ c., and sour cream, light, 1T. Uncle Ben's Flavorful Rice, Four Cheese, 1 c.
SNACK Planters Peanut Butter Cookie Crisps, 1 pack	*Red, White, Blue Parfait* (p. 292)	*Red, White, Blue Parfait* (p. 292)
36 grams fat **1,224 calories**	**46 grams fat** **1,530 calories**	**56 grams fat** **1,798 calories**

Weekday Menu PHASE ③ 30% Fat

1,200 CALORIES 40 GRAMS FAT	1,500 CALORIES 50 GRAMS FAT	1,800 CALORIES 60 GRAMS FAT
BREAKFAST *Aloha Fruit Salad w/Macadamia Crunch* (p. 167) (no lettuce) Cottage cheese, whole-milk, ½ c. Health Valley low-fat cookie, 1	*Aloha Fruit Salad w/Macadamia Crunch* (p. 167) (no lettuce) Cottage cheese, 2%, 1 c.	*Aloha Fruit Salad w/Macadamia Crunch* (p. 167) (no lettuce) Cottage cheese, whole-milk, ½ c. Pepperidge Farm Raisin Bread, 1 slice
LUNCH Bird Eye Chicken Fajita Skillet, 1½ c. Oreo Thin Crisps, 1 pack Peach, 1	Bumble Bee Chicken Salad w/Crackers Lunch Kit, 1 Oreo Thin Crisps, 1 pack Dried figs, 2	Bumble Bee Chicken Salad w/Crackers Lunch Kit, 1 Milk, fat-free, 1 c. Plums, 2
SNACK *Stuffed Celery* (p. 305)	Pear, 1 oz.	Whole fruit sorbet, ½ c.
DINNER *Tuna Kabobs* (p. 205) *Vegetable Risotto*, as side dish (p. 276), 1½ srv.	*Tuna Kabobs* (p. 205), 1½ srv. *Vegetable Risotto*, as side dish (p. 276)	*Tuna Kabobs* (p. 205), 2 srv. *Vegetable Risotto*, as side dish (p. 276), 1½ srv.
SNACK *Chocolate-Covered Strawberries*, (p. 289), 1½ srv.	*Chocolate-Covered Strawberries* (p. 289); Stella D'Oro Anisette Cookie, 1	*Chocolate-Covered Strawberries* (p. 289); Stella D'Oro Anisette Cookie, 1
38.5 grams fat **1,223 calories**	**46 grams fat** **1,524 calories**	**55 grams fat** **1,802 calories**

Weekday Menu PHASE 3 30% Fat

1,200 CALORIES 40 GRAMS FAT	1,500 CALORIES 50 GRAMS FAT	1,800 CALORIES 60 GRAMS FAT
BREAKFAST *Almond-Pumpkin Bread* (p. 139) Milk, 1%, 1 c.	*Almond-Pumpkin Bread* (p. 139) Milk, 2%, 1 c. Orange, 1	*Almond-Pumpkin Bread* (p. 139) Milk, 2%, 1 c. Orange, 1
LUNCH *Hero's Hoagie* (p. 236)	*Hero's Hoagie* (p. 236) w/turkey breast, deli, 1 oz.	*Hero's Hoagie* (p. 236) w/turkey breast, 2 oz.
SNACK Pear, 1	Newton Caramel Apple Bar, 3	Newton Caramel Apple Bar, 3
DINNER Mixed greens w/Wish-Bone Light! Parmesan Peppercorn Dressing, 2 T. Stouffer's Stuffed Pepper, 10 oz. Soft breadstick, 1	Mixed greens w/Wish-Bone Light! Parmesan Peppercorn Ranch Dressing, 2 T. Stouffer's Stuffed Pepper, 10 oz. Soft breadsticks, 2	Greens w/ranch dressing, fat-free, 2 T. Stouffer's Stuffed Peppers, 15 oz. Corn on the cob, 1 large ear Soft breadstick, 1
SNACK *Grilled Peaches* (p. 299)	*Grilled Peaches* (p. 299)	*Grilled Peaches* (p. 299) Stella D'Oro Anisette Cookies, 2
37.5 grams fat **1,213 calories**	**46 grams fat** **1,489 calories**	**54 grams fat** **1,830 calories**

Weekday Menu PHASE 3 30% Fat

1,200 CALORIES 40 GRAMS FAT	1,500 CALORIES 50 GRAMS FAT	1,800 CALORIES 60 GRAMS FAT
BREAKFAST Kellogg's Cracklin' Oat Bran Cereal, ½ c. Milk, 1%, 1 c. Strawberries, sliced, ¼ c.	Kellogg's Cracklin' Oat Bran Cereal, ¾ c. Milk, 2%, 1 c. Strawberries, sliced, ½ c.	Kellogg's Cracklin' Oat Bran Cereal, 1 c. Milk, 2%, ½ c. Strawberries, ½ c.
LUNCH Lettuce and tomato salad w/ Kraft Roasted Red Pepper w/Parmesan Dressing, 2T Lean Cuisine Deluxe French Bread Pizza	Mixed Greens w/light Italian Dressing, 2T. Lean Cuisine Pepperoni French Bread Pizza	*Field Greens w/Pears and Walnuts* (p. 175) Lean Cuisine Four Cheese Pizza Snackwell Fat-Free Cookies, 2
SNACK Plum, 1	Apple, 1	Pear, 1
DINNER *Petite Filet w/Caramelized* *Onions* (p. 241) *Lean and Mean Mashed* *Potatoes* (p. 284), ¾ srv. Steamed green beans, 1 c.	*Petite Filet w/Caramelized* *Onions* (p. 241) *Lean and Mean Mashed Pota-* *toes* (p. 284) *Baked Asparagus w/Gremolata* (p. 281)	*Petite Filet w/Caramelized Onions* (p. 241) *Lean and Mean Mashed Potatoes* (p. 284) *Creamed Spinach* (p. 277), 1½ srv.
SNACK *Chocolate-Covered Strawber-* *ries* (p. 289) Stella D'Oro Anisette Cookies, 2	*Chocolate-Covered Strawberries* (p. 289) Stella D'Oro Anisette Cookies, 2	*Chocolate-Covered Strawberries* (p. 289), 1½ srv. Stella D'Oro Anisette Cookies, 2
37 grams fat **1,203 calories**	**45 grams fat** **1,523 calories**	**57 grams fat** **1,839 calories**

Weekday Menu PHASE ③ 30% Fat

1,200 CALORIES 40 GRAMS FAT	1,500 CALORIES 50 GRAMS FAT	1,800 CALORIES 60 GRAMS FAT
BREAKFAST *Ratatouille Omelet* (p. 145) Orange juice, 6 oz.	*Ratatouille Omelet* (p. 145), 1¼ srv. Wheat toast, 1 slice Orange juice, 6 oz.	*Ratatouille Omelet* (p. 145), 1½ srv. Wheat toast, 1 slice, w/margarine, reduced-fat, 1 tsp.
LUNCH Healthy Choice Meat Loaf Dannon Light 'n Fit Yogurt, 4 oz.	Healthy Choice Meat Loaf Sourdough roll, 1 Margarine, reduced-fat, 2t.	Michelina's Authentico Meatloaf w/Mashed Potatoes Carrots, cooked, 1c. Sourdough roll, 1 Snackwell Fat-Free Cookies, 2
SNACK Grapes, 1c.	Chips Ahoy Thin Crisps, 1 pack	Dried figs, 3
DINNER Lettuce and tomato salad w/Italian dressing, light, 2 T. *Mac and Cheese* (p. 184)	Lettuce and tomato salad w/Ital- ian dressing, light, 2 T. *Mac and Cheese* (p. 184), 1¼ srv.	Lettuce and tomato salad w/*Rasp- berry-Walnut Dressing* (p. 333), and walnuts, chopped, 1 tsp. *Mac and Cheese* (p. 184), 1½ srv.
SNACK *Chocolate-Covered Strawber- ries* (p. 289) Stella D'Oro Anisette Cookie, 1	*Chocolate-Covered Strawberries* (p. 289) Stella D'Oro Anisette Cookie, 1	*Chocolate-Covered Strawberries* (p. 289) Stella D'Oro Anisette Cookie, 1
37 grams fat 1,235 calories	**46 grams fat 1,519 calories**	**55.6 grams fat 1,816 calories**

Weekday Menu PHASE ③ 30% Fat

1,200 CALORIES 40 GRAMS FAT	1,500 CALORIES 50 GRAMS FAT	1,800 CALORIES 60 GRAMS FAT
BREAKFAST Eggs, scrambled dry, 1 Wheat toast, thin, 2 slices Vegetable juice, 6 oz.	Eggs, scrambled dry, 2 Wheat toast, 2 slices Orange juice, 4 oz.	Eggs, scrambled, dry, 2 Wheat toast, 2 slices Orange juice, 8 oz.
LUNCH Campbell's Cream of Aspara- gus Soup w/fat-free milk, ½ c. *Grilled Cheese and Bacon* (p. 250)	*Asparagus Soup* (p. 149) *Grilled Cheese and Bacon* (p. 250) Health Valley Fat Free Healthy Chips Cookies, 1	*Asparagus Soup* (p. 149), 1½ srv. *Grilled Cheese and Bacon* (p. 250) Snackwell Fat-Free Cookie, 1
SNACK Chips Ahoy Thin Crisps, 1 pack	Grapes, 1c.	Jell-O Pudding Snack Cup, 1
DINNER Birds Eye Voila! Garlic Shrimp, 1¼ c. Lettuce and tomato salad w/ *Orange Vinaigrette* (p. 342)	Birds Eye Voila! Garlic Shrimp, 1½ c. Lettuce and tomato salad w/ *Basil-Cream Dressing* (p. 334) Soft breadsticks, 2	Birds Eye Voila! Garlic Shrimp, 2 c. Lettuce and tomato salad w/*Basil- Cream Dressing* (p. 334) Soft breadsticks, 2
SNACK Apple, 1	*Mixed Fruit w/Strawberry-Ginger Sauce* (p. 298)	*Mixed Fruit w/Strawberry-Ginger Sauce* (p. 298)
36 grams fat 1,216 calories	**43 grams fat 1,511 calories**	**56 grams fat 1,834 calories**

Weekday Menu PHASE ③ 30% Fat

1,200 CALORIES 40 GRAMS FAT	1,500 CALORIES 50 GRAMS FAT	1,800 CALORIES 60 GRAMS FAT
BREAKFAST Pepperidge Farm Homestyle French Toast, 1 slice, sugar-free syrup, 2 T. Milk, 1%, ½ c.	Hungry Jack Waffles, 2, w/margarine, reduced-fat, 2 tsp., and no-sugar syrup, 2T. Orange juice, 8 oz.	Hungry Jack Waffles, 2, w/margarine, reduced-fat, 2 tsp., and sugar-free syrup, 2 T. Orange juice, 6 oz
LUNCH Campbell's Cream of Potato Soup, ¾ c. Lettuce & tomato salad w/chicken breast, 4 oz., and *Creamy Italian Dressing* (p. 336)	Campbell's Cream of Potato Soup, 1 c. Lettuce & tomato salad w/chicken breast, 2 oz., and *Creamy Italian Dressing* (p. 336), 2 T.	Campbell's Cream of Potato Soup, 1 c. Lettuce & tomato salad w/chicken breast, 4 oz., and *Creamy Italian Dressing* (p. 336), 2 T. Club roll, 1, w/margarine, reduced-fat, 2t.
SNACK Dried fig, 1	Healthy Choice Ice Cream Sandwich, 1	Chips Ahoy Thin Crisps, 1 pack
DINNER *Pasta Primavera* (p. 261)	*Pasta Primavera* (p. 261) w/steamed shrimp, 8 large	*Pasta Primavera* (p. 261), 1¼ srv., w/steamed shrimp, 8 large Crisp breadstick, 1, w/*Roasted Garlic Puree* (p. 327), 1 T.
SNACK *Mixed Fruit w/Sauce* (p. 298)	*Mixed Fruit w/Sauce* (p. 298)	*Mixed Fruit w/Sauce* (p. 298)
35.4 grams fat **1,196 calories**	**44.2 grams fat** **1,531 calories**	**54.7 grams fat** **1,834 calories**

Weekday Menu PHASE ③ 30% Fat

1,200 CALORIES 40 GRAMS FAT	1,500 CALORIES 50 GRAMS FAT	1,800 CALORIES 60 GRAMS FAT
BREAKFAST *Breakfast Bread* (p. 139) Cream cheese, low-fat, 1 T. Orange juice, 4 oz.	*Breakfast Bread* (p. 139) Cream cheese, low-fat, 1 T. Milk, 2%, 1 c.; Orange, 1	*Breakfast Bread* (p. 139), 1½ srv. Cream cheese, low-fat, 1 T. Orange juice, 8 oz.
LUNCH *Watercress & Strawberry Salad* (p. 168), w/shrimp, 12 large, and feta cheese, 1 T. Whole wheat potato roll, 1	*Watercress & Strawberry Salad* (p. 168), 1½ srv., w/shrimp, 12 large, and feta cheese, 1 T. Whole wheat potato roll, 1	*Watercress & Strawberry Salad* (p. 168), 1½ srv., w/shrimp, 12 large, and feta cheese, 2 T. Club roll, 1,
SNACK Archway Oatmeal Raisin Cookie, 1	Archway Oatmeal Raisin Cookie, 1	Archway Oatmeal Raisin Cookie, 1
DINNER Rotisserie chicken, 3 oz. *Rosemary New Potatoes* (p. 280) *Glazed Carrots* (p. 279) Cranberry sauce, ½ slice	Rotisserie chicken, 4 oz. *Rosemary New Potatoes* (p. 280) *Glazed Carrots* (p. 279), 1½ srv. Cranberry sauce, 1 slice	Rotisserie chicken, 6 oz. *Rosemary New Potatoes* (p. 280) *Glazed Carrots* (p. 279) Cranberry sauce, 2 slices
SNACK Peach w/*Raspberry Sauce* (p. 300)	Peach w/*Raspberry Sauce* (p. 300)	Peach w/*Raspberry Sauce* (p. 300)
32.2 grams fat **1,217 calories**	**49 grams fat** **1,532 calories**	**57 grams fat** **1,794 calories**

Weekday Menu PHASE ③ 30% Fat

1,200 CALORIES 40 GRAMS FAT	1,500 CALORIES 50 GRAMS FAT	1,800 CALORIES 60 GRAMS FAT
BREAKFAST Blueberries and raspberries, 1 c. Cottage cheese, whole-milk, ¾ c.	Cinnamon raisin bread, 1 slice Ricotta cheese, light, ½ c.	Cinnamon raisin bread, 1 slice Ricotta cheese, light, ¾ c. Blueberries and raspberries, 1 c.
LUNCH Mixed lettuce salad w/*Raspberry-Walnut Dressing* (p. 333) Lean Cuisine Gourmet Mushroom Pizza	Mixed lettuce salad w/ *Raspberry-Walnut Dressing* (p. 333) Smart Ones Pepperoni Pizza	Mixed lettuce salad w/apple, sliced, 1, and *Raspberry-Walnut Dressing* (p. 333) Smart Ones Pepperoni Pizza
SNACK Oreo Thin Crisps, 1 pack	Plum, 1	Archway Oatmeal Raisin Cookie, 1
DINNER Baked chicken breast, 4 oz. Healthy Choice Cheddar Broccoli Potato, 1	Baked chicken breast, 4 oz. Healthy Choice Cheddar Broccoli Potato, 1, w/crumbled bacon, 2 T.	Baked chicken breast, 6 oz. Healthy Choice Cheddar Broccoli Potato, 1, w/crumbled bacon, 2 T.
SNACK Fudgesicle, 1	Healthy Choice Ice Cream Sandwich, 1	*Chocolate-Covered Strawberries* (p. 289), 1½ srv. Stella D'Oro Anisette Cookies, 2
36.3 grams fat 1,233 calories	**47.2 grams fat 1,499 calories**	**56.9 grams fat 1,800 calories**

Weekday Menu PHASE ③ 30% Fat

1,200 CALORIES 40 GRAMS FAT	1,500 CALORIES 50 GRAMS FAT	1,800 CALORIES 60 GRAMS FAT
BREAKFAST Nature Valley Granola Bars, 2 Milk, 1%, ½ c.	Nature Valley Granola Bars, 2 Milk, 2%, 1 c. *Frozen Grapes* (p. 304), ½ c.	Nature Valley Granola Bars, 2 Milk, 2%, ¾ c. Orange and grapefruit sections, 1c.
LUNCH *Warm Eggplant, Tomato, and Mozzarella Salad* (p. 165), ¾ srv., w/cooked chicken breast, boneless & skinless, 3 oz. Whole wheat potato roll, 1	*Warm Eggplant, Tomato, and Mozzarella Salad* (p. 165), w/cooked chicken breast, boneless & skinless, 4 oz. Peach, 1	*Warm Eggplant, Tomato, and Mozzarella Salad* (p. 165), w/cooked chicken breast, boneless & skinless, 6 oz. Whole wheat potato roll, 1
SNACK Health Valley Low-Fat Cookie, 1	Archway Oatmeal Raisin Cookie, 1	Nabisco Gingersnaps, 2
DINNER Lettuce & tomato salad w/*Poppy Seed Dressing* (p. 340) *Penne w/Broccoli and Cheese* (p. 264)	Lettuce & tomato salad w/*Poppy Seed Dressing* (p. 340) *Penne w/Broccoli and Cheese* (p. 264), 1¼ srv.	Lettuce & tomato salad w/*Poppy Seed Dressing* (p. 340) *Penne w/Broccoli and Cheese* (p. 264), 1¼ srv. Italian bread, 1½" piece.
SNACK *Banana Ice Cream* (p. 288) w/ walnuts, chopped, 1 T.	*Banana Ice Cream* (p. 288) w/ walnuts, chopped, 1 T.	*Banana Ice Cream* (p. 288) w/ walnuts, chopped, 1 T.
36.1 grams fat 1,213 calories	**48.3 grams fat 1,524 calories**	**55.4 grams fat 1,800 calories**

Weekday Menu PHASE ③ 30% Fat

1,200 CALORIES 40 GRAMS FAT	1,500 CALORIES 50 GRAMS FAT	1,800 CALORIES 60 GRAMS FAT
BREAKFAST Amy's Breakfast Burrito, 1	Amy's Breakfast Burrito, 1 Sour cream, 2T. Orange and grapefruit sections, ¾ c.	Hot Pockets Biscuits w/Bacon, Egg and Cheese, 1 Dannon Light and Fit, 6 oz. Orange & grapefruit sections, 1 ½ c.
LUNCH *Hero's Hoagie* (p. 236)	*Hero's Hoagie* (p. 236) *Creamy Coleslaw* (p. 286)	*Hero's Hoagie* (p. 236) *Creamy Coleslaw* (p. 286) Potato chips, baked, 1 oz.
SNACK Quaker Chewy 90 Calories Bar, 1	Dried fig, 1	Chips Ahoy Thin Crisps, 1 pack
DINNER *Grilled Swordfish* (p. 207) 1½ srv. *Garden Peas w/Fresh Mint* (p. 269)	*Grilled Swordfish* (p. 207), 1½ srv. *Tropical Rice* (p. 274), ¾ srv. *Grilled Portobello Mushrooms* (p. 271)	*Grilled Swordfish* (p. 207), 2 srv. *Creamed Spinach* (p. 277) *Grilled Portobello Mushrooms* (p. 271)
SNACK Jell-O Pudding Snack Cup, 1	*Peachy Blueberry Crisp* (p. 296)	*Peachy Blueberry Crisp* (p. 296)
37.4 grams fat **1,215 calories**	**45.4 grams fat** **1,523 calories**	**56.5 grams fat** **1,824 calories**

Weekday Menu PHASE ③ 30% Fat

1,200 CALORIES 40 GRAMS FAT	1,500 CALORIES 50 GRAMS FAT	1,800 CALORIES 60 GRAMS FAT
BREAKFAST Pepperidge Farm Raisin Cinnamon Swirl Bread, 1 slice, w/*Cranberry-Walnut* *Spread* (p. 324), 1 T. Milk, 1%, ¾ c.	Pepperidge Farm Raisin Cinnamon Swirl Bread, 1½ slices, w/ *Cranberry-Walnut Spread* (p. 324), 2 T. Dannon La Crème Mousse Yogurt, 4 oz.	Pepperidge Farm Raisin Cinnamon Swirl Bread, 2 slices, w/*Cranberry-Walnut* *Spread* (p. 324), 2 T. Dannon La Crème Yogurt, 4 oz.
LUNCH *Lunch-Box Tuna Salad* *Sandwich* (p. 218) Keebler Soft Batch Chocolate Chip Cookie, 1	*Lunch-Box Tuna Salad Sandwich* (p. 218) Keebler Soft Batch Chocolate Chip Cookies, 2	*Lunch-Box Tuna Salad Sandwich* (p. 218), 1½ srv. Keebler Soft Batch Chocolate Chip Cookies, 2
SNACK Peach, 1	Apple, 2	Peach, 1
DINNER Birds Eye Voila! Southwestern Chicken, 1 c. Sour cream, 1T. Tortilla, low-carb, 1.5 oz.	Birds Eye Voila! Chicken Fajita, 1¼ c. Tortilla, low-carb, 1.5 oz. *Key Lime Pie* (p. 290)	Campbell's Chunky Baked Potato w/Bacon Bits Soup, 1½ c. Birds Eye Voila! Chicken Fajita, 1½ c. Tortilla, low-carb, 1.5 oz.
SNACK *Key Lime Pie* (p. 290)	Chips Ahoy Thin Crisps, 1 pack	*Key Lime Pie* (p. 290)
36.1 grams fat **1,230 calories**	**47.8 grams fat** **1,528 calories**	**57.3 grams fat** **1,824 calories**

Weekday Menu PHASE ③ 30% Fat

1,200 CALORIES 40 GRAMS FAT	1,500 CALORIES 50 GRAMS FAT	1,800 CALORIES 60 GRAMS FAT
BREAKFAST Whole wheat toast, 1 slice, w/ peanut butter, reduced-fat, 1½ tsp., and low-sugar fruit preserves, 1½ tsp. Milk, 2%, ¾ c.	Whole wheat toast, 2 slices, w/peanut butter, reduced-fat, 1 T., and low-sugar fruit preserves, 1 T. Milk, 2%, ½ c.	Whole wheat toast, 2 slices, w/ peanut butter, reduced-fat, 1 T., and reduced-sugar fruit preserves, 1 T. Milk, 2%, 1 c.
LUNCH *Greek Salad* (p. 163), ½ srv., w/steamed shrimp, 8 large Cherries, 25	*Greek Salad* (p. 163), ½ srv., w/steamed shrimp, 12 large Soft breadsticks, 2 Cherries, 20	*Greek Salad* (p. 163), ¾ srv., w/steamed shrimp, 12 large Soft breadsticks, 2 Cherries, 20
SNACK *Zesty Bean Salsa* (p. 317), 6 T. Low-fat wheat crackers, 3	*Zesty Bean Salsa* (p. 317), ¼ c. Celery, 3 ribs	*Zesty Bean Salsa* (p. 317), ¼ c. Triscuits, 2
DINNER *Pasta Carbonara* (p. 262) *Garlic-Lemon Spinach* (p. 278)	*Pasta Carbonara* (p. 262) *Garlic-Lemon Spinach* (p. 278) Grated Parmesan cheese, 1T.	*Pasta Carbonara* (p. 262), 1¼ srv. *Garlic-Lemon Spinach* (p. 278) Grated Parmesan cheese, 1T
SNACK Archway Oatmeal Raisin Cookie, 1	Chips Ahoy Thin Crisps, 1 pack	Chips Ahoy Thin Crisps, 1 pack
37.5 grams fat **1,229 calories**	**45.5 grams fat** **1,490 calories**	**57 grams fat** **1,791 calories**

Weekday Menu PHASE ③ 30% Fat

1,200 CALORIES 40 GRAMS FAT	1,500 CALORIES 50 GRAMS FAT	1,800 CALORIES 60 GRAMS FAT
BREAKFAST Eggs, boiled or scrambled dry, 1 Whole wheat toast, 1 slice, w/margarine, reduced-fat, 1 tsp. Grapefruit, ½	Eggs, boiled or scrambled dry, 1 Whole wheat toast, 2 slices w/margarine, reduced-fat, 2 tsp. Orange Juice, 6 oz.	Eggs, boiled or scrambled dry, 2, w/ham, 2 oz. Whole wheat toast, 2 slices w/ margarine, reduced-fat, 2 tsp. Grapefruit, ½
LUNCH Campbell's Chunky Baked Potato w/Bacon Bits Soup, 1 c. *Tex-Mex Dip* (p. 311)	Campbell's Chunky Baked Potato w/Bacon Bits Soup, 1 c. *Tex-Mex Dip* (p. 311)	Campbell's Chunky Baked Potato w/Bacon Bits Soup, 1 c. *Tex-Mex Dip* (p. 311) *Chicken Wingettes* (p. 302)
SNACK Plum, 1	Chips Ahoy Thin Crisps, 1 pack	Chips Ahoy Thin Crisps, 1 pack
DINNER *Brook Trout* (p. 212) Uncle Ben's Ready Rice, Long Grain & Wild, ¾ c. *Baked Asparagus* (p. 281)	*Brook Trout* (p. 212) Uncle Ben's Ready Rice, Long Grain & Wild, ¾ c. *Baked Asparagus* (p. 281)	*Brook Trout* (p. 212), 1½ srv. Uncle Ben's Ready Rice, Long Grain & Wild, 1 c. *Baked Asparagus* (p. 281)
SNACK *Banana Ice Cream* (p. 288) w/blackberries, ½ c.	*Banana Ice Cream* (p. 288) w/blackberries, ½ c., and walnuts, chopped, 1T.	*Banana Ice Cream* (p. 288) w/blackberries, ½ c.
34.3 grams fat **1,210 calories**	**45.6 grams fat** **1,533 calories**	**55 grams fat** **1,833 calories**

Weekend Menu PHASE ③ 30% Fat

1,200 CALORIES 40 GRAMS FAT	1,500 CALORIES 50 GRAMS FAT	1,800 CALORIES 60 GRAMS FAT
BREAKFAST *Carrot-Raisin Bran Muffin* (p. 142) Milk, whole, ½ c. Strawberries, ½ c.	*Carrot-Raisin Bran Muffin* (p. 142) Milk, whole, 1 c. Blueberries, ½ c.	*Carrot-Raisin Bran Muffins* (p. 142), 2 Milk, whole, ¾ c.
LUNCH *Pumpkin Soup* (p. 153), ¾ srv. *Nachos* (p. 193)	*Pumpkin Soup* (p. 153), 1½ srv. *Nachos* (p. 193)	*Pumpkin Soup* (p. 153), 1½ srv. *Nachos* (p. 193), 1½ srv.
SNACK Jell-O Pudding Snack Cup, 1	Jell-O Pudding Snack Cup, 1	Oreo Thin Crisps, 1 pack
DINNER *Grilled Margarita Chicken* (p. 224) *Tropical Rice* (p. 274), ½ srv. *Cheesy Broccoli* (p. 264), ¾ srv.	*Grilled Margarita Chicken* (p. 224) *Tropical Rice* (p. 274) *Cheesy Broccoli* (p. 264)	*Grilled Margarita Chicken* (p. 224), 1½ srv. *Tropical Rice* (p. 274) *Cheesy Broccoli* (p. 264), 1½ srv.
SNACK *Grilled Peaches* (p. 299)	*Grilled Peaches* (p. 299)	*Grilled Peaches* (p. 299)
38 grams fat **1,225 calories**	**48 grams fat** **1,493 calories**	**57 grams fat** **1,825 calories**

Weekend Menu PHASE ③ 30% Fat

1,200 CALORIES 40 GRAMS FAT	1,500 CALORIES 50 GRAMS FAT	1,800 CALORIES 60 GRAMS FAT
BREAKFAST *Aloha Fruit Salad* (p. 167), no lettuce Cottage cheese, whole-milk, ½ c.	*Aloha Fruit Salad* (p. 167), no lettuce, 1¼ srv. Cottage cheese, whole-milk, ½ c.	*Aloha Fruit Salad* (p. 167), no lettuce, 1½ srv. Cottage cheese, whole-milk, ½ c.
LUNCH *Asparagus Soup* (p. 149), ¾ srv. *Grilled Shrimp w/Corn Salad*, (p. 173) Whole wheat potato roll, 1	*Asparagus Soup* (p. 149), ¾ srv. *Grilled Shrimp w/Corn Salad*, (p. 173), 1½ srv. Whole wheat potato roll, 1	*Asparagus Soup* (p. 149), 1½ srv. *Grilled Shrimp w/Corn Salad*, (p. 173), 1½ srv. Whole wheat potato roll, 1
SNACK Laughing Cow Light Cheese Wedge, 1 Grapes, ½ c.	Laughing Cow Light Cheese Wedge, 1 Grapes, 1 cup	*Sesame Cheese Balls*, (p. 304) Crisp breadsticks, 2
DINNER Grilled pork chop, 3 oz. *Braised Cabbage w/Apples* (p. 270), ½ srv. *Lean Mashed Potatoes* (p. 284), ¾ srv.	Grilled pork chop, 3 oz. *Braised Cabbage w/Apples* (p. 270) *Lean Mashed Potatoes* (p. 284)	Grilled pork chop, 4 oz. *Braised Cabbage w/Apples* (p. 270) *Lean Mashed Potatoes* (p. 284), 1½ srv.
SNACK Planters Peanut Butter Cookie Crisps, 1 pack	Planters Peanut Butter Cookie Crisps, 1 pack	Planters Peanut Butter Cookie Crisps, 1 pack
39 grams fat **1,218calories**	**47 grams fat** **1,506 calories**	**57 grams fat** **1,820 calories**

Weekend Menu (Meatless) PHASE 3 30% Fat

1,200 CALORIES 40 GRAMS FAT	1,500 CALORIES 50 GRAMS FAT	1,800 CALORIES 60 GRAMS FAT
BREAKFAST Cheese blintzes, 2 *Spiced Apples* (p. 295)	Cheese blintzes, 3 *Spiced Apples* (p. 295)	Cheese blintzes, 3, w/light sour cream, 1 T. *Spiced Apples* (p. 295), 1½ srv.
LUNCH Mixed lettuce salad w/*Garlic Vinaigrette* (p. 341) *Texas-Style Stuffed Peppers* (p. 178) Strawberries, ¾ c.	Mixed lettuce salad w/*Garlic Vinaigrette* (p. 341) *Texas-Style Stuffed Peppers* (p. 178) Sourdough roll w/reduced-fat margarine, 1 tsp. Strawberries, ¾ c.	Mixed lettuce salad w/*Garlic Vinaigrette* (p. 341) *Texas-Style Stuffed Peppers* (p. 178), 1½ srv. Sourdough roll w/reduced-fat margarine, 2 tsp.
SNACK *Stuffed Celery* (p. 305), 3	*Stuffed Celery* (p. 305), 2	*Stuffed Celery* (p. 305), 2
DINNER *Spinach-Stuffed Mushrooms* (p. 185) *Spaghetti with Summer Toma- toes, Basil, and Garlic* (p. 256), w/Parmesan, 1 T.	*Spinach-Stuffed Mushrooms* (p. 185) *Spaghetti with Summer Tomatoes, Basil, and Garlic* (p. 256), 1¼ srv., w/Parmesan, 1 T.	*Spinach-Stuffed Mushrooms* (p. 185) *Spaghetti with Summer Squash* (p. 258), 1½ srv., w/Parmesan, 1 T.
SNACK *Grilled Peaches* (p. 299)	*Grilled Peaches* (p. 299) Stella D'Oro Anisette Cookies, 2	*Grilled Peaches* (p. 299)
38 grams fat **1,216 calories**	**46 grams fat** **1,516 calories**	**57 grams fat** **1,795 calories**

Weekend Menu PHASE 3 30% Fat

1,200 CALORIES 40 GRAMS FAT	1,500 CALORIES 50 GRAMS FAT	1,800 CALORIES 60 GRAMS FAT
BREAKFAST Egg, scrambled, 1 w/ham, 1 oz. Grits, ½ c. w/reduced-fat margarine, 1 tsp.	Egg, scrambled, 1 w/ham, 1 oz. Grits, ½ c. Buttermilk biscuits, 2 w/reduced-fat margarine, 2 tsp.	Egg, scrambled, 1 w/ham, 2 oz. Grits, ½ c. Buttermilk biscuits, 2 w/reduced- fat margarine, 2 tsp.
LUNCH *Tuna Salad Sandwich* (p. 218) *Creamy Coleslaw* (p. 286) Keebler Country Oatmeal Cookie, 1	*Buttery Squash Soup* (p. 151) *Tuna Salad Sandwich* (p. 218) w/Kraft 2% Cheddar, 1 slice	*Buttery Squash Soup* (p. 151), 1½ srv. *Tuna Salad Sandwich* (p. 218) w/Kraft 2% Cheddar, 2 slices
SNACK Vitalicious Brownie, 1	Vitalicious Brownie, 1	*Raspberry Sauce* (p. 300), over Vitalicious Brownie, 1
DINNER *Veal Marsala* (p. 251) Egg noodles, ½ c. *Cheesy Broccoli* (p. 264)	*Veal Marsala* (p. 251), 1½ srv. Egg noodles, ½ c. *Cheesy Broccoli* (p. 264)	*Veal Marsala* (p. 251), 1½ srv. Egg noodles, 1 c. *Cheesy Broccoli* (p. 264), 1½ srv.
SNACK *Chambord Compote* (p. 166)	*Chambord Compote* (p. 166)	*Chambord Compote* (p. 166)
38 grams fat **1,225 calories**	**47 grams fat** **1,505 calories**	**57 grams fat** **1,807 calories**

Weekend Menu PHASE ③ 30% Fat

1,200 CALORIES 40 GRAMS FAT	1,500 CALORIES 50 GRAMS FAT	1,800 CALORIES 60 GRAMS FAT
BREAKFAST Oatmeal, 1 c. w/chopped walnuts, 　2 tsp. Milk, 1 %, ½ c.	Oatmeal, 1½ c. w/chopped 　walnuts, 1 T., and raisins, 1 T. Milk, 1 %, ½ c.	Oatmeal, 1 ½ c. w/chopped 　walnuts, 1 T., and raisins, 2 T. Milk, 2 %, ¾ c.
LUNCH Campbell's Cream of Potato 　Soup, ¾ c. w/crumbled bacon, 　1 T *Grilled Chicken Caesar Salad* 　(p. 170)	Progresso N. Eng. Clam Chowder, 　¾ c. *Grilled Chicken Caesar Salad* 　(p. 170), 1¼ srv.	Progresso N. Eng. Clam Chowder, 　1 c. *Grilled Chicken Caesar Salad* 　(p. 170), 1½ srv.
SNACK *Stuffed Celery* (p. 305), 2	*Stuffed Celery* (p. 305), 4	Plums, 2
DINNER *Chilean Sea Bass* (p. 217) Brown rice, ½ c. *Creamed Spinach* (p. 277), ¾ srv.	*Chilean Sea Bass* (p. 217) Polenta, ½ c. *Creamed Spinach* (p. 277)	*Chilean Sea Bass* (p. 217) Polenta, ¾ c. *Creamed Spinach* (p. 277), 　1½ srv.
SNACK Stella D'Oro Almond Toasts, 2	Stella D'Oro Almond Toasts, 2	Stella D'Oro Almond Toasts, 2
37 grams fat 1,211 calories	**46 grams fat 1,492 calories**	**55 grams fat 1,805 calories**

Weekend Menu PHASE ③ 30% Fat

1,200 CALORIES 40 GRAMS FAT	1,500 CALORIES 50 GRAMS FAT	1,800 CALORIES 60 GRAMS FAT
BREAKFAST *Asparagus Omelet* (p. 144) Whole wheat toast, thin,1 slice 　w/reduced-fat marg., 1 tsp. Cantaloupe, ⅛	*Asparagus Omelet* (p. 144) Whole wheat toast,1 slice 　w/reduced-fat marg., 2 tsp. Cantaloupe, ¼	*Asparagus Omelet* (p. 144) Whole wheat toast, 2 slices 　w/reduced-fat marg., 1 tsp. Cantaloupe, ¼
LUNCH *Pita Sandwiches to Go* (p. 189) 　w/Swiss cheese, 1 oz.	*Pita Sandwiches to Go* (p. 189) 　w/turkey, 4 oz., & Swiss, 1oz.	*Pita Sandwiches to Go* (p. 189) 　w/roast beef, 4 oz., & Swiss, 　1 oz. *Creamy Coleslaw* (p. 286)
SNACK Pear, 1	*Stuffed Celery* (p. 305), 3	*Stuffed Celery* (p. 305), 3
DINNER *Poached Chicken w/Avocado* 　*Sauce* (p. 225) *Tropical Rice* (p. 274), ¾ srv. *Cheesy Broccoli* (p. 264)	*Poached Chicken w/Avocado* 　*Sauce* (p. 225), 1½ srv. *Tropical Rice* (p. 274) *Cheesy Broccoli* (p. 264), 　1½ srv.	*Poached Chicken w/Avocado* 　*Sauce* (p. 225), 1½ srv. *Tropical Rice* (p. 274) *Cheesy Broccoli* (p. 264), 　1½ srv.
SNACK *Chocolate-Covered Strawberries* 　(p. 289) Stella D'Oro Anisette Cookies, 1	*Chocolate-Covered Strawberries* 　(p. 289) Stella D'Oro Anisette Cookies, 1	*Chocolate-Covered Strawberries* 　(p. 289) Stella D'Oro Anisette Cookies, 1
37 grams fat 1,193 calories	**47 grams fat 1,524 calories**	**55 grams fat 1,784 calories**

Weekend Menu (Meatless) PHASE ③ 30% Fat

1,200 CALORIES 40 GRAMS FAT	1,500 CALORIES 50 GRAMS FAT	1,800 CALORIES 60 GRAMS FAT
BREAKFAST *Eggs-and-Potato Hash* (p. 146) Whole wheat toast, 1 slice	*Eggs-and-Potato Hash* (p. 146) Whole wheat toast, 2 slices, w/margarine, reduced-fat, 2 tsp.	*Eggs-and-Potato Hash* (p. 146) 1¼ srv. Whole wheat toast, 2 slices, w/marg., reduced-fat, 2 tsp.
LUNCH Lean Cuisine Gourmet Mushroom Pizza Mixed lettuce salad, 1½ c., w/*Honey-Lime Dressing* (p. 338), 1 T.	*Watercress and Strawberry Salad* (p. 168) Lean Cuisine Gourmet Mushroom Pizza	Lean Cuisine Four Cheese Pizza *Watercress and Strawberry Salad* (p. 168)
SNACK Pear, 1	Pear, 1	Peach, 1; Plum, 1
DINNER *Grilled Swordfish* (p. 207) *Creamed Spinach* (p. 277) *Glazed Carrots* (p. 279)	*Grilled Swordfish* (p. 207) *Creamed Spinach* (p. 277) Baked potato, ½, w/margarine, reduced-fat, 1 T.	*Grilled Swordfish* (p. 207) *Creamed Spinach* (p. 277) 1¼ srv. Baked potato, w/margarine, reduced-fat, 1 T.
SNACK Breyers Light Ice Cream, ½ c.	Breyers 98% Fat-Free Ice Cream, ½ c.	Breyers Light Ice Cream, ½ c.
36 grams fat 1,221 calories	**45 grams fat 1,486 calories**	**54 grams fat 1,813 calories**

Weekend Menu PHASE ③ 30% Fat

1,200 CALORIES 40 GRAMS FAT	1,500 CALORIES 50 GRAMS FAT	1,800 CALORIES 60 GRAMS FAT
BREAKFAST *Ratatouille Omelet* (p. 145) Whole wheat toast, 2 slices Orange juice, 4 oz.	*Ratatouille Omelet* (p. 145) Whole wheat English muffin, 1	*Ratatouille Omelet* (p. 145) Whole wheat English muffin, 1, w/margarine, reduced-fat, 2 tsps. Grapefruit, ½
LUNCH *Hero's Hoagie* (p. 236)	*Hero's Hoagie* (p. 236) Baked potato chips, 1 oz.	*Hero's Hoagie* (p. 236), turkey breast, 7 oz. Baked potato chips, 1 oz.
SNACK Peach, 1	Plum, 1	Grapes, 1c.
DINNER *Stuffed Bell Peppers* (p. 244) Mixed Greens w/fat-free Italian dressing, 2T.	*Stuffed Bell Peppers* (p. 244) *Rosemary Roasted New Potatoes* (p. 280) Mixed Greens w/fat-free Italian dressing, 2T.	*Stuffed Bell Peppers* (p. 244) *Mashed Potatoes* (p. 284), w/ margarine, reduced-fat, 1 T. Mixed Greens w/avocado, ¼, and Italian dressing, fat-free, 2T
SNACK Honey Maid Graham Crackers, 1	Breyers Light Ice Cream, ½ c.	Breyers Light Ice Cream, ½ c.
30 grams fat 1,220 calories	**46 grams fat 1,502 calories**	**55 grams fat 1,813 calories**

Weekend Menu PHASE ③ 30% Fat

1,200 CALORIES 40 GRAMS FAT	1,500 CALORIES 50 GRAMS FAT	1,800 CALORIES 60 GRAMS FAT
BREAKFAST		
Eggo Special K For Your Low Carb Lifestyle Waffles, 2 *Strawberry Sauce* (p. 300)	*Pecan Waffles* (p. 138) w/ *Strawberry Sauce* (p. 300) Milk, 2%, ½ c.	*Pecan Waffles* (p. 138) w/ *Strawberry Sauce* (p. 300) Milk, 2 %, 1 c.
LUNCH		
Texas Black Bean Soup (p. 157) *Warm Eggplant, Tomato, and Mozzarella Salad* (p. 165)	*Texas Black Bean Soup* (p. 157) *Warm Eggplant, Tomato, and Mozzarella Salad* (p. 165) Club roll, 1, w/margarine, reduced-fat, 2 tsp.	*Texas Black Bean Soup* (p. 157) *Warm Eggplant, Tomato, and Mozzarella Salad* (p. 165) Club roll, 1, w/margarine, reduced-fat, 1 T.
SNACK		
Popcorn, butter flavor, ½ oz.	Popcorn, butter flavor, ½ oz.	Popcorn, butter flavor, 1 oz.
DINNER		
London Broil Two Ways w/ Savory Marinade (p. 243), 4 oz. *Lean Mashed Potatoes* (p. 284), ½ srv. *Garlic-Lemon Spinach* (p. 278) *Grilled Peaches* (p. 299)	*London Broil Two Ways w/Savory Marinade* (p. 243), 5 oz. *Lean Mashed Potatoes* (p. 284) *Garlic-Lemon Spinach* (p. 278)	*London Broil Two Ways w/Savory Marinade* (p. 243), 8 oz. *Lean Mashed Potatoes* (p. 284) *Garlic-Lemon Spinach* (p. 278) *Grilled Peaches* (p. 299)
SNACK		
Jell-O Fat-Free Pudding Snack	*Grilled Peaches* (p. 299)	Jell-O Fat-Free Pudding Snack
40 grams fat 1,157 calories	**50.6 grams fat 1,529 calories**	**60 grams fat 1,833 calories**

Weekend Menu PHASE ③ 30% Fat

1,200 CALORIES 40 GRAMS FAT	1,500 CALORIES 50 GRAMS FAT	1,800 CALORIES 60 GRAMS FAT
BREAKFAST		
Egg, fried in nonstick pan, 1 Swiss cheese, low-fat, 1 oz. Thomas' 100% Whole-Wheat English Muffin, 1	*Grilled Cheese and Bacon* (p. 250) w/egg, fried in 1 tsp. reduced-fat margarine, 1	*Grilled Cheese and Bacon* (p. 250) w/egg, fried in 1 T. reduced-fat margarine, 1
LUNCH		
Vegetarian Antipasto (p. 190) Crisp breadsticks, 2	*Vegetarian Antipasto* (p. 190) w/tuna, 2 oz. Crisp breadsticks, 2	*Vegetarian Antipasto* (p. 190) w/tuna, 2 oz. Soft breadsticks, 2, w/margarine, reduced-fat, 1 tsp.
SNACK		
Country-style oatmeal cookie, 1	Country-style oatmeal cookie, 1	Country-style oatmeal cookie, 1
DINNER		
Steak Kabobs (p. 242) *Tropical Rice* (p. 274), ½ srv. Tomato, 3 thick slices, w/*Basil-Cream Dressing* (p. 334), 2 T.	*Steak Kabobs* (p. 242), 1¼ srv. *Tropical Rice* (p. 274) Tomato, 3 thick slices, w/*Basil-Cream Dressing* (p. 334), 2 T.	*Steak Kabobs* (p. 242), 1½ srv. *Tropical Rice* (p. 274), 1½ srv. Tomato, 3 thick slices, w/*Basil-Cream Dressing* (p. 334), 2 T.
SNACK		
98% Fat-free ice cream, ½ c.	98% Fat-free ice cream, ½ c.	98% Fat-free ice cream, ½ c.
39.7 grams fat 1,200 calories	**49 grams fat 1,519 calories**	**59 grams fat 1,782 calories**

Weekend Menu PHASE 3 · 30% Fat

1,200 CALORIES 40 GRAMS FAT	1,500 CALORIES 50 GRAMS FAT	1,800 CALORIES 60 GRAMS FAT
BREAKFAST *Ratatouille Omelet* (p. 145) Whole wheat toast, very thin, 1 slice Orange Juice, 6 oz.	*Ratatouille Omelet* (p. 145) Buttermilk biscuits, 2, w/marga- rine, reduced-fat, 2 T. Orange Juice, 6 oz.	*Ratatouille Omelet* (p. 145) Buttermilk biscuits, 2 Orange and grapefruit sections, 1c.
LUNCH *Turkey Loaf* (p. 237) w/turkey gravy, canned, ¼ c. *Lean and Mean Mashed Potatoes* (p. 284), ½ srv.	*Turkey Loaf* (p. 237), 1½ srv., w/turkey gravy, canned, ¼ c. *Lean and Mean Mashed Potatoes* (p. 284)	*Turkey Loaf* (p. 237), 2 srv., w/ turkey gravy, canned, ¼ c. *Lean and Mean Mashed Potatoes* (p. 284)
SNACK *Stuffed Celery* (p. 305), 1	Chips Ahoy Thin Crisps, 1 pack	Jell-O Pudding Snack Cup, 1
DINNER *Grilled Lamb Chops w/Grilled Grapes* (p. 254) *Glazed Carrots* (p. 279), 1¼ srv. *Baked Asparagus* (p. 281)	*Grilled Lamb Chops w/Grilled Grapes* (p. 254) *Mashed Sweet Potatoes* (p. 282), ½ srv. *Baked Asparagus* (p. 281)	*Grilled Lamb Chops w/Grilled Grapes* (p. 254) *Rosemary Roasted New Potatoes* (p. 280), 2 srv. *Baked Asparagus* (p. 281), 2 srv. Club roll, 1
SNACK *Spiced Apples* (p. 295)	*Spiced Apples* (p. 295) w/walnuts, chopped, 2 tsp.	*Spiced Apples* (p. 295) w/walnuts, chopped, 1½ tsp.
38 grams fat 1,224 calories	**45 grams fat 1,515 calories**	**57 grams fat 1,801 calories**

Weekend Menu PHASE 3 · 30% Fat

1,200 CALORIES 40 GRAMS FAT	1,500 CALORIES 50 GRAMS FAT	1,800 CALORIES 60 GRAMS FAT
BREAKFAST *Poached Salmon Two Ways w/Dill Sauce* (p. 209), ½ srv. Whole wheat English muffin, 1	*Poached Salmon Two Ways w/Dill Sauce* (p. 209), ½ srv. Whole wheat English muffin, 1, w/margarine, reduced-fat, 2tsp. Grapefruit, ½	*Poached Salmon Two Ways w/ Dill Sauce* (p. 209), ¾ srv. Whole wheat English muffin, 1, w/margarine, reduced-fat, 2tsp. Grapefruit, ½
LUNCH *Chili Mac* (p. 245), ¾ srv. Mixed lettuce salad w/*Honey- Lime Dressing* (p. 338)	*Chili Mac* (p. 245) Mixed lettuce salad w/*Honey- Lime Dressing* (p. 338)	*Chili Mac* (p. 245), 1¼ srv. Mixed lettuce salad w/*Honey-Lime Dressing* (p. 338)
SNACK Plum, 1	Plum, 1	Plum, 1
DINNER *Chicken Fajitas* (p. 222)	*Chicken Fajitas* (p. 222) Uncle Ben's Ready Rice, Spanish, Style, ½ c.	*Chicken Fajitas* (p. 222) Sour cream, 2 T. Uncle Ben's Ready Rice, Spanish, Style, ¾ c.
SNACK Archway Oatmeal Raisin Cookie, 1	Archway Oatmeal Raisin Cookie, 1	Nabisco Chips Ahoy Thin Crisps, 1 pack
36 grams fat 1,204 calories	**46 grams fat 1,505 calories**	**56 grams fat 1,792 calories**

Weekend Menu (Meatless) PHASE 3 30% Fat

1,200 CALORIES 40 GRAMS FAT	1,500 CALORIES 50 GRAMS FAT	1,800 CALORIES 60 GRAMS FAT
BREAKFAST		
Smoked trout, 2 oz., w/*Chile Mayonnaise* (p. 328), 2 T. Whole wheat English muffin, ½	Smoked trout, 3 oz., w/*Chile Mayonnaise* (p. 328), 2 T. Whole wheat English muffin, 1 Citrus sections, ½ c.	Smoked trout, 2 oz., w/*Chile Mayonnaise* (p. 328), 1 T. Whole wheat English muffin, 1 Citrus sections, ½ c.
LUNCH		
Mac and Cheese (p. 184), ¾ srv. Mixed lettuce salad w/*Raspberry-Walnut Dressing* (p. 333)	*Mac and Cheese* (p. 184) Mixed lettuce salad w/raspberries, ¼ c., and *Raspberry-Walnut Dressing* (p. 333)	*Mac and Cheese* (p. 184), 1¼ srv. Mixed lettuce salad w/raspberries, ¼ c., and *Raspberry-Walnut Dressing*, (p. 333)
SNACK		
Archway Oatmeal Raisin Cookie, 1	Archway Oatmeal Raisin Cookie, 1	Archway Oatmeal Raisin Cookie, 1
DINNER		
Sesame Fried Tofu (p. 187) *Tropical Rice* (p. 274) *Glazed Carrots* (p. 279)	*Sesame Fried Tofu* (p. 187), 1½ srv. *Tropical Rice* (p. 274) *Glazed Carrots* (p. 279)	*Sesame Fried Tofu* (p. 187), 2 srv. *Tropical Rice* (p. 274), 1½ srv. *Glazed Carrots* (p. 279)
SNACK		
Mixed Fruit w/Sauce (p. 298)	*Mixed Fruit w/Sauce* (p. 298)	*Mixed Fruit w/Sauce* (p. 298)
35.6 grams fat 1,211 calories	**46 grams fat 1,509 calories**	**55 grams fat 1,818 calories**

Weekend Menu PHASE 3 30% Fat

1,200 CALORIES 40 GRAMS FAT	1,500 CALORIES 50 GRAMS FAT	1,800 CALORIES 60 GRAMS FAT
BREAKFAST		
Whole wheat English muffin, 1, w/*Cranberry-Walnut Spread* (p. 324), 1 T. Dannon La Crème yogurt, 4 oz.	Sara Lee Croissant, 1, w/*Cranberry-Walnut Spread* (p. 324), 1 T. Blueberries, ½ c.	Sara Lee Croissant, 1, w/*Cranberry-Walnut Spread* (p. 324), 2 T. Blueberries, ½ c., w/Dannon La Crème Yogurt, 6 oz.
LUNCH		
Pumpkin Soup (p. 153), ½ srv. *Watercress and Strawberry Salad* (p. 168) w/shrimp, 12 large	*Pumpkin Soup* (p. 153) *Watercress and Strawberry Salad* (p. 168) w/shrimp, 12 large Crisp breadstick, 1	*Pumpkin Soup* (p. 153) *Watercress and Strawberry Salad* (p. 168), 1½ srv., w/shrimp, 12 large
SNACK		
Peach, 1	Peach, 1	Archway Oatmeal Raisin Cookie, 1
DINNER		
Petite Filet w/Onions (p. 241) *Wild Rice Salad* (p. 275), ¾ srv. Tomato, 3 thick slices, w/*Basil-Cream Dressing* (p. 334), 2 T.	*Petite Filet w/Onions* (p. 241) *Wild Rice Salad* (p. 275), ¾ srv. *Creamed Spinach* (p. 277)	*Petite Filet w/Onions* (p. 241) *Wild Rice Salad* (p. 275) *Creamed Spinach* (p. 277), 1½ srv.
SNACK		
Healthy Choice Ice Cream Sandwich, 1	*Pineapple-Mango Topping w/Frozen Yogurt* (p. 297)	Healthy Choice Ice Cream Sandwich, 1
37 grams fat 1,226 calories	**46 grams fat 1,511 calories**	**57 grams fat 1,815 calories**

No-Cook Menu PHASE ③ 30% Fat

1,200 CALORIES 40 GRAMS FAT	1,500 CALORIES 50 GRAMS FAT	1,800 CALORIES 60 GRAMS FAT
BREAKFAST		
Amy's Breakfast Burrito, 1	Amy's Breakfast Burrito, 1 Canteloupe, ¼ Milk, 2%, 1 c.	Amy's Breakfast Burrito, 1 Canteloupe, ¼ Milk, whole, ¾ c.
LUNCH		

Birds Eye Chicken Fajita Skillet,
  1½ c.
Archway Fat Free Oatmeal
  Raisin Cookie, 1
Plum, 1
	Bumble Bee Chicken Salad
	  w/Crackers Lunch Kit, 1
	Archway Fat Free Oatmeal Raisin
	  Cookie, 1
	Nectarine, 1
		Bumble Bee Chicken Salad
		  w/Crackers Lunch Kit, 1
		Archway Fat Free Oatmeal Raisin
		  Cookies, 2
		Pear, 1

SNACK		
Dole Individual Fruit Bowl	Pear, 1	Healthy Choice Ice Cream Sandwich, 1
DINNER		

Lean Cuisine Stuffed Cabbage
  w/Whipped Potatoes, 2
Mixed lettuce salad,1½ c., w/
  Italian dressing, light, 2 T.
	Stouffer's Stuffed Pepper
	Mixed lettuce salad,1 c., w/Italian
	  dressing, fat-free, 2 T.
	Club roll,1, w/marg. fat-free,
	  2 tsp.
		Stouffer's Stuffed Pepper
		Mixed lettuce salad,1½ c., w/
		  Italian dressing, fat free, 2 T.
		Soft Breadsticks, w/marg.,
		  reduced-fat, 2 tsp.
		Jell-O Pudding Snack Cup, 1

SNACK		
Nabisco Sugar Snaps, 2	Edy's Light Ice Cream, ½ c.	Low-fat popcorn, 1 bag
36 grams fat **1,209 calories**	**46 grams fat** **1,518 calories**	**54 grams fat** **1,817 calories**

No-Cook Menu PHASE ③ 30% Fat

1,200 CALORIES 40 GRAMS FAT	1,500 CALORIES 50 GRAMS FAT	1,800 CALORIES 60 GRAMS FAT
BREAKFAST		

English muffin, 1, w/natural
  peanut butter, 2 tsp.
Strawberries, ½ c
	English muffin, 1. w/natural
	  peanut butter, 1 T.
	Smucker's Simply Fruit, 2 T.
	Milk, 2%, ½ c.
		English muffin, 1, w/natural
		  peanut butter, 2 T.
		Smucker's Simply Fruit, 1½ T.
		Citrus sections 1 c.

LUNCH		

Smart Ones Meatloaf
Archway Oatmeal Raisin
  Cookie, 1
	Smart Ones Meatloaf
	Archway Oatmeal Raisin Cookie, 1
		Smart Ones Meatloaf
		Archway Oatmeal Raisin
		  Cookies, 2
		Pear, 1

SNACK		
Jell-O Pudding Snack Cup, 1	Jello Pudding Snack Cup, 1	Jello Pudding Snack Cup, 1
DINNER		

Rotisserie chicken (with skin),
  ¼
Mixed greens w/Italian
  dressing, fat-free, 2 T.
	Rotisserie chicken (with skin), ¼
	Mixed greens w/Italian dressing,
	  fat-free, 2 T.
	Club roll, 1, w/marg., reduced-fat,
	  1 tsp.
		Rotisserie chicken (with skin), ¼
		Mixed greens w/ranch dressing,
		  fat-free, 2 T.
		Club roll, 1, w/marg. reduced-
		  fat, 2 tsp.

SNACK		

Planter's Peanut Butter Cookie
  Crisps, 1 pack
	Planter's Peanut Butter Cookie
	  Crisps, 1 pack
		Planter's Peanut Butter Cookie
		  Crisps, 1 pack

37 grams fat **1,206 calories**	**47.6 grams fat** **1,493 calories**	**54 grams fat** **1,788 calories**

No-Cook Menu PHASE ③ 30% Fat

1,200 CALORIES 40 GRAMS FAT	1,500 CALORIES 50 GRAMS FAT	1,800 CALORIES 60 GRAMS FAT
BREAKFAST		
Eggo Nutrigrain Waffles w/sugar free syrup, 2T. Citrus sections, ½ c.	Eggo Nutrigrain Waffles w/sugar free syrup, 2T. Citrus sections, 1 c. Milk, 1%, ½ c.	Eggo Nutrigrain Waffles w/sugar free syrup, 2T. Citrus sections, 1 c. Milk,1%, ½ c.
LUNCH		
Campbell's Chunky Chili, 1 c. Kraft Shredded Cheddar, 2%, 1 T. Club roll, 1	Campbell's Chunky Chili, 1 c. Kraft Shredded Cheddar, 2%, 2 T. Uncle Ben's Ready Rice, 1 c.	Campbell's Chunky Chili, 1 c. Kraft Shredded Cheddar, 2%, ¼ c., and sour cream, light, 1 T. Uncle Ben's Ready Rice, 1 c. Dole Individual Fruit Bowl
SNACK		
Dried Fig, 1	Pear, 1	Healthy Valley Granola Bar, 1
DINNER		
Healthy Choice Cheddar Broccoli Potato, 1 pack w/bacon bits, 1T. Mixed greens w/low-fat ranch dressing, 2 T.	Mixed greens w/turkey breast, 2 oz., & low-fat ranch dressing, 2 T. Healthy Choice Cheddar Broccoli Potato, 1 pk. w/bacon bits, 2 T.	Healthy Choice Cheddar Broccoli Potato, 1 pk. w/bacon bits, 1T. Mixed greens w/low-fat ranch dressing. 2 T. Club roll, 1
SNACK		
Jell-O Pudding Snack Cup, 1	Jell-O Pudding Snack Cup, 1	Jell-O Pudding Snack Cup, 1
36.5 grams fat **1,230 calories**	**46.5 grams fat** **1,534 calories**	**56.5 grams fat** **1,810 calories**

No-Cook Menu PHASE ③ 30% Fat

1,200 CALORIES 40 GRAMS FAT	1,500 CALORIES 50 GRAMS FAT	1,800 CALORIES 60 GRAMS FAT
BREAKFAST		
Mixed tropical fruit in juice w/walnuts, chopped, 1 T. Quarker Chewy 90 Calories Bar, 1	Pillsbury Toaster Scramblers, Cheese, Egg & Bacon, 1 Milk, fat free, ¾ c.; Orange, 1	Pillsbury Toaster Scramblers, Cheese, Egg & Bacon, 1 Milk, fat free, 1c.; Orange, 1
LUNCH		
Dr. Praeger's Frozen Fish Sticks, 3, w/Kraft Tartar Sauce, 1 T. Mixed greens, 2 c., w/feta, 2 T., and fat-free Caesar dressing, 2 T. Cherries, 20	Moosewood Broccoli & Pasta Parmesan Del Monte Sliced Peaches in 100% Juice Keebler Oatmeal Cookie, 1	Campbell's Cream of Asparagus Soup w/fat-free milk, ¾ c. Lean Cuisine Mushroom Pizza Mixed greens, w/feta, 2 T., and fat-free Caesar dressing, 2 T. Keebler Oatmeal Cookie, 1
SNACK		
Honey Maid Graham Crackers, 1	Laughing Cow Wedge, 1, w/low-fat wheat crackers, 3	Jell-O Pudding Snack Cup, 1
DINNER		
Lean Cuisine Roasted Pork McCain's Premium Golden Crisp Sweet Potato Fries, 6 oz.	Healthy Choice Beef Stroganoff Mixed greens, 2 c., w/feta, 2 T., and fat-free Caesar dressing, 2 T.	Stouffer's Roasted Pork Entree Green Giant Broccoli & Three Cheese Sauce, ¾ c. Smart Ones Key Lime Pie
SNACK		
Jell-O Pudding Snack Cup, 1	Jell-O Pudding Snack Cup, 1 .	Nabisco Chips Ahoy Thin/Crisps, 1 pack
37 grams fat **1,213 calories**	**49 grams fat** **1,550 calories**	**56 grams fat** **1,802 calories**

recipe substitutes

Recipe	Substitute	Fat (g)	Cals.
Almond-Pumpkin Breakfast Bread	2 slices Pepperidge Farm Cinnamon Swirl Bread	5	180
Aloha Fruit Salad w/ Macadamia Crunch	1 banana	0	110
	1 T. chopped walnuts	5	50
Arizona Jerk Turkey	4 oz. turkey breast, deli	3	120
	2 T. fat-free mayo	0	20
Artichokes and Dip	1 c. baby carrots	0	60
	1 T. Wish-Bone Light! Blue Cheese Dressing	1	25
Asparagus Omelet w/Summer Herbs	1 egg	5	75
	1 slice whole wheat toast	1	80
Asparagus Soup	¾ c. Campbell's Cream of Asparagus Soup, fat-free milk	5	150
Autumn Bean and Squash Stew	Amy's Whole Meals Chili & Cornbread	6	340
Baby Greens w/Avocado, Strawberries, and Walnuts	2 c. mixed salad greens	0	15
	2 T. dried cranberries	0	50
	1 T. chopped walnuts	5	50
	2 T. Newman's Own Lighten Up! Raspberry &Walnut Dressing	5	70
Baked Apples	½ c. Mott's Cinnamon Applesauce	0	120
	1½ t. chopped walnuts	2.5	25
Baked Asparagus w/Gremolata	6 asparagus spears	0	25
	1 t. reduced-fat margarine	1.6	17
Baked Halibut w/Red Pepper and Parsley Crust	Lean Cuisine Baked Lemon Pepper Fish	6	220
Baked Stuffed Acorn Squash	½ c. Green Giant Candied Sweet Potatoes	4	160
Balsamic Mustard Dressing	2 T. Kraft Free Italian Dressing	0	15
Banana Chutney	1 T. Crosse and Blackwell's Major Grey's Chutney	0	60
Banana-Nut Hotcakes	2 slices Aunt Jemima Homestyle French Toast	6	240
Basil-Cream Dressing	1 T. Wish-Bone Light! Blue Cheese Dressing	1	25
Bean and Red Pepper Spread	2 T. Amy's Organic Black Bean & Corn Salsa	0	15
Beef and Vegetable Stew	1 c. Birds Eye Voila! Beef Steak & Garlic Potato	7	190
Beef Stroganoff	Healthy Choice Beef Stroganoff	9	330
Blueberry Banana Split	½ c. Ben & Jerry's Cherry Garcia Low Fat Frozen Yogurt	3	170
	1 small banana	0	90
Blueberry Muffins	1 low-fat coffee cake	2	110

Recipe	Substitute	Fat (g)	Cals.
Blueberry Salsa	2 T. Newman's Own Chunky Peach Salsa	0	25
Boston Baked Beans	½ c. Bush's Best Boston Recipe Baked Beans	1.5	170
Boston Clam Chowder	2 c. Campbell's Select 98% Fat Free New England Clam Chowder	3	200
Braised Cabbage with Apples	1½ c. Glory Foods Seasoned Country Cabbage	4.5	135
	1½ t. chopped walnuts	2.5	25
Brook Trout with Tomato and Red Onion Relish	4 oz. smoked trout	10	200
	¼ c. Hunt's Diced Tomatoes w/Sweet Onions	0	23
Brown Sugar-Grilled Peaches	½ c. Del Monte Sliced Peaches in 100% Juice	0	60
	2 tsp. chopped walnuts	3.4	35
Buttery Squash Soup	1 c. Campbell's Select Golden Butternut Squash Soup	2	90
California Fruit Salad	½ c. mixed tropical fruit in juice	0	80
	2 c. mixed lettuce	0	15
	2 T. Newman's Own Lighten Up! Raspberry & Walnut Dressing	5	70
	2 T. chopped walnuts	10	100
Carrot Cake	⅛ Sara Lee Free & Light Pound Cake	2	100
Carrot-Raisin Bran Muffins	1 Quaker Breakfast Bar	2.5	130
Chambord Compote	½ c. mixed tropical fruit in juice	0	80
	2 tsp. chopped walnuts	3.4	35
Cheddar-Stuffed Acorn Squash	1½ c. Green Giant Cinnamon Spiced Squash	0	240
	1 T. sunflower seeds	5	50
	1 T. chopped walnuts	5	50
	2 T. dried cranberries	0	50
Cheesy Broccoli	1 c. Green Giant Broccoli & Three Cheese Sauce	5	100
Chicken Fajitas	1 c. Birds Eye Voila! Southwestern Chicken	6	250
	2 T. Calavo Fiesta Guacamole	5	60
	1 Cedar's Low Carb Whole Wheat Wrap	1.5	70
Chicken Fingers	3 oz. Perdue Home Style Breaded Chicken Breast Strips	6	170
Chicken Fingers with Honey Mustard Sauce	3 oz. Perdue Home Style Breaded Chicken Breast Strips	6	170
	2 T. Boar's Head Brand Honey Mustard	0	60
	2 T. fat-free mayonnaise	0	20
Chicken Paprikash	Smart Ones Chicken Carbonara	5	260

Recipe	Substitute	Fat (g)	Cals.
Chicken Pot Pie	1¼ c. Green Giant Chicken Cheesy Pasta Skillet Meal	4	215
	2 Pillsbury Buttermilk Biscuits	2	100
Chicken Soup with Soba Noodles	2 c. Campbell's Chunky Chicken Noodle Soup	5	200
Chicken Wingettes	3 Perdue Frozen Hot & Spicy Chicken Wings	10	170
Chilean Sea Bass en Papillote	2 pieces Gorton's Classic Grilled Salmon	7	200
	1 T. Kraft Hot & Spicy Tartar Sauce	3	35
Chili Bean Dip	½ c. Old El Paso Traditional Refried Beans	1	100
Chili Mac	Stouffer's Macaroni & Beef	13	360
Chili Mayonnaise	1½ t. French's Smoked Chipotle GourMayo	2.5	25
Chili-Spiced Tuna Steaks with Grilled Tomato Sauce	Lean Cuisine Salmon w/Lemon Dill Sauce	6	240
Chocolate-Covered Strawberries	1 square Dove Dark Chocolate	2.6	42
	½ c. sliced strawberries	0	23
Classic Spinach Salad	2 c. raw spinach	0	15
	1 T. Hormel Real Crumbled Bacon	2	30
	2 T. fat-free ranch dressing	0	50
Cod and Tomato Stew	1 c. Birds Eye Voila! Shrimp Scampi	2.5	190
Cornish Hens with Apricot Stuffing	2 c. Glory Foods Chicken & Dumplings	14	500
Crab Cakes with Red Pepper Sauce	3 Dr. Praeger's Lightly Breaded Frozen Fish Sticks	6	158
	¼ c. Contadina Recipe Ready Diced Tomatoes with Roasted Red Peppers	0	30
Cranberry Muffins	1 Health Valley Cobbler Cereal Bar	2	130
Cranberry-Walnut Spread	2 T. Philadelphia Fat Free Strawberry Cream Cheese	0	40
	1 tsp. chopped walnuts	1.7	17
Creamed Spinach	1 c. Green Giant Creamed Spinach	5	140
Creamy Coleslaw	Lettuce and tomato salad	0	20
	2 T. Kraft Free Ranch Dressing	0	50
Creamy Dijon Dressing	2 T. Cains Fat Free Honey Dijon Dressing	0	35
Creamy Italian Dressing	2 T. Wish-Bone Fat Free! Italian Dressing	0	20
Creamy Onion Dip	¼ c. fat-free sour cream	0	60
	1 t. dry onion soup mix	0	10
Creamy Raspberry Dressing	2 T. Wish-Bone Fat Free! Ranch Dressing	0	30
Crispy Beer Batter Onion Rings	3 oz. McCain's Premium Golden Crisp Sweet Potato Fries	3	120

Recipe	Substitute	Fat (g)	Cals.
Curried Grape Salsa	2 T. Newman's Own Chunky Peach Salsa	0	25
Drunken Pork Chops	Lean Cuisine Roasted Pork	6	180
Eggs-and-Potato Hash	1 large egg	5	75
	1 t. reduced-fat margarine	1.6	17
	1 c. Cascadian Farm Country Style Potatoes	0	70
Field Greens with Pears and Walnuts	2 c. mixed lettuce	0	15
	½ sliced pear	0.5	55
	2 t. chopped walnuts	3.4	35
	2 T. Wish-Bone Lemon Garlic and Herb Vinaigrette	6	70
Fish Sticks	4 Mrs. Paul's Healthy Selects Fish Sticks	8	152
Fisherman's Stew	¾ c. Birds Eye Voila! Garlic Shrimp	6	165
French Onion Soup	1 c. Progresso Vegetable Classics French Onion Soup	1.5	50
	1" slice French bread	1	100
	1 t. grated Parmesan	0.5	10
Fresh Raspberry Sauce	1 T. Smucker's Low Sugar Raspberry Preserves	0	25
Frozen Grapes	1 c. grapes, pineapple chunks, or watermelon chunks	0	60
Garden Peas with Fresh Mint	⅔ c. Birds Eye Petite Peas & Mushrooms w/Chives	3.5	90
Garlic-Lemon Spinach	¾ c. Green Giant Cut Leaf Spinach & Butter Sauce	1.5	45
Garlic Vinaigrette	1 T. Wish-Bone Garlic Ranch	7.5	70
Glazed Carrots	½ c. Del Monte Savory Sides Honey Glazed Carrots	0	70
Greek Lamb Kabobs	1 c. Birds Eye Voila! Beef Steak & Garlic Potato	7	190
Greek Salad	2 c. mixed lettuce	0	15
	1 hard-cooked egg	5	75
	1 tomato	0	35
	2 T. crumbled feta cheese	3.5	45
	3 kalamata olives	4	45
	2 T. Wish-Bone Italian Dressing	8	80
Green Olive Tapenade	1 T. Cantare Olive Tapénade	2	30
Gremolata	1 T. Progresso Parmesan Bread Crumbs	0.5	27
Grilled Cheese and Bacon	1 Cheeseburger Lean Pockets	7	280
Grilled Chicken Caesar Salad	1 c. Perdue Short Cuts Carved Chicken Breast, Original Roasted	4	180
	2 c. Romaine lettuce	0	15
	2 T. Cains Fat Free Caesar Dressing	0	30
	1 T. grated Parmesan	2	30

Recipe	Substitute	Fat (g)	Cals.
Grilled Chicken Salad Véronique	½ c. Perdue Short Cuts Carved Chicken Breast, Original Roasted	2	90
	2 c. mixed lettuce	0	15
	½ c. seedless grapes	0	30
	2 T. Kraft Free Honey Dijon Dressing	0	50
Grilled Citrus-Scented Swordfish with Ginger	Lean Cuisine Baked Lemon Pepper Fish	6	220
Grilled Cowboy Steaks w/Secret Sauce and Tomato Topping	Lean Cuisine Steak Tips Portabello	7	180
Grilled Lamb Chops with Grilled Grapes	Stouffer's Roasted Pork	11	350
Grilled Margarita Chicken	1¼ c. Birds Eye Voila! Southwestern Chicken	7.5	312
Grilled Marinated Eggplant	2 c. Birds Eye Tuscan Vegetables in Herbed Tomato Sauce	4	100
Grilled Marinated Swordfish	2 Gorton's Classic Char-Grilled Fillets	6	200
Grilled Pineapple Chicken Sandwich	Lean Cuisine Chicken Teriyaki	4.5	300
Grilled Portobello Mushrooms	3 Brew City Beer Battered Mushrooms	4	75
Grilled Shrimp with Corn-and-Tomato Salad	⅔ c. Birds Eye Steamfresh Specially Seasoned Southwestern Corn	2	90
	12 large steamed shrimp	1.5	120
	2 T. Kraft Light Done Right! Italian Dressing	3	40
Grilled Tofu Burgers	1 Morningstar Farms Garden Veggie Patty	2.5	100
	1 slice Cheddar Kraft Singles	4.5	60
	3½" hard roll	2.5	170
Grilled Vegetables with Garlic Vinaigrette	2 c. Birds Eye Tuscan Vegetables in Herbed Tomato Sauce	4	100
	1 baked potato	0	220
Guacamole	2 T. Calavo Fiesta Guacamole	5	60
Hero's Hoagie	1 Turkey & Ham w/Cheese Hot Pockets	13	300
Hoagie Dressing	2 T. Kraft Free Italian Dressing	0	15
Honey-Lime Dressing	2 T. Cains Light French Dressing	3.5	50
Horseradish Dip	2 T. fat-free mayonnaise	0	20
	1 t. prepared horseradish	0	0
Hot and Cold Melon Soup	¼ cantaloupe or	0	50
	honeydew melon	0	45
Hot Grilled Tuna Kabobs	Lean Cuisine Salmon w/ Lemon Dill Sauce	6	240
Hot-Hot Sauce	2 t. French's Chipotle Chili GourMayo	3.3	33
Key Lime Pie	1 Smart Ones Key Lime Pie	6	200

Recipe	Substitute	Fat (g)	Cals.
Lean and Mean Mashed Potatoes	1 c. prepared Barbara's Bakery Mashed Potatoes	0	140
Linguine with Clam Sauce	2 c. Birds Eye Voila! Shrimp Scampi	5	380
Little Caesar Salad	2 c. Romaine lettuce	0	15
	2 T. Cains Fat Free Caesar Dressing	0	30
	1 T. grated Parmesan	2	30
	6 Pepperidge Farm Fat Free Caesar Croutons	0	30
London Broil Two Ways	Lean Cuisine Oven Roasted Beef	8	210
Low-Fat Hummus	1 T. Cedar's Hommus	1	25
Lunch-Box Tuna Salad Sandwich	StarKist Lunch To-Go Kit	9	210
Mac 'n' Cheese	1½ c. Kraft Deluxe Macaroni & Cheese Dinner w/Original Cheddar Cheese Sauce	10	320
Make Your Own Tortilla Chips	1 oz. Baked Tostitos	1	110
Mashed Sweet Potatoes	¾ c. Princella Fancy Mashed Sweet Potatoes	0	135
Mini Pizzas Two Ways	Lean Cuisine Gourmet Mushroom Pizza	7	280
Mixed Fruit with Strawberry-Ginger Sauce	1½ c. frozen mixed berries	0	105
Moroccan Vegetable Stew	1 c. Glory Foods Seasoned Black Beans and Rice	3	180
	1 c. Green Giant Cinnamon Spiced Squash	0	160
Mussels Marinière	1 c. Progresso Traditional Manhattan Clam Chowder	2	110
Nachos	¾ c. Campbell's Chunky Roadhouse Chili	6	165
	1 oz. Baked Tostitos	1	110
Navy Bean Soup	1 c. Campbell's Select Savory Lentil Soup	1	140
Orange Vinaigrette	2 T. Litehouse Fat Free Raspberry Vinaigrette	0	25
Oriental Ginger Dressing	2 T. Annie's Naturals Low Fat Gingerly Vinaigrette	2	40
Orzo with Cherry Tomatoes, Capers, and Pine Nuts	Lean Cuisine Angel Hair Pasta Marinara	4	260
Oven-Fried Chicken	3 oz. Perdue Home Style Breaded Chicken Breast Strips	6	170
Pan-Seared Red Snapper with Olive Crust	Healthy Choice Herb Baked Fish	8	360
	1 T. Kraft Tartar Sauce	3	35
Pasta Carbonara	Moosewood Broccoli & Pasta Parmesan	12	340
Pasta Primavera	Birds Eye Vegetables & Shells in Garlic Butter Sauce	13	270

Recipe	Substitute	Fat (g)	Cals.
Pasta with Cherry Tomatoes and Parsley	Lean Cuisine Penne Pasta w/ Tomato Basil Sauce	3	270
Peach Chutney	1 T. Crosse and Blackwell's Major Grey's Chutney	0	60
Peach-Nectarine Salsa	2 T. Newman's Own Chunky Peach Salsa	0	25
Peachy Blueberry Crisp	½ c. sliced peaches in juice	0	60
	½ c. blueberries	0	40
	½ c. Edy's or Light Ice Cream	4.5	130
Pecan Waffles with Strawberry Sauce	2 Eggo Apple Cinnamon Waffles	6	190
	1 T. chopped walnuts	5	50
	2 T. Smucker's Strawberry Topping	0	100
Penne with Broccoli and Cheese	1 c. cooked penne pasta	1	200
	1 c. Birds Eye Broccoli & Cheese Sauce	10	180
Petite Filet with Caramelized Onions	Stouffer's Beef Pot Roast Entrée	11	260
Pineapple-Mango Topping with Frozen Yogurt	½ c. Edy's Frozen Yogurt Fat Free Vanilla	0	90
	½ c. crushed pineapple in juice	0	70
Pineapple Salsa	3 T. Newman's Own Chunky Peach Salsa	0	25
Pita Sandwiches to Go	Green Giant Rice Pilaf	3	200
Poached Chicken with Avocado Sauce	1 cup Perdue Short Cuts Carved Chicken Breast, Fajita Style	5	180
	¼ c. Calavo Frozen Avocado Sauce	1	30
Poached Salmon Two Ways (w/Balsamic Tomato Sauce)	2 pieces Gorton's Classic Grilled Salmon	7	200
	2 T. Zatarain's Remoulade Sauce	4	50
Poached Salmon Two Ways (w/Dill Sauce)	2 pieces Gorton's Classic Grilled Salmon	7	200
	2 T. Kraft Tartar Sauce	6	70
Poppy Seed Dressing	2 T. Annie's Naturals Raspberry Vinaigrette	1.5	35
Portobello Burgers	3 oz. BinB Mushrooms	1.5	40
	1 c. Birds Eye Rice Pilaf in Herbed Butter Sauce	4	190
Raisin Bran Muffins with Orange Glaze	2 Nutri-Grain Blueberry Cereal Bars	6	280
Raspberry-Walnut Dressing	2 T. Newman's Own Lighten Up! Raspberry & Walnut Dressing	5	70
Ratatouille Omelet	½ c. Birds Eye Tuscan Vegetables in Herbed Tomato Sauce	1	25
	2 scrambled eggs	10	150
Red, White, and Blue Parfaits	6 oz. Stonyfield Farm Lowfat Luscious Lemon Yogurt	1.5	140
	½ c. blueberries	0	40

Recipe	Substitute	Fat (g)	Cals.
Roast Chicken with Winter Vegetables	Lean Cuisine Chicken & Vegetables	5	230
Roasted Chicken Salad with Raspberry Vinaigrette	1 cup Perdue Short Cuts Carved Chicken Breast, Original Roasted	4	180
	2 c. mixed lettuce	0	15
	2 T. Annie's Naturals Raspberry Vinaigrette	1.5	35
Roasted Garlic Puree	1 tsp. Lawry's Ready to Spread Garlic Spread	3.3	33
Rosemary Roasted New Potatoes	¾ c. Birds Eye Baby Red Potatoes w/ Rosemary	4	110
Sauteed Chicken with Cider Sauce	1 Perdue Short Cuts Carved Chicken Breast, Honey Roasted	2.5	90
	6 oz. Stouffer's Harvest Apples	2.5	190
Seafood au Gratin	Lean Cuisine Lemon Garlic Shrimp	7	350
Seafood Jambalaya	1 cup Zatarain's Ready-to-Serve New Orleans Style Red Beans & Rice	6	280
	8 large steamed shrimp	1	80
Seared Scallops with Asparagus and Ginger	¾ c. Birds Eye Voila! Shrimp Scampi	2	142
Sesame Cheese Balls	2 T. Fritos Chili Cheese Dip	3	45
Sesame Fried Tofu	½ package TofuTown Grilled Tofu Tenders, Sesame Ginger Teriyaki	9	240
Shrimp Caesar Salad	12 large steamed shrimp	1.5	120
	2 c. Romaine lettuce	0	15
	2 T. Cains Fat Free Caesar Dressing	0	30
	1 T. grated Parmesan	2	30
	6 Pepperidge Farm Fat Free Caesar Croutons	0	30
Shrimp Salad Sandwiches	1 c. Birds Eye Voila! Shrimp Scampi	2.5	190
Sizzlin' Shrimp with Black-Eyed Peas	¾ c. Birds Eye Voila! Garlic Shrimp	6	165
Skinny Chef's Salad	3 oz. deli turkey breast	2	90
	2 c. mixed lettuce	0	15
	½ c. mandarin oranges in juice	0	50
	2 T. Annie's Naturals Raspberry Vinaigrette	1.5	35
Southern Red Beans and Rice	Lean Cuisine Three Bean Chili	7	270
Spaghetti and Meatballs	12 oz. Stouffer's Spaghetti w/ Meat Sauce	11	400
Spaghetti w/Fresh Mushrooms and Red Sauce	Smart Ones Spaghetti Bolognese	6	310
Spaghetti with Summer Squash	2¼ c. Birds Eye Rotelle & Vegetables in Herbed Butter Sauce	10	400
Spaghetti with Summer Tomatoes, Basil, and Garlic	Smart Ones Three Cheese Ziti Marinara	7	290
Spiced Apples	1 c. unsweetened applesauce w/ ½ tsp. cinnamon	0	100

Recipe	Substitute	Fat (g)	Cals.
Spinach Pesto with Penne and Peas	2 c. Birds Eye Pasta & Vegetables in a Creamy Cheese Sauce	8	340
Spinach Risotto	Green Giant Rice Medley	3.5	240
Spinach-Stuffed Mushrooms	2 Dr. Praeger's Spinach Pancakes	4	80
Stir-Fried Pork and Greens	Lean Cuisine Roasted Pork	6	180
Stir-Fried Pork with Apples and Figs	¼ c. Lloyd's Barbeque Original BBQ Shredded Pork	2	90
	1 c. Glory Foods Sensibly Seasoned Tomatoes, Okra & Corn (canned)	0	75
Strawberry Sauce	1 T. Smucker's Strawberry Topping	0	50
Stuffed Bell Peppers	15.5 oz. Stouffer's Stuffed Peppers	14	360
Stuffed Celery	2 ribs celery	0	12
	1 T. Wish-Bone Fat Free! Chunky Blue Cheese Dressing	0	18
Super-Quick Pumpkin Soup	1 c. Campbell's Select Creamy Portobello Mushroom Soup	4	100
Sweet and Spicy Shrimp	Smart Ones Shrimp Marinara	2	180
Sweet Potato Jacks with Cinnamon-Apple Topping	2 slices whole wheat toast	2	160
	1 T. Smucker's Low Sugar Apricot Preserves	0	25
	¼ c. unsweetened applesauce	0	25
Tartar Sauce	2 T. Kraft Fat Free Tartar Sauce	0	25
Texas Black Bean Soup	1 c. Progresso Hearty Black Bean Soup w/Bacon	1.5	170
Texas-Style Stuffed Peppers	Lean Cuisine Three Bean Chili	7	270
Tex-Mex Dip	2 T. Cedarlane Five Layer Mexican Dip	3	60
	1 oz. Baked Tostitos	1	110
Thousand Island Dressing	2 T. Kraft Free Thousand Island Dressing	0	45
Tomato and Zucchini Gratin	½ c. Glory Foods Tomato, Okra & Corn Casserole (frozen)	4.5	110
Tomato and Zucchini Gratin with Rice	½ c. Glory Foods Tomato, Okra & Corn Casserole (frozen)	4.5	110
	1 c. Success Boil-in-Bag Brown Rice	2	300
Tomato Chutney	¼ c. Del Monte Diced Tomatoes w/Basil, Garlic & Oregano	0	25
Tomato-Corn Bisque	1 c. Progresso Vegetable Classics Hearty Tomato Soup	1	110
	¼ c. Del Monte Summer Crisp Sweet Corn	0.5	35
Tomato-Pepper Salsa	2 T. Pace Lime & Garlic Chunky Salsa	0	15
Trail Mix	¼ c. raisins	0	110
	2 t. chopped walnuts	3.4	35

Recipe	Substitute	Fat (g)	Cals.
Tropical Rice	½ c. Lundberg Rice Sensations Thai Coconut Ginger	2	114
Tuna Burgers with Wasabi Mayonnaise	Healthy Choice Herb Baked Fish	8	360
Tuna Noodle Casserole	Healthy Choice Macaroni & Cheese	6	270
Turkey Burgers	1 Dr. Prager's California Veggie Burger	4.5	110
	1 hamburger roll	2.5	120
	1 slice 2% Cheddar Kraft Singles	3	50
Turkey Loaf	Lean Cuisine Meatloaf w/Gravy and Whipped Potatoes	7	250
Turkey Sloppy Joes	Lean Cuisine Roasted Turkey Breast	2.5	270
Two-Potato Bisque	1 c. Walnut Acres Organic Autumn Harvest Soup	2	100
Ukrainian Borscht	1 cup Progresso 99% Fat Free Minestrone Soup	1	100
Veal Marsala	Lean Cuisine Pork w/Cherry Sauce	5	260
Veal Scallops with Fennel and Grapes	Lean Cuisine Beef Burgundy	7	300
Vegetable Risotto	Green Giant Rice Pilaf	3	200
Vegetarian Antipasto	Amy's Non-Dairy Vegetable Pot Pie	13	360
Vegetarian Chili	Lean Cuisine Three Bean Chili	7	270
Waffles with Strawberry Sauce	2 Eggo Homestyle Waffles	6	190
	2 T. Smucker's Strawberry Topping	0	100
Warm Eggplant, Tomato, and Mozzarella Salad	5 oz. Cedarlane Eggplant Parmesan	8	160
Warm Potato and Tuna Salad	¾ c. Birds Eye Baby Red Potatoes with Rosemary	4	110
	3 oz. tuna in water	1	70
	1 tomato	0	35
Watercress and Strawberry Salad	2 c. mixed lettuce	0	15
	1 T. Kraft Special Collection Creamy Poppy Seed Dressing	5	65
	½ c. sliced strawberries	0	25
	1½ t. chopped pecans	2.5	25
Wild Rice Salad	1 c. Uncle Ben's Long Grain & Wild Rice Original Recipe	0	200
Wilted Spinach Salad	2 c. raw spinach	0	15
	1 T. Hormel Real Crumbled Bacon	2	30
	2 T. Kraft Free Ranch Dressing	0	50
Yogurt Cheese	1 T. fat-free sour cream	0	18
Zesty Bean Salsa	2 T. Amy's Organic Black Bean & Corn Salsa	0	30

FOOD, AMOUNT	FAT (g)	CALS.
Fruit Snacks: 0–1 gram fat		
Apple, 1	0	80
Applesauce, unsweetened, ½ c.	0	50
Apricots, Fresh, 3	1	60
Banana, 1	0.5	110
Blackberries, ½ c.	0	30
Blueberries, ½ c.	0	40
Cantaloupe, ¼	0	50
Cherries, Fresh, 20	0	90
Dried apricots, 5 pieces	0	100
Dried figs, 2 pieces	1	120
Dried plums, 5 pieces	0	100
Fig, fresh, 1	0	40
Grapefruit, ½	0	50
Grapes, 1 c.	0	60
Honeydew melon, ¼	0	90
Kiwifruits, 2	1	100
Mandarin oranges (in juice), ½ c.	0	60
Mango, ½	0	55
Nectarine, 1	0	0
Orange, 1	0	60
Papaya cubes, 1 c.	0	70
Peach, 1	0	40
Pear, 1	1	100
Pineapple chunks, 1 c.	0	70
Plum, 1	0.5	40
Pomegranate, 1	0	100
Raisins, ¼ c.	0	125
Raspberries, ½ c.	0.5	30
Strawberry slices, ½ c.	0	25
Tangerine, 1	0	50
Watermelon chunks, 1 c.	0	50

FOOD, AMOUNT	FAT (g)	CALS.
Variety Snacks: 0–1 gram fat		
Apple w/Philadelphia Fat Free Strawberry Cream Cheese, 2 T.	0	120
Archway Fat Free Oatmeal Raisin Cookie, 1	0.5	106
Archway Fat Free Devil's Food Cookie, 1	0.2	68
Baby carrots, 1 c., w/Wish-Bone Fat Free! Chunky Blue Cheese Dressing, 2 T.	0	35
Baked Tostitos, 1 oz.	1	110
Campbell's Soup at Hand, Classic Tomato, 1	0	140
Celery, 2 ribs, w/Wish-Bone Fat Free! Chunky Blue Cheese Dressing , 2 T.	0	35
Cottage cheese, fat-free, w/pineapple chunks, ½ c.	0	110
Crisp breadsticks, 2	1	75
Dannon Light 'n Fit Creamy Yogurt, 6 oz.	0	100
Dannon Light 'n Fit Nonfat Yogurt, 6 oz.	0	60
Dannon Light 'n Fit Smoothie, 7 oz.	0	70
Dole Individual Fruit Bowls, 1	0	75
8th Continent Light Premium Soy Milk, Vanilla, 8 oz.	1	60
Fat Free Blueberry Crunch Cake, 1 oz.	0	70
Frozen yogurt, nonfat, vanilla, ½ c.	0	90
FrozFruit Bar, 1	0	80
Fruit Roll-Up, 1	1	50
Health Valley Low Fat Healthy Chips Double Chocolate Cookie, 1	0	35
Health Valley Low Fat Stoned Wheat Crackers, 5	1	60

Food, Amount	Fat (g)	Cals.
Health Valley Moist n' Chewy Granola Bar, Wild Berry or Dutch Apple, 1	1	100
Healthy Choice Ice Cream Vanilla Bar w/Fudge Coating, 1	1	80
Healthy Choice Premium Fudge Bar, 1	1	80
Honey Maid Low Fat Graham Crackers, 2 squares	1	60
Ice cream, fat-free, ½ c.	0	100
Jell-O Fat Free Pudding Snack, 1	0	100
Jell-O Gelatin, ½ c.	0	80
Jell-O Gelatin, Sugar Free, ½ c.	0	10
Laughing Cow Light Gourmet Cheese Bites, 2	0.4	15
Light Golden Loaf Cake, 2 oz.	0	160
Minute Maid Frozen Juice Bar, 1	0	60
Nabisco Fat Free Fig Newton Cookies, 2	0	90
Pepperidge Farm 100% Whole Wheat Mini Bagel, 1	0.5	100
Pretzels, 1 oz.	0	120
Quaker Quakes Rice Snacks, Apple Cinnamon or Caramel Corn, 8	0	60
Quaker Rice Cakes, Apple Cinnamon or Caramel Corn, 1	0	50
Quaker Rice Cakes, Chocolate Crunch or Peanut Butter Chocolate Chip, 1	1	60
Sara Lee Free & Light Pound Cake, ⅛ cake	0.5	100
Sargento Fat Free Ricotta Cheese, ¼ c.	0	50
Shrimp, steamed, 5 large, w/cocktail sauce, 2 T.	0.5	100
Smucker's Low Sugar Preserves, 1 T., w/saltines, 3	1	60

Food, Amount	Fat (g)	Cals.
Snackwell's Fat Free Cookie Cakes, Devil's Food, 1	0.2	50
StarKist Tuna Creations, Hickory Smoked, 2 oz.	1	60
Stella D'oro Anisette Sponge Cookies, 2	1	90
Triscuit, 1	0.7	20
V8 100% Vegetable Juice, 8 oz.	0	50
Vitalicious VitaMuffin, Bran, 2 oz.	0	100
Whole-fruit sorbet, ½ c.	0	140
Yoplait Light or Light Thick & Creamy Yogurt, 6 oz.	0	100
Yoplait Light Smoothie, 8 oz.	0	90

Variety Snacks: 1.5–4 grams fat

Food, Amount	Fat (g)	Cals.
Act II 94% Fat Free Butter Popcorn, 1 bag	2.5	130
Archway Oatmeal Raisin Cookie, 1	3.5	107
Ben & Jerry's Cherry Garcia Low Fat Frozen Yogurt, ½ c.	3	170
Breakstone's Cottage Doubles, 1	2.5	150
Breyers Creme Savers Smoothie, 10 oz.	3	190
Breyers Double Churned Extra Creamy or Dreyer's/ Edy's Slow Churned Rich & Creamy Light Ice Cream, Chocolate, ½ c.	3.5	110
Bumble Bee Fat Free Tuna Salad w/crackers, 3.5 oz.	1.5	150
Dannon Natural Flavors Yogurt, 6 oz.	2.5	150
Fig Newtons, 100% Whole-Grain, 2	2	110
Fudgsicle, 1 bar	2	100
Guiltless Gourmet Tortilla Chips, 1 oz., w/Pace Chunky Salsa, ¼ c.	2	130

Food, Amount	Fat (g)	Cals.	Food, Amount	Fat (g)	Cals.
Health Valley Cobbler Cereal Bar, 1	2	130	Post Raisin Bran Cereal Bar, 1	2	120
Healthy Choice Caramel Swirl Ice Cream Sandwich, 1	3	140	Potato Chips, Baked, 1 oz.	1.5	110
Healthy Choice Vanilla Ice Cream Sandwich, 1	3	130	Quaker Chewy 90-Calorie Granola Bar, 1	2	90
Honey Maid Graham Crackers, 2 squares	1.5	65	Quaker Quakes Rice Snacks, Cheddar Cheese, Nacho Cheese, or Ranch, 9	2.5	70
Jell-O Pudding Snack, 1	4	140	Sargento Light Ricotta Cheese, ¼ c.	2.5	60
Kashi GoLean Crunchy! Bar, Chocolate Caramel, 1	3	150	Sargento Light String Cheese, 1 piece	2.5	50
Keebler Country Style Oatmeal Cookie, 1	3	60	Silk Live! Soy Smoothie, 1	4	220
Keebler Soft Batch Chocolate Chip Cookie, 1	3.5	80	Silk Soymilk, Very Vanilla or Chocolate, 8 oz.	4	140
Kraft Cheese Nips Thin Crisps, 1 pack	3	100	Smart Ones Chocolate Chocolate Chip Muffin, 1	2	190
Laughing Cow Light Cheese Wedge, 1	2	35	Soymilk, light, chocolate, 8 oz.	1.5	120
Laughing Cow Mini Babybel Light Cheese, 1 piece	3	50	Stella D'oro Almond Toast Cookies, 2	2.5	110
Low Fat Coffee Cake, 1	2	110	Stella D'oro Breakfast Treat, 1 cookie	3	90
Nabisco Chips Ahoy Thin Crisps, 1 pack	3	100	Stonyfield Farm Lowfat Yogurt, 6 oz.	1.5	130
Nabisco Ginger Snaps, 4	2.5	120	Thomas' Sahara Pita Bread, 100% Whole-Wheat, w/ Cedar's Hommus, 1 T.	1.75	95
Nabisco Oreo Thin Crisps, 1 pack	2	100	Vitalicious VitaBrownie, 1	2.5	100
Newman's Own 94% Fat Free Butter Popcorn, 1 bag	1.5	110	Vitalicious VitaMuffin, Bran, 4 oz.	0	200
Newton Caramel Apple Bars, 2 cookies	2.5	130	Vitalicious VitaMuffin, Deep Chocolate, 2 oz.	1.5	100
Nilla Wafers, Reduced-Fat, 8	2	120	Wheat Thins Minis, 1 pack	3	100
Planter's Peanut Butter Cookie Crisps	3	100	Yoplait Whips! Yogurt, 4 oz.	2.5	140

eating out with alli™

When you prepare meals at home, you are in control of the amount of fat and calories that go into a dish as well as your portion size. Eating at restaurants, however, is a completely different experience. There it is the chefs and their penchant for using oil, butter, and cheese who make the decisions. A little extra wrist action with the oil bottle can push your calorie and fat intake well over the edge—and you'll never even know it.

This doesn't mean you have to avoid all sit-down and fast-food restaurants. There are plenty of ways to dine confidently on the alli™ diet. All it takes is a little menu savvy. On the following pages are some tips on how to read between the lines of a menu to understand what's in the food you order and how it is prepared. We have also included a list of smart choices at 100 chain eateries.

Restaurant Eating Made Diet Friendly

These dining out rules will help you through a restaurant meal.

- **Don't go to the restaurant too hungry.** Remember, you need to limit your fat intake to no more than 15, 20, or 30 percent of calories from fat, depending on which phase of the plan you're in. You also need to keep track of your overall calorie intake. Eating a mid- or late-afternoon snack with less than 30 percent calories from fat will satisfy you so that you're not tempted to overeat.

- **Know before you go.** If possible, pick a familiar restaurant so you can decide what to order before you even get there. This helps you avoid being tempted by other items on the menu. If you are unfamiliar with the restaurant, make a decision quickly and then close the menu to avoid temptation.

- **Order first.** This will prevent you from being swayed by someone else's meal choice and changing your order to something not on your diet.

- **Order soup.** This is a smart tactic if you're dining with friends and know it's going to be a long evening. A study at Pennsylvania State University found that people who order hot soup at the start of a restaurant meal actually end up eating fewer calories and fat grams than those who don't—even fewer than those who pass on the first course completely—but forgo cream soups in favor of broths and consommés. While you're sipping soup, odds are you will be less tempted to dip into the bread basket and butter dish.

- **Dare to be different.** Who says you have to order an entrée? You can create your own meal by choosing side dishes and appetizers. This tactic puts you in control of your portions. Plus you get to sample a little bit of everything, making for a more interesting meal. Just make sure you stay within your calorie and fat targets for that meal.

- **Split an entrée.** When eating with a friend, share a main dish. Some restaurants will charge to share a meal, but the cost for two will still be less expensive than buying two whole entrées. And more important, you are saving half the calories and fat!

- **When in doubt, dress yourself.** If you choose a restaurant that does not offer low-fat salad dressing, take your own. A few tablespoons of dressing in a tiny container takes up very little room in your purse or pocket. And you needn't worry about being boorish; just pour it discreetly. Failing that, order salad dressing on the side or use lemon wedges or olive oil and vinegar.

- **Avoid all-you-can-eat buffets.** The variety of food on display at buffets just offers too much opportunity to sample and splurge. It's also human nature to want to get your money's worth, so you may overload your plate … many times.

- **Don't "clean your plate."** A study at the University of North Carolina found that portion sizes in restaurants have increased considerably over the last 20 years. Be aware of this and eat accordingly. Take home what you don't finish and eat it for lunch or dinner the next day. In fact you even might want to ask for the take-out container when you order and place half the food in the box before you start eating.

A World of Good Food

Dining on a variety of cuisines can help keep you from getting bored with your food choices. In fact some ethnic cuisines offer great choices for weight loss and health. For example, studies show that people who live in Asia and regions near and around the Mediterranean (and eat their native diets) are among the slimmest and healthiest people in the world. Vegetables, fruit, and fish are staples of their diets. When they eat meat, it complements, rather than stars in, a meal. Many ethnic restaurants bring these good qualities to their menus. But it can be tricky knowing what to order when you're experimenting with unfamiliar cuisines. Use these guidelines.

Chinese

Go for:
- Appetizers with lettuce wraps
- Steamed dumplings
- Steamed rice
- Szechwan dishes with sauces made from chicken stock
- Whole steamed fish for sharing

Pass on:
- Fried rice
- Fried wontons and spring rolls
- Sweet-and-sour dishes

French

Go for:

- Broth-based stews such as bouillabaisse, which is made with different types of fish
- Coq au vin, which is chicken simmered in wine
- *Salade niçoise,* which is made with tuna, green beans, and salad ingredients

Pass on:

- Au gratin dishes, which are made with cheese, butter, and sometimes cream
- Anything with hollandaise or béarnaise sauces
- Dessert pastries
- Quiches, which are usually made with cream and also have butter-rich crusts

Greek

Go for:

- Fish baked with garlic and tomato-based *plaki* sauce
- Shish kebab or any grilled lamb dish
- *Torato,* a cold soup made with eggplant, peppers, and yogurt
- *Tzatziki,* a yogurt, garlic, and cucumber dip or dressing

Pass on:

- *Avgolemono,* a soup made with egg yolks
- *Baklava,* a traditional ultrasweet dessert
- *Moussaka,* a casserole covered in a cheese-and-egg-enriched cream sauce

Italian

Go for:

- Florentine dishes, usually chicken or veal dressed with spinach
- Pastas with tomato-based sauces
- Primavera made with a medley of fresh vegetables

Pass on:

- Alfredo, a rich sauce based on butter and heavy cream
- Pasta carbonara, traditionally containing cream, eggs, Parmesan cheese, and bacon
- Pizza topped with sausage and pepperoni

Japanese

Go for:

- *Miso* soup
- Sukiyaki, a mixture of noodles, vegetables, and thinly sliced meat in a fish-based broth or a thin stock
- Sushi and sashimi

Pass on:

- Anything described as crispy
- California sushi rolls (made with mayonnaise)
- Meat fried and glazed with a sweet sauce
- Tempura, which are deep-fried vegetables and seafood

Mexican

Go for:

- Chicken enchiladas without cheese
- Salsas served with baked chips
- *Seviche*, which is seafood marinated in citrus juices
- Soft tacos
- Veracruz dishes, which are made from tomatoes, onions, and chiles

Pass on:

- Anything made with sour cream and cheese
- Fried chips and taco shells
- Guacamole

Middle Eastern

Go for:

- Anything made with couscous or *tabbouleh*
- *Lavash*, a thin flatbread
- Lentil dishes
- Moroccan stew, which is made with meat, vegetables, lemons, and garlic

Pass on:

- *Baba ghanoush* and hummus spreads
- Dips floating in oil
- Falafel, which are deep-fried chickpea croquettes
- Stuffed grape leaves, which usually come bathed in oil

Thai

Go for:

* Chicken saté (dip into the peanut sauce sparingly)
* Hot and spicy soups
* Noodle bowls
* Steamed or grilled fish

Pass on:

* Coconut curries
* Pad thai, a stir-fried noodle dish

Listen to Your Food Talk

Many of the cooking terms you'll see on menus can tell you whether or not a dish has been prepared in a diet-friendly way or is likely loaded with fat.

Go for dishes that are:

* **Baked**—cooked in a hot oven without added fat

* **Braised**—slow-cooked in a hot oven in liquid

* **Char-broiled, grilled, or barbecued**—cooked over hot coals so the fat drips off

* **En papillote**—cooked in parchment paper without added fat

* **Poached**—gently cooked in liquid heated to just below the boiling point

* **Stir-fried**—rapidly cooked in a pan or wok using very little oil

* **Steamed**—cooked over hot water with no added oil

Avoid dishes that are:

* **Battered or breaded**—coated and then usually fried

* **Deep-fried**—speaks for itself

* **En croûte (also called Wellington)**—cooked in a pastry shell; fat can't escape, and the pastry contains more fat

* **Roasted**—cooked in its own drippings

* **Sauteed**—fried in shallow oil

* **Au Gratin**—with cheese

* **Alfredo**—with cream

Eating Out Options

Americans spend an estimated $1.4 billion a day eating meals and snacks away from home. That's a lot of spaghetti!

Fast food, all-you-can-eat campaigns, and super-sized portions have become part of the American landscape. Fortunately many eating establishments, including fast-food restaurants, are making efforts to accommodate healthy eaters. It is unrealistic to expect you not to want to eat a taco, doughnut, or burger again. You can find a place for them on your diet if you make this style of dining the exception rather than the rule and seek out items that are lowest in fat and calories. *The alli™ Diet Plan* can help steer you in a diet-smart direction. Listed are 100 popular eateries that are part of national chains that provide nutritional information about their menus. Their inclusion in no way implies an endorsement. The list is only a random sampling of eateries. Likewise, the meals and foods listed do not necessarily include all the low-fat foods a particular restaurant offers. The list should help you choose a meal that does not exceed the highest calorie limit of the diet and does not go over 30 percent of calories from fat.

Let's say you visit Au Bon Pain for lunch and order the Tuna Niçoise. You'll see, according to the following list, that the salad contains 270 calories and 13 grams of fat. These 13 grams of fat mean you will get 43 percent of calories from fat if you ate only the salad as served—this is too much fat. But wait: If you are on a 1,500-calorie-per-day diet, then your lunch should total 450 calories and 15 grams of fat. To balance the meal you might choose the raspberry vinaigrette dressing to top the salad (80 calories and 0 grams of fat) and also order the garden vegetable soup (100 calories and 2 grams of fat). The entire meal now totals 450 calories and 15 grams of fat—meaning you get exactly 30 percent of calories from fat.

Make sure not to forget vegetables and fruit. If you have a slice of pizza, round it out with a salad topped with low- or no-fat dressing to help make it more nutritious. The goal of the alli™ diet is to eat smart, in moderation, and within a healthy range of fat and calories. You'll have the most freedom to use this list during Phase 3 of the diet.

SERVING	FAT (g)	CALS.

Applebee's
Entrées
Grilled Shrimp Skewer Salad	2	210
Mesquite Chicken Sandwich	4	250
Sizzling Chicken Skillet		
with salsa and tortillas	4	360
Cajun Lime Tilapia	6	310
Grilled Tilapia with		
Mango Salsa and Rice	6	320
Confetti Chicken	7	370
Teriyaki Steak and		
Shrimp Skewer	7	370
Onion Soup au Gratin	8	150
Southwest Cobb Salad	8	440
Blackened Chicken Salad	8.5	424
Tango Chicken Sandwich	9	370
Tortilla Chicken Melt	13	430

Dessert
Chocolate Raspberry Layer Cake	3	230

Arby's
Plain Baked Potato with Light		
Buttermilk Ranch Dressing	6	305
Martha's Vineyard Salad with		
Fat Free Italian Dressing,		
no almond	8	280
Junior Roast Beef	9	280
Arby Q Sandwich	11	375
Regular Roast Beef	13	320

Atlanta Bread Company
Tangy Roast Beef Sandwich	4	390
Veggie Sandwich on 9-Grain		
Bread	5	340
Honey Maple Ham		
on Honey Wheat Bread	5	410
Roasted Turkey Breast on		
9-Grain Bread	7	430
Grilled Cheese on French Bread	11	390

Salads (without dressing)
House Salad	0	50
Fruit Salad	0	130
Caesar Salad with Grilled		
Chicken	12	260
Chopstix Chicken Salad	13	280

Dressings (serving size: 2 tablespoons)
Fat-Free Raspberry Vinaigrette	0	85

Soups (serving size: 10 oz.)
Garden Vegetable	1.5	100
Classic Chicken Noodle	2.5	140
French Onion, no toppings	2.5	80
Chicken Gumbo	2.5	120
Pasta Fagioli	6	170

SERVING	FAT (g)	CALS.

Breakfast Items
Blueberry muffin, plain	1	270
Cinnamon raisin bagel, plain	1	270
with 2 oz. plain light cream		
cheese	11	390
Low-fat pumpkin muffin	4.5	320
Low-fat apple muffin	5	340

Au Bon Pain
Salads (without dressings)
Large Garden Salad	2	110
Artichoke Salad	5	70
Thai Chicken Salad	5	190
Riviera Chopped Salad	5	200
Asian Chicken Lettuce Cups	7	150
Steak Salad with Cranberries		
and Mandarin Oranges	7	290
Chicken Caesar Asiago Salad	12	320
Tuna Nicoise	13	270
Sonoma Salad	13	300

Salad Dressings (serving size: 2.5 oz.)
Fat-Free Raspberry Vinaigrette	0	80

Soups
Old-Fashioned Tomato Rice		
(12 oz.)	1	120
Jamaican Black Bean (12 oz.)	1	180
Garden Vegetable (12 oz.)	1.5	80
Vegetarian Minestrone (12 oz.)	1.5	120
Vegetarian Lentil (12 oz.)	1.5	140
Old-Fashioned Tomato Rice		
(16 oz.)	1.5	170
Southern Black-Eyed Pea		
(12 oz.)	1.5	180
Vegetarian Lentil (16 oz.)	1.5	190
Split Pea with Ham (12 oz.)	1.5	210
Black Bean-Low Fat (12 oz.)	1.5	240
Jamaican Black Bean (16 oz.)	1.5	240
Garden Vegetable (16 oz.)	2	100
Curried Rice and Lentil (12 oz.)	2	150
Vegetarian Minestrone (16 oz.)	2	160
Southern Black-Eyed Pea (16 oz.)	2	250
French Moroccan Tomato Lentil		
(12 oz.)	2	280
Split Pea with Ham (16 oz.)	2	280
Black Bean-Low Fat (16 oz)	2	320
Tomato Florentine (12 oz.)	2.5	120
Vegetable Barley (12 oz.)	2.5	140
Curried Rice and Lentil (16 oz.)	2.5	190
French Moroccan Tomato		
Lentil (16 oz.)	2.5	240
Mediterranean Pepper (12 oz.)	3	100
Southwest Vegetable (12 oz.)	3	100
Chicken Noodle (12 oz.)	3	140

Serving	Fat (g)	Cals.
Vegetarian Chili (12 oz.)	3	170
Vegetarian Chili (16 oz.)	3	230
Southwest Vegetable (16 oz.)	3.5	140
Tomato Florentine (16 oz.)	3.5	160
Vegetable Barley (16 oz.)	3.5	190
French Onion (12 oz.)	4	120
Mediterranean Pepper (16 oz.)	4	140
Chicken Noodle (16 oz.)	4	190
Red Lentil and Mango Stew (12 oz.)	4.5	230
French Onion (16 oz.)	5	160
Tuscan Vegetable (12 oz.)	5	170
Red Beans, Italian Sausage & Rice (12 oz.)	5	240
Chicken Chili with Beans (12 oz.)	5	260

Breakfast Items

Serving	Fat (g)	Cals.
Cholesterol and Fat free egg, 1	0	25
Small fruit cup	0.5	70
Large fruit cup	1	140
Bagel, plain	1	280
Fresh fruit and yogurt salad	1.5	170
Low-fat triple berry muffin	2	290
Oatmeal	3	150

Auntie Anne's Pretzels

Values are for 1 pretzel without butter.

Serving	Fat (g)	Cals.
Jalapeño Pretzel	1	270
Sour Cream & Onion	1	310
Garlic Pretzel	1	320
Original Pretzel	1	340
Stix, 6	1	340
Almond Pretzel	1.5	350
Whole Wheat Pretzel	1.5	350
Cinammon Sugar Pretzel	2	350

Dips

Serving	Fat (g)	Cals.
Sweet Dip (1.25 oz.)	0	40
Sweet Mustard (1.25 oz.)	0	40
Marinara Sauce (1.3 oz.)	0.5	30

Baja Fresh

Serving	Fat (g)	Cals.
Original Baja Taco (Shrimp)	5	200
Original Baja Taco (Chicken)	5	210
Baja Ensalada with Shrimp	6	230
Original Baja Taco (Carnitas, i.e., pork)	7	220
Baja Ensalada with Chicken, no dressing	7	310
Original Baja Taco (Steak)	8	230
Soft Veggie Taco	8	310
Egg & Cheese Taco (flour), refried	9	200
Grilled Mahi Mahi	9	230
Classic Soft Chicken Taco	10	230

Serving	Fat (g)	Cals.
Classic Soft Mahi Mahi Taco	10	240
Classic Soft Breaded Fish Taco	11	240
Classic Soft Carnitas (pork) Taco	12	250
Baja Fish Taco	13	250
Classic Soft Beef Taco	13	260

Dressing *(serving size: 2.5 oz.)*

Serving	Fat (g)	Cals.
Fat Free Salsa Verde	0	15

Baskin Robbins

(serving size: 4-ounce scoop of Truly Free No Sugar Added)

Serving	Fat (g)	Cals.
Nonfat Soft Serve Yogurt (all flavors)	0	90
Peppermint Nonfat Soft Serve Yogurt	0	110
Red Raspberry Nonfat Soft Serve Yogurt	0	110
Vanilla Nonfat Soft Serve Yogurt	0	110
Chocolate Nonfat Soft Serve Yogurt	0	120
Daiquiri Ice	0	130
Margarita Ice	0	130
Watermelon Ice	0	130
Pineapple Ice/Sorbet	0	140
Vanilla Nonfat Yogurt	0	150
Berries 'n Banana No Sugar Added Low Fat Ice Cream	2	110
Blueberry Swirl Ice Cream	2	130
Pineapple Coconut No Sugar Added Low Fat Ice Cream	2	150
Blue Raspberry Sherbet	2	160
Orange Sherbet	2	160
Rainbow Sherbet	2	160
Red Raspberry Sherbet	2	160
Tin Roof Sundae No Sugar Added Low Fat Ice Cream	3	150
Wild 'N Reckless Spirit Sherbet	3	160
Twisted Chip Sherbet	3	180
Rock 'n Pop Swirl Sherbet	3	190

Ben and Jerry's

(serving size: 1 half-cup)

Serving	Fat (g)	Cals.
Berried Treasure™ Sorbet	0	110
Strawberry Kiwi Swirl Sorbet	0	110
Jamaican Me Crazy Sorbet	0	130
Chocolate Fudge Brownie™ Low Fat Frozen Yogurt	2.5	190
Cherry Garcia® Low Fat Frozen Yogurt	3	170
Half Baked® Low Fat Frozen Yogurt	3	190

Big Apple Bagels

Regular Bagels

Serving	Fat (g)	Cals.
Vegetable	2	318
Honey Oat	2	320
Tomato Basil	2	322
Salt	2	324
Egg	2	328
Blueberry	2	330
Garlic	2	330
Wheat	2	330

Cream Cheese (serving size: 2 tablespoons)

Serving	Fat (g)	Cals.
Santa Fe Vegetable Lite	4	60
Plain Garden Vegetable Lite	5	60
Plain Lite	5	70
Strawberry Lite	6	80

Muffins (serving size: about ⅓ jumbo-size muffin or 2 mini-muffins)

Serving	Fat (g)	Cals.
Fat Free Blueberry	0	108
Fat Free Cherry Pie	0	109
Fat Free Chocolate Éclair	0	120
Fat Free Chocolate Marble	0	125
Fat Free Raspberry Amaretto	0	127

Gourmet Salads (w/no dressing, separate values for dressings not specified)

Serving	Fat (g)	Cals.
Garden Mix Cafe Salad (w/o egg)	2	63
Garden Mix Salad (w/o egg)	4	123
Garden Mix Cafe Salad	5	100

Soups (serving size: 8 oz.)

Serving	Fat (g)	Cals.
Hearty Vegetable Beef	1	100
Garden Vegetable	1	110
Country Bean	1.5	140
French Onion	2	60
Split Pea with Ham	2	90
Navy Bean with Ham	2	110
Beef Barley Mushroom	3	100
Vegetable Beef	3	110
Chicken Gumbo	3	130
Minestrone	3	150
Beef Pot Roast	4	110
Chicken Noodle	4	110
Sirloin Beef with pasta	7	190

Specialty Drinks (serving size: 16 oz. prepared with fat-free milk, on request)

Serving	Fat (g)	Cals.
Americano	0	12
Italiano	1	89
Vanilla Crème Latte	1	132
Cappuccino	1	133
Latte	1	145

Bob Evans

Serving	Fat (g)	Cals.
Grilled Chicken, 1 piece (Lunch Savors Menu)	6	93
Specialty Side Salad, no dressing	9	156
Meatless Green Pepper and Onion Pasta, seniors' portion	11	400
Grilled Chicken Dinner, plain	13	232
Grilled Chicken Dinner with Wildfire BBQ sauce	13	294

Dressings

Serving	Fat (g)	Cals.
Hot Bacon (1.5 oz)	3	106
Vinegar and Oil (3 oz.)	6	54

Soups (serving size: 8 oz.)

Serving	Fat (g)	Cals.
Bean Soup, 1 cup	3	144
Hearty Bean Soup, 1 bowl	5	205
Vegetable Beef Soup, 1 bowl	8	180

Breakfast Items

Serving	Fat (g)	Cals.
Strawberry Yogurt, 1 cup (breakfast a la carte menu)	1	145
French Toast, 1 slice	2	65
Smoked Ham, 1 slice (breakfast a la carte menu)	2	99
Oatmeal, plain, 1 cup (breakfast a la carte menu)	3	172
Mush, 1 slice	4	43
Hardcooked Eggs, Egg Beaters	4	60
One Egg Over Easy	8	101

Bojangles'

Serving	Fat (g)	Cals.
Green Beans	0	25
Potatoes without gravy	1	80
Marinated Cole Slaw	3	136
Cajun Fillet, without mayo	11	337
Biscuit (plain)	12	243

Bonanza

Nutrtitional information was not available as of this writing.

Boston Market

Values are for an individual serving.

Serving	Fat (g)	Cals.
Roasted Turkey	3	180
Caesar Salad Entrée, no dressing	8	140
Quarter White Rotisserie Chicken, no skin	8	250
Quarter White Rotisserie Chicken	12	330
Quarter Dark Rotisserie Chicken, no skin	13	260

Side Dishes

Serving	Fat (g)	Cals.
Fresh Steamed Vegetables	2	50
Garlic Dill New Potatoes	3	140
Cinnamon Apples	3	210

Serving	Fat (g)	Cals.
Green Beans	5	90
Fresh Vegetable Stuffing	8	190
Mashed Potatoes	9	210
Condiments		
Poultry Gravy, 2 oz.	1	25
Cranberry Walnut Relish	2	140
Corn Bread, 1	3.5	130
Salads		
Fresh Fruit Salad	0	60
Caesar Side Salad, no dressing	2	40
Chopped Salad, no dressing	9	220
Soups		
Chicken Tortilla Soup w/out toppings	5	90
Chicken Noodle Soup	7	180

Bruegger's Bagels

Bagel Sandwiches

Serving	Fat (g)	Cals.
Garden Veggie Sandwich	2.5	400
Supreme Club Sandwich	9	470
Santa Fe Turkey Sandwich	9	490
Smoked Salmon	10	490
Plain Bagels		
Everything	2	320
Garlic	2	320
Onion	2	320
Plain	2	320
Salt	2	320
Sundried Tomato	2	320
Blueberry	2	330
Cinnamon Raisin	2	330
Cranberry Orange	2	330
Jalapeño	2	330
Pumpkin	2	330
Sourdough	2	340
Cinnamon Sugar	2	350
Spreads (for 1 scoop)		
Garden Veggie Light cream cheese	6	90
Herb and Garlic Light cream cheese	6	90
Plain Light cream cheese	6	100
Soups (serving size: 1 cup)		
Mushroom Barley	2	110
Minestrone	2	120
Moroccan Stew	2.5	140
Chicken Spaetzle Soup	5	120
Italian Wedding	8	160

Burger King

Entrées

Serving	Fat (g)	Cals.
Grilled Chicken Filet Sandwich with honey mustard	6	340
Tendergrill Chicken Caesar Salad	7	220
BK Veggie Burger without mayo	7	310
Hamburger	13	330
Side Dishes		
Garden Salad, no dressing	0	25
Strawberry Applesauce	0	90
Salad Dressings and Sauces		
Honey Mustard	0	20
BBQ or Sweet and Sour Sauce	0	45
Ken's Fat Free Ranch	0	60
Breakfast Items		
Pancake Platter (3 pancakes) plain	4	240
Pancake Platter (3 pancakes) with 1 oz. syrup	4	330
Bagel with egg, cheese and ham	12	410

Captain D's

Serving	Fat (g)	Cals.
Baked Chicken Dinner (1 piece)	3.5	350
Shrimp Scampi Dinner (10 pieces)	5	370
Baked Fish Dinner (3 pieces)	5	390
Baked Salmon Dinner (1 piece)	8	470

Carl's Jr.

Serving	Fat (g)	Cals.
Side Salad (no dressing)	3	50
Charbroiled BBQ Chicken Sandwich	4	370
French Toast Dips (no syrup, 5 pieces)	5	370
Charbroiled Chicken Salad, no dressing	7	300
Dressings		
Fat Free French (no serving size specified)	0	60
Low Fat Balsamic (2 oz. packet)	2	35

Carvel

Serving	Fat (g)	Cals.
No Fat Chocolate Ice Cream, 4 oz	0	120
No Fat Vanilla Ice Cream, 4 oz	0	120
No Fat Parfait	0	190
Grand Central Cooler	0	250
Broadway Banana Smoothie	0	270
No Fat Soda Float	0	270
Rockefeller Raspberry Smoothie	0	270
Staten Island Berry Smoothie	0	270
No Fat Classic Strawberry Sundae	0	290
No Fat Ice Cream Soda	0	290
No Fat Old Fashioned Sundae	0	300
Sherbet, 7 oz	1.5	180

SERVING	FAT (g)	CALS.
98% Fat Free Flying Saucer	1.5	190
No Sugar Added Miniature Sundae	2.5	200
No Sugar Added Parfait	2.5	200

Chevy's Fresh Mex

Grande Salads

SERVING	FAT (g)	CALS.
Santa Fe Chopped Salad, no cheese, bacon, or avocado	6	258
Santa Fe Chopped Salad, no cheese or bacon	13	338

Chick-Fil-A

SERVING	FAT (g)	CALS.
Chargrilled Chicken Filet, no bun	1.5	100
Chick-Fil-A Chargrilled Chicken Sandwich	3.5	270
Spicy Chicken Cool Wrap	6	380
Chargrilled Chicken Cool Wrap	7	390
Chicken Caesar Cool Wrap	10	460
Chargrilled Chicken Club Sandwich	11	380
Chick-Fil-A Chicken Sandwich	13	380

Side Dishes

SERVING	FAT (g)	CALS.
Fruit Cup	0	70
Side Salad	3	60

Soups

SERVING	FAT (g)	CALS.
Hearty Breast of Chicken Soup	3.5	140

Condiments

SERVING	FAT (g)	CALS.
Barbecue Sauce, 1 packet	0	45
Honey Mustard Sauce	0	45
Light Italian Salad Dressing (2 tablespoons)	0.5	15

Breakfast Items

SERVING	FAT (g)	CALS.
Sunflower Multigrain Bagel, plain	3	220

Chili's Grill

The following values are for Guiltless Grill Selections.

SERVING	FAT (g)	CALS.
Chicken Sandwich	8	490
Chicken Pita	9	550
Chicken Platter	9	580
Salmon	14	480

Salads

SERVING	FAT (g)	CALS.
Dinner House Salad w/o dressing	7	140
Grilled Caribbean Salad	10	440

Salad Dressings (serving size: 2 oz.)

SERVING	FAT (g)	CALS.
Balsamic Vinaigrette (low-fat)	0	50
Honey Mustard Dressing (nonfat)	1	90
Ranch (low-fat)	6	110

Soups

SERVING	FAT (g)	CALS.
Chicken Noodle (1 cup)	1	50
Chicken Noodle (1 bowl)	2	90
Southwestern Vegetable (1 cup)	5	110
Chicken Tortilla (1 cup)	7	140
Broccoli Cheese (1 cup)	9	160
Southwestern Vegetable (1 bowl)	9	220
Chili w/ Cheese (1 cup)	9	250

Kids' Entrées (without sides)

SERVING	FAT (g)	CALS.
Grilled Chicken Platter (1 serving)	1	140
Grilled Chicken Sandwich (1 sandwich)	1	140
Pepper Pal Pasta w/marinara	5	290

Chuck E. Cheese's

(serving size: one slice of a small pie)

SERVING	FAT (g)	CALS.
Cheese	6	192
Vegetarian	6	194
Canadian Bacon and Pineapple	6	199
BBQ Chicken	6	214
Pepperoni	8	215
Super Combo	8	220

Church's Fried Chicken

Values are for one piece of chicken.

SERVING	FAT (g)	CALS.
Original Leg	6	110
Spicy Fish Fillet	9	160
Spicy Leg	11	180
Original Breast	11	200

Side Dishes

SERVING	FAT (g)	CALS.
Collard Greens	0	100
Mashed potatoes and gravy, regular size	2	70
Corn on the cob, 1 ear	3	140
Cajun rice, regular size	7	130
Macaroni and Cheese	11	150

Corner Bakery

Salads

SERVING	FAT (g)	CALS.
Fruit Medley	0	110
Mixed Berry Salad	1	70
Cucumber Tomato Salad	2	120
Tuscan Pesto Salad	9	230

Soups

SERVING	FAT (g)	CALS.
Mom's Chicken Noodle	4	170
Roasted Tomato Basil	5	160
Black Bean	5	260

Breakfast Items

SERVING	FAT (g)	CALS.
Fruit Medley	0	110
Oatmeal	2	230
Swiss Oatmeal	3	350
Mixed Berry Parfait	5	360

Cosi

Serving	Fat (g)	Cals.
Mixed Green Salad with fat-free dressing	1	90
Bombay Salad with fat-free dressing	3	220
Caesar Salad with fat-free dressing	8	225
Hummus and Fresh Veggie Sandwich	8	435
Shanghai Chicken	9	265
Turkey Light Sandwich	9	475
Sesame Ginger Chicken Sandwich	11	510

Cousin's Subs

Better Bunch Sandwiches

Serving	Fat (g)	Cals.
4" Garden Veggie	1	136
4" Mini Hot Veggie	1	144
4" Mini Chicken Breast	1	185
4" Mini Turkey Breast	2	177
4" Mini Ham	2	178
4" Mini Roast Beef	2	205
7½" Garden Veggie	2	266
7½" Hot Veggie	2	287
7½" Chicken Breast	2	366
4" Mini Club	3	193
7½" Roast Beef	3	335
7½" Ham	4	336
7½" Club	5	381
7½" Roast Beef	6	405

Regular Subs

Serving	Fat (g)	Cals.
4" Mini Garden Veggie	7	216
4" Mini Hot Veggie	10	254
7½" Garden Veggie Sub	12	390

Salads (without dressing)

Serving	Fat (g)	Cals.
Chicken Sedona Salad	5	232
Side Salad	6	135
Garden Salad	11	241
Seafood Salad	11	320
Garden Salad with Chicken Breast	12	335

Soups

Serving	Fat (g)	Cals.
Tomato Basil with Raviolini, regular	1	96
Eight Bean Soup with Ham, regular	1	105
Vegetable Beef, regular	2	70
Beef Steak and Noodle, regular	3	105
Vegetable Beef, large	3	110
New England Clam Chowder, regular	3	149
Chicken Noodle, regular	4	114

Serving	Fat (g)	Cals.
Chicken and Dumplings, regular	4	149
Cheddar Cauliflower, regular	5	114
Fiesta Tortilla Soup with Chicken, regular	5	114

Culver's

Serving	Fat (g)	Cals.
Blackened Chicken Sandwich	8	370

Side Dishes

Serving	Fat (g)	Cals.
Mashed Potatoes (168 g serving size)	2	132

Salads

Serving	Fat (g)	Cals.
Caesar Salad, no dressing	4	79
House Salad, no dressing	5	86
Garden Fresco Salad, no dressing	12	247

Dressings (serving size: 2 oz.)

Serving	Fat (g)	Cals.
Raspberry Vinaigrette	0	50
Sesame Ginger Dressing	0	70

Soups (serving size: 10.58 oz.)

Serving	Fat (g)	Cals.
Minestrone	1	100
Tomato Florentine	1	112
Fire Roasted Vegetable	2	72
Chicken Noodle	2	112
Seven Bean Medley	2	150
Tomato Basil Ravioletti	3	112
Stuffed Green Pepper with Beef	3	150
Vegetable Beef & Barley	4	112
Chicken Gumbo	6	120
Lumberjack Mixed Vegetable	6	150

D'Angelo's Sandwich Shops

D'Lite Sandwiches

Serving	Fat (g)	Cals.
Turkey	4	364
Roast Beef	5	353
Chicken Stir Fry D'Lite	6	426
Fresh Veggie	7	348
Classic Veggie	7	362
Chicken Caesar Salad Wrap	7	378
Grilled Chicken Breast	7	388

Small Subs

Serving	Fat (g)	Cals.
Salad	3	281
Turkey	4	317
Roast Beef	5	234
Grilled Chicken	7	369
Turkey Club	8	362
Ham and Cheese	10	377

Wraps

Serving	Fat (g)	Cals.
Salad	2	324
Roast Beef	3	360
Turkey	3	369

Pokket® Sandwiches

Serving	Fat (g)	Cals.
Classic Veggie No Cheese	1	238
Salad	2	222

Roast Beef	3	273
Turkey	3	282
Grilled Chicken	5	329
Turkey Club	8	356

Salads *(entrée size without dressing)*

Tossed	1	49
Turkey	2	157
Roast Beef	3	146
Chicken Stir Fry	3	168

Salad Dressings *(serving size: 1 oz.)*

Fat Free Caesar	0	20

Soups

Hearty Vegetable, 8 oz.	0	40
Hearty Vegetable, 12 oz.	1	60
Chicken Noodle, 8 oz.	2	130
Chicken Noodle, 12 oz.	4	195
Beef Stew, 8 oz.	8	220
Beef Stew, 12 oz.	12	330

Kidz Meals

Turkey D'Lite	3	217
Ham and Cheese Sub	4	214

Dairy Queen

(Serving size: ½ cup)

DQ® Vanilla Soft Serve	4.5	140
DQ® Chocolate Soft Serve	5	150

Del Taco

Chicken Taco Del Carbon	5	170
Soft Taco	8	160
Carne Asada Taco	8	237
Steak Taco Del Carbon	11	220
Big Fat Taco™	11	320
Chicken Soft Taco	12	210

Denny's

Grilled Chicken Dinner	5	200
Roast Turkey and Stuffing with Gravy	10	435
Fried Shrimp Dinner	11	258
Tilapia platter (with rice, green beans, tomato)	11	410
Boca Burger with Fruit Bowl	11	508
Grilled Chicken Sandwich w/o dressing	14	476

Salads

Side Green Salad w/o dressing	7	113
Turkey Breast Salad w/o dressing	8	248
Grilled Chicken Breast Salad	11	259
Chef's Salad	16	365

Salad Dressings *(serving size: 1 oz.)*

Fat Free Caesar	0	20

| Fat Free Ranch | 0.2 | 25 |
| Fat Free Italian Dressing | 0.5 | 15 |

Side Dishes

Sliced Tomatoes	0	13
Applesauce	0	60
Baked potato, plain, w/skin	0	220
Green beans	1	40
Corn	2	110
Cottage Cheese	3	72
Vegetable pilaf	3	173
Mashed potatoes, plain	7	168

Soups

Vegetable Beef Soup	1	79
Chicken Noodle Soup	6	110

Breakfast Items

EggBeaters Egg Substitute (4 oz.)	0	56
Grits (4 oz.)	0	80
Bagel (dry)	1	310
Oatmeal	2	100
English muffin (dry)	2	150
Pancakes (3) w/ 1.5 oz. of sugar-free maple syrup	5	443
Egg (1), grilled ham, and 1 slice toast, dry	6	285
Veggie Eggbeaters Omelette w/ English muffin	8	330
Slim Slam Breakfast w/o topping	11	490

Seniors' Items

Senior Grilled Chicken Breast	5	200
Senior Grilled Fried Shrimp	6	149
Senior Turkey and Stuffing	9	360
Senior Grilled Tilapia	10	248
Senior Chicken Strips	10	285

Domino's Pizza

Salads, no dressing

Garden Fresh Salad	4	70
Grilled Chicken Caesar	4	105

Salad Dressings

Light Italian Dressing	1	43

Don Pablo's

Appetizers

Chicken Flauta (1)	3	65
Beef Taquito (1)	4	63

Salads and Soups

Chicken Chili, 1 cup	11	234

Primo Enchiladas

Mama's Skinny Enchiladas (3)	14	368

Enchiladas *(serving size: 1)*

Chicken	13	210
Spinach and Poblano	13	258

Rellenos *(serving size: 1)*

	FAT (g)	CALS.
Chicken Relleno	11	235
Chicken	13	210

Sides

	FAT (g)	CALS.
Mexican Rice, 3 oz.	1	107
Charra Beans, 5 oz.	2	96
Black Beans, 4 oz.	2	119
Garden Vegetables, 6 oz.	5	98
Saffron Rice (3 oz.)	7	150

Donato's Pizza

	FAT (g)	CALS.
Ham 'N Cheese Sub with Lite Italian Dressing	14	534
14" Original Crust Chicken Veggy Medley, ¼ pie	19	500

Side Dishes

	FAT (g)	CALS.
Side Tuscan Salad	6	87
Side salad, no dressing	7	106
Side Italian Salad	8	108
Entrée Tuscan Chicken Caesar	8	198

Salad Dressings *(serving size: 1.5 oz.)*

	FAT (g)	CALS.
Fat Free Ranch	0	45
Lite Italian	5	20

Dunkin Donuts

Donuts

	FAT (g)	CALS.
Sugar Raised Donut	8	170
Apple N' Spice Donut	8	200
Black Raspberry Donut	8	210
Jelly Filled Donut	8	210
Strawberry Donut	8	210

Bagels *(plain, no topping)*

	FAT (g)	CALS.
Plain Bagel	2.5	320
Salt	2.5	320
Blueberry	2.5	330
Cinnamon Raisin	3	330
Onion	3.5	320
Wheat	4	330
Everything	6	370
Multigrain	6	380
Poppyseed	7	370
Sesame	8	380
Reduced Carb with Cheese	12	380

Muffins

	FAT (g)	CALS.
English Muffin	1.5	160
Reduced Fat Blueberry Muffin	5	400

Sandwiches

	FAT (g)	CALS.
Egg Cheese English Muffin	9	280
Ham Egg Cheese English Muffin	10	310
Southwestern Chicken Panini	10	420
Ham and Swiss Sandwich	11	360
Steak Panini	12	450

Soups

	FAT (g)	CALS.
Chicken Noodle	3.5	140
Timberline Chili with Beans	8	230

Hot Drinks *(serving size: 10 oz., except where indicated)*

	FAT (g)	CALS.
Espresso, 2 oz.	0	0
Espresso with Sugar, 2 oz.	0	30
Hot Latte Lite	0	70
Vanilla Latte Lite	0	80
Cappuccino with Soy Milk	2.5	70
Cappuccino with Soy Milk and Sugar	2.5	120

Eat'N'Park

Bakery *(1 item)*

	FAT (g)	CALS.
Corn Bread	4	108
Corn Muffin	7	212
Blueberry Muffin	7	242
Apple Raisin Muffin	7	249
Pumpkin Raisin Muffin	7	259
Mocha Java Muffin	8	222
Crumby Bun	9	193
Cranberry Muffin	9	266
Strawberry Crème Muffin	9	273
Strawberry Filled Muffin	9	280
Oat Bran Apple Raisin Muffin	10	296
Oat Bran Muffin	12	333

Breakfast Items

	FAT (g)	CALS.
Fruit Cup	0.5	60
English Muffin, plain	1	133
Bagel, plain	2	312
Raisin Bagel, plain	2	320
Oatmeal, plain	3	154
Poached egg, 1	5	77
French Toast, 1 slice	5	128
Oatmeal with Milk	5	224
Cereal with milk	5	363
Oatmeal with Bananas	6	317
Oatmeal with Fruit	10	424

Salads *(no dressing)*

	FAT (g)	CALS.
Garden	3	102
Fruit with Sherbet	3	308
Chicken and Strawberry	6	216
Chicken Portabella	12	331

Salad Dressings *(serving size: 2 tbsp.)*

	FAT (g)	CALS.
Italian Fat-Free	0	12
French Fat-Free	0	70

Sandwiches

	FAT (g)	CALS.
Hot Turkey	5	260
Turkey Pita	5	444
Classic Gardenburger	6	250
Hot Roast Beef	6	309

Chargrilled Chicken	6	318	**Salads** *(no dressing)*		
Chicken Fiesta	11	324	Monterrey Pollo Salad w/o		
Dinner Items			dressing,	6	176
Chesapeake Crab Stuffed Cod	9	286	Caesar Pollo	9	221
Rosemary Chicken	10	322	**Salad Dressings** *(serving size: 1.5 oz.)*		
Seniors Meals			Fat Free Italian	0	25
Floridian Scrod	1.5	119	Fat Free Honey Mustard	0	60
Chargrilled Chicken	4	139	**Side Dishes**		
Hot Turkey Sandwich	4	175	Corn Cobbette	0	42
Spaghetti Marinara	4	311	Mashed Potatoes & Gravy	1	122
Rosemary Chicken	5	161	Garden Salad	7	111
Hot Roast Beef Sandwich	6	183	**Dressings**		
Fried Jumbo Shrimp	6	187	Light Italian Dressing (1.5 oz.)	1	20
Spaghetti with Meat Sauce	9	410			

Einstein Bros Bagels

Bagels *(plain, without topping)*

Fazoli's

Sandwiches

Jalapeño	1	310	7" Grilled Chicken Submarino	8	390
Honey Whole Wheat	1	320	Grilled Chicken Panini	8	390
Plain	1	320	**Salads**		
Pumpernickel	1	320	Garden Side Salad	0	25
Sun-Dried Tomato	1	320	Grilled Chicken Salad	1.5	100
Chopped Onion	1	330	Caesar Side Salad	5	110
Everything	2	340	**Build Your Own Pasta**		
Poppy Dip	2	350	Whole Wheat Penne, small	1.5	420
Egg	3	340	Fettuccine, small	2	370
Asiago	3	360	Penne, small	2	370
Chocolate Chip	3	370	Spaghetti, small	2	370
Potato	4.5	350	**Sauce**		
Sesame Dipped	5	380	Marinara, small	1	80
Cinnamon Raisin Swirl	10	350	Spicy Marinara, small	1.5	60
Cranberry	10	350	Parmesan Alfredo Tomato,		
Toppings *(serving size: 2 tbsp.)*			small	3	80
Garden Veggie	5	60	Hearty Meat, small	3	110
Honey Almond	5	60	**Toppings**		
Jalapeño salsa	5	60	Garlic Shrimp	0	80
Maple Raisin and Walnut	5	60	Peppery Chicken	1.5	70
Reduced Fat Plain	5	60	Broccoli	2	45
Sundried Tomato	5	60	Broccoli & Tomatoes	2	50
Blueberry	5	70	Zesty Peppers & Onions	4.5	80
Strawberry	5	70			
Smoked Salmon	6	60			

Godfather's Pizza

Values are for one-quarter of a 10-in. pizza.

Onion and Chives	6	70	Original Cheese	4	150
Plain	7	70	Original Hawaiian	4	160
Sandwiches			Original Veggie	4.5	160
Veg Out on Sesame Bagel	13	500	Original Pepperoni	5	160
			Original Super Hawaiian	6	180
			Original Combo	8	210

El Pollo Loco

Healthy Dining Menu

Hardee's

Taco al Carbon (1)	3	134	Pancake Platter	5	300
Flame-Grilled Chicken Breast	4	153	Charbroiled BBQ Chicken		
Pollo Bowl	10	543	Sandwich	5	415
BRC Burrito	15	528	Regular Hamburger	12	310
Chicken Guacamole Burrito	17	535			

Hungry Howie's Pizza

Pizza *(serving size: 1 restaurant slice of a 14-in. large pizza)*

	FAT (g)	CALS.
Cheese	4.9	208
Green Peppers	4.9	210
Mushroom	4.9	210
Banana Peppers	5.0	216
Ham	5.3	215
Black Olives	5.3	218
Green Olives	5.3	218
Bacon	5.4	234
Pineapple	5.5	213
Onions	5.8	211
Sausage	6.6	234
Beef	6.6	237
Pepperoni	6.9	230
Anchovies	8	263

Sub Sandwiches, half

	FAT (g)	CALS.
Turkey Sub	12.9	466
Ham & Cheese Sub	15	475
Steak & Cheese Sub	15	491
Turkey Club Sub	15	556

Salads

	FAT (g)	CALS.
Garden, small	0.8	40
Garden, large	1.2	68
Chef, small	13.4	228
Antipasto, small	14	230

Dressings

	FAT (g)	CALS.
Fat Free Italian (1.5 oz)	0	25
French Style (1 oz),	0	30
Fat Free Ranch (1.5 oz)	0	45

In-N-Out Burger

	FAT (g)	CALS.
Hamburger with onion, mustard, and ketchup	10	310

Jack in the Box

	FAT (g)	CALS.
Southwest Chicken Pita, no salsa	3.5	230
Chicken Fajita Pita, no salsa	10	300

Salads

	FAT (g)	CALS.
Asian Chicken Salad	1	140
Side Salad	3	60

Dressings *(serving size: 2.5 oz.)*

	FAT (g)	CALS.
Low Fat Balsamic	2	20

Jamba Juice

Smoothies *(serving size: 16 oz.)*

	FAT (g)	CALS.
Strawberry Nirvana	0	160
Grape Escape	0	190
Strawberry Whirl	0	200
Berry Fulfilling	0.5	160
Mango Mantra	0.5	170
Raspberry Rainbow™	0.5	190

	FAT (g)	CALS.
Tropical Awakening™	0.5	190
Mega Mango	0.5	220
Tahiti Green Tea™	1	240
Caribbean Passion®	1.5	290

Yogurt Blends

	FAT (g)	CALS.
Sunrise Strawberry	0.5	300
Bright Eyed and Blueberry™	1	280

Matcha Green Tea Shots *(serving size: 4 oz.)*

	FAT (g)	CALS.
Matcha with Orange Juice	0	60
Matcha Dream™	0	70
Matcha w/Soy Milk	0	80

Other Beverages

	FAT (g)	CALS.
Wheatgrass (1 oz. shot)	0	5

Baked Goods

	FAT (g)	CALS.
Pizza Protein Stick (1)	6	230
Blueberry Cinnamon Swirl	6	320
Honey Berry Bran	12	320

Jimmy John's Gourmet Subs

	FAT (g)	CALS.
Turkey Tom	0	326
Slim Tom	0	406
Baked Turkey Breast Slim French Bread	1	399
Slim John	1.6	418
Rare Roast Beef Unwich Slim	3	91
Rare Roast Beef, Slim French Bread	3	431
Baked Turkey Breast, Slim 7-Grain Wheat Bread	5	419
Rare Roast Beef, 7-Grain Wheat Bread	7	451
Slim Bacon	8	488
Ham & Cheese, Slim French Bread	12	524
Slim Pepe	12	538

Juicestop

	FAT (g)	CALS.
Knockout	1	252
Touchdown	1	299

KFC

	FAT (g)	CALS.
Honey BBQ Sandwich	2.5	220
Tender Roast Chicken Sandwich, no sauce	5	260
Tender Roast Chicken Filet Meal	7	360
Roast BLT Caesar Salad	9	220

Sides

	FAT (g)	CALS.
BBQ Beans	1	230
Green Beans	1.5	50
Corn on the Cob	1.5	70
Mashed Potatoes with Gravy	4.5	120

Koo Roo Roo

SERVING	FAT (g)	CALS.
1 Original Breast	5.5	287
Spicy Ginger Garlic Bowl	6	485
Sliced Turkey Breast	8	182
BBQ Chicken Sandwich	12	562

Salads *(without dressings)*

House Salad	4	113
Chicken Caesar Salad	11	286

Dressings

BBQ Vinaigrette (2 oz.)	4	101
House (1.5 oz.)	6	90

Side Dishes

Butternut Squash	0.1	66
Tossed Salad, no dressing	0.2	16
Cucumber Salad	0.2	41
Steamed Vegetables	0.3	38
Cantaloupe & Honeydew	0.3	50
Italian Vegetable	2.2	47
Green Beans	3	62
Tangy Tomato Salad	3.9	60

Soups

Ten Vegetable Soup	2	94
Chicken Noodle Soup	3	71
Chicken Tortilla Soup	6	112

Krispy Kreme Doughnuts

Beverages *(12 oz.)*

Reduced Calorie Double Chocolate Blend	1	99
Reduced Calorie Latte Blend	1	99

Krystal

Krystal, regular burger	7	160

Little Caesar's

Values are for one-quarter of a 12-inch pizza.

Cheese, thin crust	12	360

Salads

Caesar Salad	3	90
Tossed	3	100

Dressing

Fat-Free Italian	0	25

The Lone Star

Entrées

Shrimp Dinner (3.45 oz.)	1.7	103
Texas Rice, 1 serving (served with Shrimp Dinner above)	2	80
Grilled Chicken (6 oz.)	2	186

Side Dishes

Steamed vegetables (1 serving)	1	71

Salads

El Paso Shrimp	3	207

SERVING	FAT (g)	CALS.
Dinner Caesar	4	158
El Paso Salmon	9	200
Chicken Caesar	10	457

Dressings

Lite Italian (1 serving)	5	50

Soups and Chili *(serving size: 6 oz.)*

Black Bean Soup	4	189

Long John Silver

Baked Cod	4.5	120
Shrimp & Seafood Salad (1)	12	260

Dressing

Lite Italian Dressing (1 pouch)	1	43

Luby's Inc.

Entrées

Roasted Turkey w/o skin or gravy	3	280
Blackened Tilapia	11	270
Carved Ham	11	300
Pan Grilled Fillet	12	330

Sides

Holiday Rice	3	165
Spinach	4	65
Cauliflower, Peas, and Carrots	4	67
Broccoli	4	80
Carrots	4	94
Cabbage	5	70
Blue Lake Green Beans	5	83
Green Beans	5	92

Salads and Fruits

Mixed Field Greens	0	34
Grapefruit	0	46
Pineapple	0	48
Mixed Melons	0	67
Spinach Salad	2	47

Dressing *(serving size: 1 tablespoon)*

Greek	3	31

Soups

Chicken Noodle Soup	9	235

Breads

White Roll	3	130
Whole Wheat Roll	5	170

Manchu Wok

Values are for a 5-ounce serving.

Garlic Green Beans	7	117
Butterfly Shrimp	7	235
Mixed Vegetables	9	130
Oriental Grilled Chicken	9	255
Black Mushroom Tofu	10	159

McDonald's

Bacon Ranch Salad with Chicken	9	260

SERVING	FAT (g)	CALS.
Hamburger	9	260
Premium Grilled Chicken		
Classic Sandwich	9	420
Salads		
Caesar Salad with Grilled		
Chicken	6	220
Asian Salad with Grilled		
Chicken	10	290
Dressings *(1.5 oz.)*		
Newman's Own Low Fat		
Italian	2.5	60
Newman's Own Low Fat		
Sesame Ginger	2.5	90
Newman's Own Low Fat		
Balsamic Vinaigrette	3	40
Desserts		
Apple Dippers with Low Fat		
Caramel Dip	0.5	100
Kiddie Cone (1 oz.)	1	45
Fruit 'n Yogurt Parfait w/o		
granola (5 oz.)	2	130
Fruit 'n Yogurt Parfait	2	160
Vanilla Reduced Fat Ice Cream		
Cone	3.5	150
Breakfast Items		
English muffin, plain	4.5	170
Scrambled eggs (2)	12	190
Egg McMuffin	12	300
Condiments		
Grape or strawberry jam,		
1 package	0	35

Miami Subs
Sandwiches

6" Original Cheesesteak	11	408
6" Classic Cheesesteak	11	420
Chicken Pita	13	392

Mimi's Cafe

Classic Beef Dip	15	521
Salads		
Soup and Dinner Salad	4	114
Salad Dressings		
Non Fat French	0	65
Soups		
Vegetarian Vegetable	0	60
Split Pea	3	195
Corn Chowder	9	196
Red Bean and Andouille	9	252

Noodles & Co.

Shrimp Curry Saute	6	190
Bangkok Curry	10	400

SERVING	FAT (g)	CALS.
Salads		
Cucumber Tomato Salad	0	100
Mediterranean Mixed Grill		
Salad	2	190
Salad Dressing		
Reduced-calorie, low-fat dressing may not		
be available.		
Soup		
Chicken Noodle Soup	9	290

The Old Spaghetti Factory
Lunch Menu Items

Spaghetti w/Tomato Sauce	3.5	300
Spaghetti w/Tomato and		
Meat Sauce	3.5	300
Spaghetti w/Meat Sauce	3.5	310
Spaghetti w/Mushroom &		
Meat	4	310
Spaghetti w/Mushroom Sauce	5	310
Spaghetti with Meat & Clam	11	380
Spaghetti w/Tomato and		
Clam Sauce	11	380
Spaghetti w/Mushroom &		
Clam	12	380
Dinner Menu Items		
Spaghetti w/Tomato Sauce	5	440
Spaghetti w/Tomato & Meat		
Sauces	5	460
Spaghetti w/Rich Meat Sauce	5	470
Spaghetti w/Mushroom &		
Meat Sauces	6	460
Spaghetti w/Mushroom		
Sauce	7	460
Spinach & Cheese Ravioli	15	480
Spaghetti w/Meat & Clam		
Sauce	17	580
Spaghetti w/Mushroom &		
Clam Sauces	18	570
Spaghetti Vesuvius	18	590
Salads		
Orzo Salad	3	80
Salad Dressings *(serving size: 1.5 oz.)*		
Fat Free Honey Mustard	0	60
Reduced Calorie French	6	100
Soups *(serving size: 9 oz.)*		
Chicken Orzo	2.5	90
Mediterrean White Bean	6	150

Olive Garden
Values are for the Garden Fare Menu.

Minestrone Soup, lunch portion	1	164
Linguine alla Marinara, lunch		
portion	6	340

Serving	Fat (g)	Cals.
Linguine alla Marinara, dinner portion	8	551
Capellini Pomodoro, lunch portion	9	450
Grilled Chicken, kids' entrée	11	349
Shrimp Primavera, lunch portion	11	483
Chicken Giardino, lunch portion	12	408
Chicken Giardino, dinner portion	15	560

On the Border
Entrées
Margarita Chicken	11	290
Crispy Chicken Taco	12	240
Lunch Fajitas, chicken	12	310

Side Dishes
Grilled Vegetables	1	50
Black Beans	7	180
Mexican Rice	7	180

Dressings
Fat-free Balsamic Vinaigrette	0	50

P. F. Chang's China Bistro
Appetizers
Seared Ahi Tuna Appetizer	6	260
Harvest Spring Rolls (4)	7	350
Vegetable Dumplings (steamed)	8	330
Shrimp Dumplings (steamed)	9	290

Soups
Wonton Soup (1 bowl)	10	350

Entrées
Buddha's Feast Steamed Vegetarian Plate	1.5	200
Chow Mein Vegetables	4.5	470
Shanghai Cucumbers	6	120
Spinach Stir-Fried with Garlic	6	140
Sicilian Asparagus	6	200
Buddha's Feast (stir-fried vegetables)	6	430
Garlic Snap Peas (stir-fried)	10	210
Cantonese Scallops	16	400

Panda Express
Mixed Vegetables	1.5	50
Steamed Rice	2.5	380
Tangy Shrimp with Pineapple	5	150
Chicken with Mushroom	6	130
Beef with Broccoli	7	150
Mongolian Chicken	7	170
Mixed Vegetables with Tofu	8	120
Chicken Breast with String Beans	8	160
Fire Cracker Beef	8	160
Mongolian Shrimp	9	150
Chicken Breast with Sacha Sauce	9	170
Kung Pao Cashew Chicken Breast	9	200
Eggplant and Tofu in Garlic Sauce	10	180
Chicken with Potato	10	200
Mandarin Chicken	10	255
Mongolian Beef	11	180
Black Pepper Chicken	12	200

Soups
Egg Flower Soup	2.2	88
Hot and Sour Soup	3.5	110

Panera Bread
Bagels and Muffins
Everything	1.5	300
Plain	1.5	300
Blueberry	2	330
Dutch Apple	2	330
Low fat triple berry muffin	3	300

Sandwiches and Salads
Fruit Cup, Small	0	70
Fruit Cup, Large	0	150
Strawberry Poppyseed and Chicken Salad	3.5	320
California Mission Chicken Salad	12	350
Smoked Turkey Breast	14	430

Salad Dressings (serving size: 2 oz.)
Fat Free Poppyseed Dressing	0	30
Fat Free Raspberry Vinaigrette	0.5	50

Soups (serving size: 8 oz.)
Garden Vegetable	0.5	90
Vegetarian Black Bean	1	160
Chicken Noodle Soup	2	100
French Onion Soup without Cheese and Croutons	3	80
Roasted Turkey Vegetable	3.5	110
Tuscan Vegetable and Ditalini	4	130

Papa Gino's
Pizzas (serving size: 1 restaurant slice of a large pizza)
Plain	1.5	300
Cheese, Thin Crust	5	238
Buffalo Chicken, Thin Crust	6	256
BBQ Chicken, Thin Crust	6	285
Super Veggie, Thin Crust	7	259
Chicken Pepper, Thin Crust	9	296
Garlic Chicken, Thin Crust	9	302

Sandwiches

Turkey sub, 1	1	408

Salad *(entrée size w/o dressing)*

Garden	6	176
Chicken Caesar	8	324
Chicken Tender	10	282

Salad *(side dish size w/o dressing)*

Garden	2	65
Caesar	3	72

Dressings

Fat Free Honey Dijon	0	59

Papa John's

Pizzas *(serving size: 1 restaurant slice of a 14-inch pizza)*

Garden Special, Original Crust	9	287
Cheese, Original Crust	10	290
Garden Special, Thin Crust	11	228
Chicken Club, Original Crust	11	320
Cheese, Thin Crust	12	238
Spinach Alfredo, Original Crust	12	303
Chicken Alfredo, Original Crust	12	310

Pei Wei Asian Diner

Appetizers *(values are for 1 serving; typical servings per dish: 2)*

Pei Wei Spring Rolls, values for 2	5	90
Crispy Potstickers, values for 4	7	130
Edamame	8	156

Soups

Won Ton Soup, 1 cup	1.5	110
Won Ton Soup, 1 bowl	4.5	260

Salads *(values are for 1 serving, no dressing; typical servings per dish: 2)*

Pei Wei Spicy Chicken Salad	2.5	210
Vietnamese Chicken Salad Rolls	4	80
Asian Chopped Chicken Salad	8	200

Sauces and Sides *(serving size: 2 oz. unless otherwise noted)*

Fortune Cookie	0	30
Sweet Chile Sauce	0	140
Lettuce Wrap Sauce	4.5	70

Rice and Noodles *(values are for 1 serving; typical servings per dish: 2)*

Udon Noodles	0	101
Rice Noodles	0	130
Egg Noodles	2.5	210

Entrées

Mongolian Scallops	6	190

Lemon Pepper Vegetables and Tofu	10	230

Kid's Wei® *(values are for 1 serving; typical servings per dish: 2)*

Kid's Wei Teriyaki Chicken	5	240
Kid's Wei Lo Mein Chicken	7	180

Perkin's

Fruit Cup	1	50
Lite 'N Healthy Dinner	2	105
Harvest Grain Short Stack (3)	2	270
Fish Dinner	7	470
Pita Stir Fry	9	410
Mini Chef Salad	11	215
Buttermilk Pancakes (3)	12	440

Condiments

Low Cal Syrup (3 tablespoons)	0	25
Lemon Pepper Vegetables and Tofu	10	230

Peter Piper Pizza

Pizzas *(values are for 1 slice of a 14-inch pie)*

California Veggie, thin crust	4.5	130
Chicago Classic, thin crust	6	150
California Veggie, Original Crust	6	200
The Werx, thin crust	7	160
California Veggie, Hand-tossed	7	270
California Veggie, Pan	7	300
5 Meat Supreme, thin crust	8	180
Smokehouse, thin crust	9	200
New York 3 Cheese with Pepperoni, thin crust	10	200
Chicago Classic, Hand-tossed	10	300
Chicago Classic, Original Crust	10	300
Chicago Classic, Pan	10	340
The Werx, Hand-tossed	11	310
The Werx, Original Crust	11	320
The Werx, Pan	11	350

Most Popular Pizzas

Ham and Pineapple, Hand-tossed	7	280
Ham and Pineapple, Original	7	280
Ham and Pineapple, Pan	7	310
Cheese, Hand-tossed	9	290
Cheese, Pan	9	290
Cheese, Original Crust	9	300

Piccadilly Restaurant

Entrées

Mesquite Smoked Chicken Breast (1)	8	212

Serving	Fat (g)	Cals.
Mesquite Chicken Breast w/ BBQ sauce (1)	9	240
Grouper Filet, baked (6 oz.)	9	305
Grouper Filet, baked (8 oz.)	9	330
Turkey breast, carved	10	267
Baked Tilapia	11	210
Pork Loin, bone-in roast	13	373

Salads
Serving	Fat (g)	Cals.
Spring Bowl	0	15
Spring, small	0	15
Piccadilly Bowl	0	27
Cucumber and Tomato	0	41
Tomato, Cucumber and Onion	0	44
Piccadilly Fruit	0	78
Louisianne Bowl	3	44
Mexican	3	58
Cucumber Mix	4	61
Vegetable Combination with Cherry Tomato	4	68
Cucumber and Celery	4	74
Combination	5	73
Asparagus and Tomato	5	88

Salad Dressings (serving size: 2 tbsp.)
Serving	Fat (g)	Cals.
Fat Free Ranch	0	36

Pizza Hut

Pizzas (serving size: ¼ of a 12-inch Fit n' Delicious™ pizza)
Serving	Fat (g)	Cals.
Diced Red Tomato, Mushroom & Jalapeño	8	300
Green Pepper, Red Onion & Diced Red Tomato	8	300
Ham, Pineapple & Diced Red Tomato	9	320
Ham, Red Onion & Mushroom	9	320
Diced Chicken, Mushrooms & Jalapeño	10	340
Diced Chicken, Red Onion & Green Pepper	10	340

Planet Smoothie
Serving	Fat (g)	Cals.
Leapin' Lizard	1	209
Thelma & Louise	1	226
Zeus Juice	1	248
Werewolf	1	261
Yo' Adriane	1	263
Spazz	1	266
Road Runner	1	279
2 Piece Bikini-Strawberry	1	286
Twig & Berries	1	297
Captain Kid	2	194

Pollo Campero

Chicken
Serving	Fat (g)	Cals.
Drumstick	9	164

Side Dishes
Serving	Fat (g)	Cals.
Dinner Roll (1)	1	80
Corn Tortillas (2)	2	120
Tostones (3)	2	170
Sweet Plantains (2)	3	116
Campero Rice (5 oz.)	3	188

Sauces
Serving	Fat (g)	Cals.
Sliced Jalapeño	0	5
Chipotle Salsa	0	10
Salsa Margarita	0	10

Pollo Tropical
Serving	Fat (g)	Cals.
Chicken Breast Wrap, plain	2	160
Chicken Tropi-Chop w/yellow rice and vegetables	5	341

Side Dishes
Serving	Fat (g)	Cals.
Balsamic tomato combo	0	88
Black beans, combo side	2.5	90

Soups
Serving	Fat (g)	Cals.
Tropical Shrimp Soup, 8 oz.	0.5	134
Tropical Shrimp Soup, 16 oz.	1.1	280

Popeye's Chicken & Biscuits

Entrées
Serving	Fat (g)	Cals.
Naked Chicken Strips	5	170
Chicken Etoufee	6	151
Smothered Chicken	8	210

Side Dishes
Serving	Fat (g)	Cals.
Mashed Potatoes, no gravy	4	120

Qbdoba Mexican Grill
Serving	Fat (g)	Cals.
Garlic Herb Grilled Veggie Naked Taco Salad	3	170
Naked Taco Salad	12	340

Quizno's Subs
Serving	Fat (g)	Cals.
Turkey Lite, small	6	334
Honey Bourbon Chicken, small	6	360
Sierra Smoked Turkey, small	6	360

Red Lobster

Values are for Lighthouse Selections menu. Items can change, according to location.

Entrées
Serving	Fat (g)	Cals.
Live Maine Lobster (1½ lbs.)	1	145
Grilled Jumbo Shrimp	3	142
Rock Lobster Tail	3	260
Jumbo Shrimp Cocktail Dinner	4	228
Snow Crab Legs	4.5	262

Serving	Fat (g)	Cals.
Broiled Flounder	5	240
Rainbow Trout (half portion)	6	186
Tilapia (half portion)	6	186
Grilled Chicken	8	314
Lobster Chops	8.5	320
Roasted Tilapia in a Bag (half portion)	9	297
King Crab Legs	9	490
Tilapia (full portion)	10	346
Salmon (half portion)	12	258

Side Dishes

Serving	Fat (g)	Cals.
Seasoned Fresh Broccoli	0	56
Baked potato (w/o topping)	2	179
Baked potato (w/ pico de gallo topping)	2	185
Wild Rice Pilaf	5	204

Salads

Serving	Fat (g)	Cals.
Garden Salad with Shrimp	3	82
Garden Salad with Red Wine Vinaigrette	5	102

Dipping sauces *(in place of butter)*

Serving	Fat (g)	Cals.
Large cocktail sauce	2	87

Romano's Macaroni Grill

Entrées

Serving	Fat (g)	Cals.
Pollo Magra "Skinny Chicken"	5	310
Kid's Menu Grilled Chicken and Broccoli	5	380
Kid's Menu Spaghetti and Meatballs w/Meat Sauce	10	550
Chicken Caesar Salad, without dressing	15	380

Side Dishes

Serving	Fat (g)	Cals.
Grilled Asparagus	1	30
House Salad without dressing	5	130

Salad Dressings *(serving size: 1.5 oz.)*

Serving	Fat (g)	Cals.
Fat Free Creamy Italian Dressing	0	30
Low Fat Caesar Dressing	2	30

Soups

Serving	Fat (g)	Cals.
Lentil Bean Soup, cup	5	180
Lentil Bean Soup, bowl	9	380

Round Table Pizza

Pizzas *(serving size: 1 restaurant slice of a 14-inch pizza)*

Serving	Fat (g)	Cals.
Guinevere's Garden Delight, Skinny Crust	7	170
Hawaiian, Skinny Crust	7	180
Guinevere's Garden Delight Thin Crust	7	210
Hawaiian, Thin Crust	7	210
Cheese, Skinny Crust	8	180
Veggie Gourmet, Skinny Crust	8	190
Cheese, Thin Crust	8	210
Chicken & Garlic Gourmet, Skinny Crust	9	200

Rubio's Fresh Mexican Grill

Entrées

Serving	Fat (g)	Cals.
HealthMex Chicken Salad	2	260
HealthMex Chicken Taco	3	170
HealthMex Mahi Mahi Taco	3	180
Chicken Street Taco	3.5	110
Carnitas Street Taco	5	110
Carne Asada Taco	6	130
Corn Tortilla Carnitas	9	230
Corn Tortilla Carne Asada	10	250
HealthMex Chicken Burrito	10	530

Dressings

Serving	Fat (g)	Cals.
Fat Free Serrano Grape Dressing	1	80

Side dishes

Serving	Fat (g)	Cals.
Rice	1.5	160
Black Beans	2	170
Pinto Beans	3	190

Ruby Tuesday

Steaks

Serving	Fat (g)	Cals.
Petite Sirloin	5	206
Top Sirloin	6	256

Side Dishes

Serving	Fat (g)	Cals.
Premium Baby Green Beans	5	85
Fresh Tomato and Mozzarella Salad	7	112
Fresh Steamed Broccoli	8	129

Salad Dressings and Sauces *(serving size: 1 oz.)*

Serving	Fat (g)	Cals.
Barbecue Sauce	0	50
Light Ranch Dressing	5	55

Soups

Serving	Fat (g)	Cals.
Garden Vegetable Soup	7	183
White Bean Chicken Chili	8	218

Sbarro

Salads, no dressing

Serving	Fat (g)	Cals.
Mixed Garden Salad	0	35
Fruit Salad	1	130
Stringbean and Tomato Salad	7	100

Schlotzsky's

Sandwiches

Serving	Fat (g)	Cals.
Zesty Albacore Tuna Wrap	7	315
Asian Almond Chicken Wrap	7	445

Soups

Serving	Fat (g)	Cals.
Minestrone Soup	1	90
Chicken Noodle Soup	2	120

SERVING	FAT (g)	CALS.
Chicken Tortilla Soup	3	165
Chicken Gumbo Soup	5	110

Salads

Garden Salad with Light Italian Dressing	9	140
Chicken Caesar Salad with Light Italian Dressing	11	195
Chinese Chicken Salad with Light Italian Dressing	11	220

Sizzler Steak House

Entrées

Hibachi Chicken w/Broccoli	6	290

Skippers

Original Shrimp (9 shrimp)	1.5	220
Grilled Halibut	4	40
Grilled Chicken Breast	4	190
Grilled Salmon	6	200

Salads

Small Green Salad w/o dressing	0	25
Large Green Salad w/o dressing	0	45
Small Caesar	13	150

Side Dishes

Grilled Vegetables	0	35
Baked Potato w/o condiments	0	210
French Fries	6	180
Clam Strips	6	270

Sonic

Grilled Chicken Sandwich	11	330
Grilled Chicken Wrap	11	380

Souplantation/Sweet Tomatoes

Salads *(serving size: 1 cup)*

Watercress & Orange, non-vegetarian	4	90
Honey Minted Fruit Toss	6	140
Crunchy Island Pineapple,	7	140

Salads *(serving size: ½ cup)*

Aunt Doris' Red Pepper Slaw	0	70
Marinated Summer Vegetables	0	80
Oriental Ginger Slaw with Krab	3	70
Carrot Raisin	3	90
Moroccan Marinated Vegetables	3	90
Southwestern Rice & Beans	3	90
Summer Barley with Black Beans	3	110
German Potato	3	120
Mandarin Noodles with Broccoli	3	120
Mandarin Shells with Almonds	3	120
Southern Dill Potato	3	120

Dressings *(serving size: 2 tbsp.)*

Italian Dressing (Fat-free)	0	20
Honey Mustard Dressing (Fat-free)	0	45
Ranch Dressing (Fat-free)	0	50

Pasta

Oriental Green Bean & Noodle	3	240
Vegetarian Marinara w/ Basil	4	260
Vegetable Ragu	5	250
Roasted Eggplant Marinara	10	340
Pasta Florentine	10	360
Linguini w/ Clam Sauce	10	380

Muffins *(serving size: 1)*

Apple Cinnamon Bran	5	80
Carrot Pineapple with Oat Bran	6	150
Georgia Peach Poppyseed	6	150
Pumpkin Raisin Muffin	6	150

Soups and Chilis *(serving size: 1 cup)*

Autumn Root Vegetable w/ Wild Rice	0	80
Ratatouille Provencale	0	110
Vegetable Medley	1	90
Garden Fresh Vegetable	1	110
Vegetarian Lentils & Brown Rice	1	130
Asian Ginger Broth	2	50
Old Fashion Vegetable	2	100
Classical Minestrone	2	120
Hungarian Vegetable	2	120
Sweet Tomato Onion	3	90
Chicken Tortilla w/ Jalapeno Chiles & Tomatoes	3	100
Tomato Parmesan & Vegetables	3	120
Spicy 4-Bean Minestrone	3	140
Vegetarian Chili	3	150
New Orleans Jambalaya	11	210
Savory Turkey Harvest	11	210

Starbucks

Beverages, Grande *(serving size: 16 oz.)*

Coffee of the Week	0	10
Decaf Coffee of the Week	0	10
Caffè Americano	0	15
Iced Caffè Americano	0	20
Tazo® Black Iced Tea	0	80
Tazo® Green Iced Tea	0	80
Tazo® Passion™ Iced Tea	0	80
Cafe au lait (fat-free milk)	0	90

Croissants, Bagels and Breads

Plain Bagel	0	260
Cinnamon Raisin Bagel	0	280

SERVING	FAT (g)	CALS.
Everything Bagel	1	260
Blueberry Bagel	1	280

Pastry

	FAT (g)	CALS.
Petite Cookie	2	40
Crisp Cinnamon Twist	2	60
Madeline	3.5	80
Low-Fat Blueberry Muffin	5	280
Reduced-Fat Cinnamon Swirl Coffee Cake	8	330
Cranberry Orange Muffin	9	340
Reduced-Fat Marble Coffee Cake	11	340
Reduced-Fat Blueberry Coffee Cake	11	350

Steak Escape

7-inch sandwiches (without cheese or condiments)

	FAT (g)	CALS.
Vegetarian	1	300
Grand Gobbler	2	380
Hambrosia	2	380
Turkey Club	2	390
Rajun Cajun	5	420
Grandest Chicken	5	425
Great Escape	6	430
Grand Escape	6	435
Wild West BBQ	6	470

Salads (w/o cheese or dressing)

	FAT (g)	CALS.
Grilled Salad with Ham	2	130
Grilled Salad with Turkey	2	130
Grilled Salad with Chicken	5	175
Grilled Salad with Steak	6	185

Smashed Potatoes (serving size: 14 oz.)

	FAT (g)	CALS.
Smashed Potatoes, plain	0	245
Smashed Potatoes with Ham	2	335
Smashed Potatoes with Turkey	2	340
Smashed Potatoes with Chicken	4	380
Smashed Potatoes with Steak	5	390

Sub Station II

Sandwiches

	FAT (g)	CALS.
Ham and Capicola Lite	4	275
Ham Lite Sandwich	4	277
Turkey Lite Sandwich	5	296
Roast Beef & Turkey Lite	6	297
Roast Beef & Ham Lite	6	303

Salads

	FAT (g)	CALS.
Ham & Cheese Salad	7	170
Turkey & Cheese Salad	8	190
Ham, Turkey, & Cheese Salad	8	192

Subway

6-inch sandwiches

	FAT (g)	CALS.
Veggie Delite	3	230
Turkey Breast	4.5	280
Turkey Breast and Honey Mustard and Cucumbers	4.5	310
Ham	5	290
Roast Beef	5	290
Turkey Breast and Ham	5	290
Oven Roasted Chicken Breast	5	330
Bourbon Chicken	5	350
Sweet Onion Chicken Teriyaki	5	370
Subway Club	6	320

Salads

	FAT (g)	CALS.
Veggie Delite	1	60
Turkey Breast	2.5	120
Ham	3	120
Turkey Breast and Ham	3	130
Grilled Chicken Breast and Baby Spinach	3	140
Grilled Chicken Breast Strips	3	140
Roast Beef	3.5	130
Subway Club	4	160

Dressings

	FAT (g)	CALS.
Fat Free Italian, 2 oz.	0	35

Soups (serving size: 11 oz.)

	FAT (g)	CALS.
Tomato Garden Vegetable with Beef	0.5	90
Minestrone	1	90
Vegetable Beef	1.5	100
Roasted Chicken Noodle	2	90
Spanish Style Chicken with Rice	2.5	110
Chicken and Dumpling	3.5	140
Cream of Broccoli	5	140
New England Style Clam Chowder	5	150

Breakfast Sandwiches

	FAT (g)	CALS.
Honey Mustard Ham and Egg on Deli Roll	5	270
Cheese and Egg on Deli Roll	9	270

Taco Bell

Items from the Fresco Style menu

	FAT (g)	CALS.
Ranchero Chicken Soft Taco	4	135
Grilled Steak Soft Taco	5	126
Chicken Enchirito	5	206
Gordita Baja-Chicken	6	153
Tostada	6	177
Gordita Baja-Steak	7	153
Spicy Chicken Soft Taco	7	180
Steak Enchirito	7	206
Fiesta Chicken Burrito	8	198

Taco John's

	FAT (g)	CALS.
Chicken Softshell Taco	6	190
Bean Burrito, no cheese	7	320

Serving	Fat (g)	Cals.
Steak Softshell Taco	8	190
Mexican Rice	8	240
Chili, no cheese	8	310
Taco Burger, no cheese	9	250
Refried Beans	9	340

Taco Maker

Serving	Fat (g)	Cals.
Soft Taco	6	180
Chicken Fajita	7	230
Bean Burrito	9	293
Chicken Burrito [1]	12	374
Chicken & Rice Burritos	12	377

Taco Time

Serving	Fat (g)	Cals.
Soft Bean Burrito	10	380
Chicken Fiesta Salad	16	390

TCBY

Serving	Fat (g)	Cals.
Raspberry Delite (smoothie w/o yogurt, 32 oz.)	0	300
Tropical Replenisher (smoothie w/o yogurt, 32 oz.)	0	350
Raspberry Revitalizer (20 oz.)	3	370

Uno Chicago Grill

Items exclude breadstick served with the following items, which has 220 calories and 14 grams of fat.

Serving	Fat (g)	Cals.
BBQ Grilled Shrimp	2	250
BBQ Pork Stick	8	280
Grilled Simple Chicken Breast	9	240
Chicken Lettuce Wraps	10	470
Veggie Burger	11	500

Sides

House Salad	1	100
Steamed Vegetables	2	60
Roasted Vegetables	5	100

Dressing

Fat-Free Vinaigrette	0	30

Soups

Veggie Soup	1.5	110
Windy City Chili	12	360

Wendy's

Entrées

Serving	Fat (g)	Cals.
Ham and Cheese Sandwich, Kids' Meal	6	240
Turkey and Cheese Sandwich, Kids' Meal	6	250
Jr. Hamburger	9	289

Salads, no dressing, no toppings:

Side salad	0	35
Mandarin Chicken	2	170
Caesar Chicken	5	190

Side dishes:

Fresh Fruit Cup	0	80
Mandarin Oranges	0	80
Plain Baked Potato	0	270
Sour Cream & Chives Baked Potato	4	320
Chili (8 oz.)	6	220
Chili (12 oz.)	9	340

Salad Dressings and Condiments

Barbecue Nugget Sauce, 1	0	45
Sweet and Sour Nugget Sauce, 1	0	50
Fat Free French Dressing, 1	0	80
Reduced Fat Sour Cream	3.5	45

Wienerschnitzel

Serving	Fat (g)	Cals.
Healthy Choice Kraut Dog	4	210
Healthy Choice Mustard Dog	4	210
Healthy Choice Deluxe Dog	4	220
Healthy Choice Relish Dog	4	220
Healthy Choice Chili Dog	5	240
Healthy Choice Chili Cheese Dog	10	290
Deluxe Dog	12	270
Healthy Choice BBQ Bacon Dog	12	320

getting fit

Once they begin to lose weight, people often find themselves becoming more interested in exercising. And it is no different on the alli™ diet. The changes your body experiences through weight loss make exercise not only easier but also more enjoyable. The program is dieter friendly because it consists of walking and toning exercises that start out easy and gradually increase in intensity. Exercise is an integral element of *The alli™ Diet Plan* because fitness and healthy eating go hand in hand.

Starting a diet and exercise program at the same time can be overwhelming, so it's important not to begin both ventures at the same time. In fact you should wait a minimum of two weeks, and preferably four weeks, after you begin dieting to start an exercise program. Also be sure to consult with your health care provider before you start any exercise regimen—especially if you've been doing little or no physical activity, you are over age 40, or you are being treated for a health condition of any kind.

If you already exercise, by all means continue. And if walking is your main source of exercise, keep in mind that you'll see greater results if you add the toning program to your routine. Once you experience the accelerated weight loss fueled by exercise, you'll want to make physical activity an important part of your new healthy lifestyle, just as the successful dieters with whom I work do.

The Benefits of Exercise

Regular exercise doesn't just burn calories and help you lose weight—it offers a host of other benefits, such as reducing your risk for high blood pressure, type 2 diabetes, heart disease, some cancers, arthritis, and osteoporosis. It can also reduce stress and anxiety and even boost your memory.

If you haven't been exercising at all, simply walking slowly will help give you these desired effects. The more you walk, the more your body will grow accustomed to activity. Soon you'll be able to pick up the pace to a moderate speed and then, in time, to a brisk one.

Walking is the only aerobic exercise that is required on the alli™ diet, but I encourage you do more. Once you can maintain a moderate walking pace, try other types of aerobic activities, such as bike riding, jogging, or taking an aerobics class. Swimming is an excellent form of aerobic exercise because it doesn't put stress on your joints and muscles in the same way that running or riding a bicycle does. Plus swimming is a full-body workout. The more variety you put into your exercise program, the more you'll enjoy it.

For calorie burning, walking 40 to 60 minutes, five to seven days a week is ideal. If that sounds like a lot, don't worry, because you'll build up to that level. Even if you've never exercised before, you can achieve this on the alli™ program. The goal is to make exercise a regular part of your life, as routine as brushing your teeth.

Walking, however, is only half of the program. Toning is the other half.

This means working out with weights, but it doesn't require "pumping iron" or going to a gym—that is, unless you want to. Toning is part of the program (and is important to any exercise program) because strengthening your muscles is important during weight loss, especially if you have a lot of weight to lose. Toning will make muscle tissue firmer and will give your new body a more sculpted look. Firm muscles also help the body burn calories more efficiently.

The eight toning exercises you'll find here are most effective for dieters. They are easy to learn, easy to follow, and can be performed anywhere, anytime. You can even do them in your living room while you're watching television, if you like. Now that isn't too much to ask, is it?

For optimal fitness, the American College of Sports Medicine recommends performing toning exercises two or three times a week. You'll get all the benefits you need in two sessions, but if you can manage to do three sessions a week, you'll see faster results. Be sure to schedule toning exercises on nonconsecutive days, because your muscles need to rest and recover between workouts. And if, by chance, you're having a hectic week and can't fit in two sessions, remember that one session is certainly better than doing nothing at all.

You can do both the aerobic and toning workouts at a gym, if you choose to join one. Health clubs offer stair-steppers, stationary bikes, rowing machines, and elliptical trainers that will add diversity to your routines, as well as a complete range of weights that will enable you to increase the intensity of the toning regimens when the time is right. The beauty of this program, however, is that it is designed so that you can do everything at home with no fuss. All you have to do to get started is lace up your sneakers and take the first step.

Walk Yourself Fit

To begin, get some comfortable clothes and a pair of lightweight, breathable walking shoes with good support. Shop for shoes at an athletic shoe store and have them carefully fitted. Go at the end of the day when your feet will be a bit swollen and wear athletic socks when you try them on. To avoid blisters, break in your new shoes by wearing them around the house for a few days before hitting the road or treadmill.

When you're good to go, all you have to do is put one foot in front of the other. Stand tall, look straight ahead, and keep your hips aimed forward—avoid swaying from side to side. Land on your heel and push off from the ball of your foot through your toes. Keep your elbows bent at a 90-degree angle and drive your arms forward and back.

Warming up before your workout and cooling down afterward are essential. You can do both by easing into and out of your exercise time by walking at a slower, comfortable pace. The longer and harder you plan to work out, the longer you need to warm up.

If you're not very fit, your muscles won't be accustomed to working hard, and it will take more time for them to get into exercise mode. If you're a beginner or very overweight, any exercise will be high intensity. You need to gradually ease into exercise. Maintain a gentle pace for the first few days and then, over the next few weeks, slowly increase the length and speed of your walks. For fat burning, your pace should leave you a bit winded, but as a rule of thumb, you should still be able to carry on a conversation.

The calendar, beginning on page 113, illustrates one way in which you might organize your walking program. Follow it to the letter or simply use it as a template. If you already walk for exercise, start at a pace that matches your current level of fitness. If you're a beginner, this program is designed to turn you into a fitness walker in eight weeks.

Practical Tips for Walkers

Walking is generally a very safe form of exercise, but you do need to take some sensible precautions.

- When heat and humidity are soaring, walk in the early morning or in the evening. Wear light clothing, sunglasses, and a wide-brimmed hat and carry a water bottle. Wear sunscreen when necessary. Avoid pavements that reflect heat. If possible, walk in parks or on shady streets. Reduce your pace, if necessary, and be sure not to skip your warm-up and cooldown.

- Cold weather can be challenging. Three layers of clothing works best to keep you warm. Your underwear should fit snugly and be lightweight. Go for softness and warmth in the middle layer—a cotton, fleece, or wool sweater is recommended. Your outer layer needs to be windproof and rainproof. Don't forget gloves, absorbent socks, and a hat; most body heat is lost through the extremities, especially the head. In extreme cold, wear a scarf over your nose and mouth. Lip balm or petroleum jelly will protect your lips from chapping. There's a natural tendency to tense muscles in the cold, so double the time you spend warming up. A thorough warm-up will reduce the risk of injury.

- Drink water before, during, and after your walk, regardless of the temperature. You can become dehydrated as easily in cold weather as in hot. Don't waste your money on sports or energy drinks; many are loaded with sugar—often in the form of unhealthy corn syrup, which just adds calories you don't need (unless you are running a marathon). Plain water is your best option.

- A pedometer (step counter) is a great motivator. You can buy one for about $15. Wear it all day long—not just in your walks—to see how far you walk in a day. A mile is about 2,000 steps.

- Protect your legs from shin splints—leg soreness around the shins that can occur when you've been walking on hard surfaces or on hills—by never neglecting your warm-up and by stretching your calf muscles at the end of your workout. One effective stretch: Stand about 18 inches from a wall. Place both hands on the wall at shoulder height and lean forward. Step one foot back and bend the front knee. Press the heel of the back foot toward the floor. Hold for 15 to 20 seconds. Switch legs and repeat. If you do experience shin splints, take an over-the-counter painkiller and apply an ice pack to your shins for up to 30 minutes at a time.

Your 8-Week Walking Plan

Week One

Tip! No matter where you live, you can find somewhere to walk. If weather, traffic, or safety concerns keep you from getting outside, consider walking at the mall. Many malls around the country open early to let individual walkers and walking clubs take advantage of the safe and sheltered environment. (Just hotfoot it past the food court!) Also consider the indoor tracks at a local high school or college or the corridors of your office or apartment building.

Monday & Tuesday – Walk at a comfortable pace for 20 minutes. Simply clock 10 minutes out, then turn around.

Wednesday – Day off.

Thursday & Friday – Walk at a comfortable pace for 30 minutes.

Saturday – Walk at a comfortable pace for 10 minutes. Step it up to a moderate pace for 10 minutes. You should become slightly winded, break into a light sweat, and feel your heartbeat accelerate. Return to a comfortable pace for 10 minutes.

Sunday – Day off.

Week Two

Tip! Well-fitting shoes, good-quality athletic socks that are more padded than other types of socks, and moleskin padding placed where your shoes rub your feet should help prevent blisters. If you do develop blisters, don't pop them. Cover them with a bandage. If you puncture the skin, you'll break the protective barrier that has formed and risk possible infection.

Monday – Walk at a comfortable pace for 10 minutes. Step it up to a moderate pace for 10 minutes. Slow back down to a comfortable pace for 10 minutes.

Tuesday – Warm up at a comfortable pace for 5 minutes. Speed it up for 20 minutes. Slow back down for 5 minutes.

Wednesday – Walk at a comfortable pace for 30 minutes. Just clock 15 minutes out, then turn around.

Thursday – Warm up at a comfortable pace for 5 minutes. Step it up to a moderate pace for 20 minutes. Cool down for 5 minutes.

Friday – Warm up at a comfortable pace for 5 minutes. Step it up to a moderate pace for 25 minutes. Slow back down for 5 minutes.

Saturday – Warm up at a comfortable pace for 5 minutes. Step it up for 30 minutes. Slow back down for 5 minutes.

Sunday – Day off.

Week Three

Tip! Don't be deceived by the simplicity of walking. It not only burns calories and improves the efficiency of your heart and lungs but also helps decrease blood pressure and cholesterol levels. It also tones the muscles in your buttocks and thighs.

Monday, Thursday & Saturday – Warm up at a comfortable pace for 5 minutes. Step it up to a moderate pace for 30 minutes. Slow back down for 5 minutes.

Tuesday & Friday – Walk at a comfortable pace for 30 minutes. Simply clock 15 minutes out, then turn around.

Wednesday & Sunday – Days off.

Week Four

Tip! Listening to music can inspire you to keep going, so give it a try. Program a mix of music that includes selections for your warm-up, workout, and cooldown. Revise your playlist frequently to keep it fresh. In a six-month study at New Jersey's Fairleigh Dickinson University, overweight to moderately obese women who were on a reduced-calorie diet and walked three times a week were divided into two groups—those who listened to music while they exercised and those who worked out without any music. The findings: The group who listened to music followed the walking program more closely and lost twice as much weight.

Monday, Thursday & Saturday – Warm up at a comfortable pace for 5 minutes. Step it up to a moderate pace for 30 minutes. Slow back down for 5 minutes.

Tuesday & Friday – Walk at a comfortable pace for 35 minutes. Just clock 17½ minutes out, then turn around.

Wednesday & Sunday – Days off.

At this point, you should be seeing and feeling the results of being more fit, finding that both your day-to-day and exercise-related activities are easier to perform. So enjoy your new strength and energy and try not to be a couch potato between your workouts. Play ball with the kids or the dog. Swim a few laps in a pool. Or take a gentle hike before lunch.

Week Five

Tip! Thanks to the longer walks you're taking each week, you're burning more calories and increasing your endurance. Walk for even longer than the program requires, if you feel up to it. An extra 10 minutes a day on your workouts can burn an additional 275 calories a week.

Monday, Thursday & Saturday – Warm up at a comfortable pace for 5 minutes. Step it up to a brisk pace for 30 minutes. Aim for really getting into a good clip here, breaking into a sweat and significantly raising your heart rate. Cool down for 5 minutes.

Tuesday & Friday – Walk at a comfortable pace for 35 minutes. Simply clock 17½ minutes out, then turn around.

Wednesday & Sunday – Days off.

Week Six

Tip! Routine is good—it keeps you on track—but it can lead to boredom. You might want to experiment with different kinds of aerobic activities now to find out what excites you. You might break up the week with swimming, bike riding, or taking a step class at the gym. This is all about you, so find activities that you enjoy and that you'll want to stick with over the long run.

Monday, Thursday & Saturday – Warm up at a comfortable pace for 5 minutes. Step it up for 30 minutes. Cool down for 5 minutes.

Tuesday & Friday – Walk at a comfortable pace for 35 minutes. Just clock 17½ minutes out, then turn around.

Wednesday & Sunday – Days off.

Week Seven

Tip! You are doing quite a lot of exercising now. Make sure to eat properly— three meals and two snacks each day. I designed the alli™ meal plans to give you the right balance of nutrients. Generally, it's a good idea to eat an hour or two before your walk. If you are hungry and tired, you are more likely to cut your walk short or, worse, not walk at all.

Monday, Thursday & Saturday – Warm up at a comfortable pace for 5 minutes. Step it up for 35 minutes. Slow back down for 5 minutes.

Tuesday & Friday – Walk at a comfortable pace for 35 minutes. Simply clock 17½ minutes out, then turn around.

Wednesday & Sunday – Days off.

Week Eight

Tip! You've made it! At the end of the week, give yourself a fitness-related treat: perhaps a pedicure for your hardworking feet, a massage for your tired muscles, or a new workout outfit. You deserve it.

Monday, Thursday & Saturday – Warm up at a comfortable pace for 5 minutes. Step it up for 40 minutes. Cool down for 5 minutes.

Tuesday & Friday – Walk at a comfortable pace for 40 minutes. Just clock 20 minutes out, then turn around.

Wednesday & Sunday – Days off. No formal exercise scheduled for these days, but consider planning something fun and active.

After eight weeks, you should feel the benefits and see the results of committing to an exercise program. From this point forward, if you choose to maintain walking as your primary source of exercise, you can continue to increase your fitness level in two ways. You can lengthen the duration of your walks incrementally as you did in the previous eight weeks, or you can add interval training to the mix. Intervals are short bursts of fast walking (about 2 minutes) worked intermittently into your regular walking routine. For example, walk as fast as you can for one block out of every three or four you cover with the goal being that, slowly and over time, you increase your interval training so you walk an equal number of blocks at the fast pace as you walk at the regular pace. Intervals help burn more calories and can be particularly effective for overcoming a plateau in weight loss. Whatever you decide, just keep moving.

Toning: Sculpting Your New Body

Don't be intimidated about working out with weights. Very likely you can already lift more than you think. If you've picked up a baby, grabbed a gallon jug of milk from the supermarket shelf, carried in groceries, taken out the trash, or hefted a handbag onto your shoulder, you've already lifted considerable weight.

The eight toning exercises in this regimen will efficiently work all the main muscles of your body in 30 minutes. Think of the routine as the ideal multi-tasker. You'll be combining a series of exercises that work different muscle groups simultaneously. Doing them three times a week on nonconsecutive days is ideal.

Always start toning workouts with a 5- to 10-minute warm-up. Perform a light aerobic activity, such as walking, using a cardio machine, or just rocking to the beat of your favorite music with freestyle dancing. These few minutes of movement will warm up your muscles and decrease your risk of injury.

Do the toning exercises on a firm floor. Concrete, wood, or tile is better than plush carpet, which can be slippery. Make sure the chair or any other furniture you use for balance is sturdy enough to support your weight.

If you've never worked out with weights, practice the routine a few times without them so you can concentrate on maintaining correct form. When you feel comfortable with the routine, it's time to add weights. You can use cans from your pantry—a 15-ounce can of beans in each hand will suffice at the outset—but you should graduate to traditional hand weights as soon as you can. Many national chain discount stores sell fairly inexpensive weights. I recommend handheld weights, as opposed to weights that fasten around your wrists, which can stress your joints.

The right weight for you will be the amount that offers appropriate resistance. Your goal is to be able to do all of the required repetitions and be fatigued by the time you get to the last few. For women, this might mean 2 to 8 pounds in each hand. Men might need 10 pounds or more per hand. What's important is starting with the right amount of weight for you.

Don't change the sequence of the exercises. These toning exercises are designed to work all the major muscle groups, from largest to smallest. Each movement is called a repetition (rep), and the number of reps in an exercise is called a set. To begin, you will be doing one set of 10 reps of each exercise. As you progress, you'll increase to two sets of 10 reps.

Rest for 30 to 60 seconds between exercises and between sets. Use the time to stretch gently and mentally prepare for the next set. Stay focused. If you get distracted, you'll lose momentum.

Every rep should be smooth and controlled. Slowly raise and lower the weight. Slower movements use more muscle fibers and build body awareness. Inhale as you lift and exhale as you lower.

After each workout, stretch your whole body. Stretching increases blood flow to the muscles. The right way to stretch is to reach gently, as far as you can, to a point of mild tension. Then hold that place for 20 to 30 seconds. Breathe.

As you exhale, relax a little more into the stretch. Never bounce when you stretch—it's a surefire way to pull a muscle or tendon.

You might feel some muscle soreness after your weight workouts. This soreness sometimes kicks in most noticeably on the second day after you've exercised. It can last for a couple of days but will diminish gradually. This is normal and to be expected. Stretching after your workouts can reduce soreness. If you do wake up a bit stiff and sore, don't stop moving: Walking will help loosen your muscles. Aspirin or other over-the-counter analgesics can also provide some relief.

1. Squat and Press (buttocks, thighs, upper back, and shoulders)
Tip! Press your body weight into your heels as you squat. Keep your abdominal muscles tightly pulled in to stabilize your lower back. Lower your body as though you are about to sit in a chair. Don't scrunch your shoulders when you lift the weights above your head. Keep them down and relaxed.

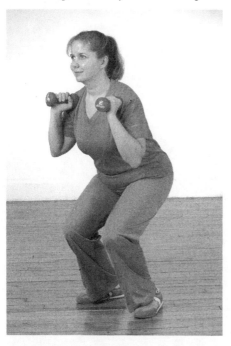

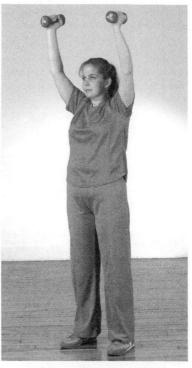

Stand with your feet hip width apart and rest a weight on each shoulder, elbows bent, palms facing in. Contract your abdominal muscles and draw your shoulder blades down and together. Lower your hips until your knees are bent at about a 90-degree angle.

Return to a standing position. Extend your arms to press the weights directly overhead. Bend your arms, returning the weights to the starting position.

2. One-Arm Row (back, shoulders, and front upper arms)

Tip! Make sure you keep your back level to the floor and don't twist your shoulder as you raise your arm.

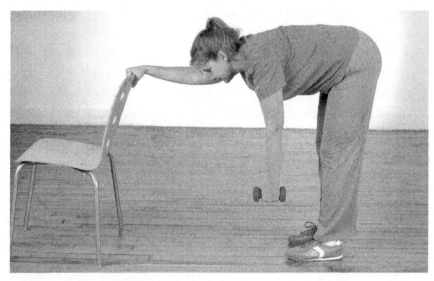

Stand with your feet hip width apart, knees slightly bent, 2 to 3 feet from the back of a chair. Hold a weight in your left hand. With your right hand, hold the back of the chair for support. Pull in your abdominal muscles and bend forward until your back is parallel to the floor. Let your left arm hang down in line with your shoulder, palm facing in.

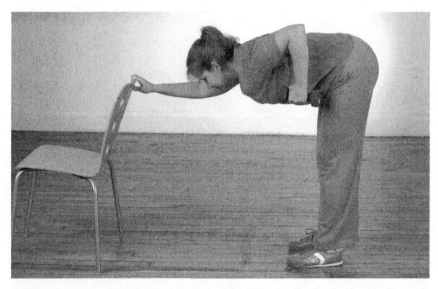

Bring your elbow up toward your rib cage. Straighten your arm. Perform 10 reps. Switch sides and repeat with your right arm.

3. Lunge (buttocks, thighs, and calves)

Tip! Both feet should point straight ahead; neither should turn in or out. Also be sure that the forward foot is flat on the floor—don't come down on your toes.

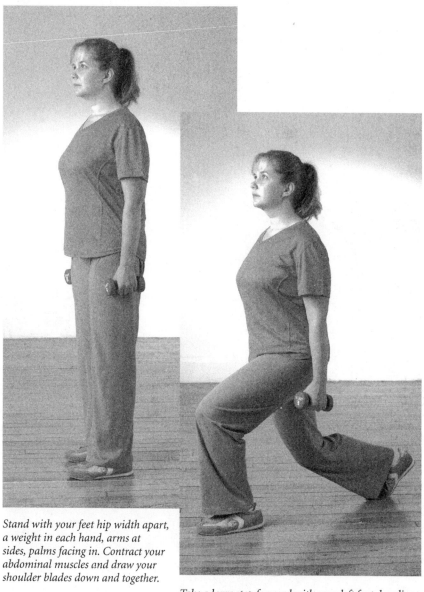

Stand with your feet hip width apart, a weight in each hand, arms at sides, palms facing in. Contract your abdominal muscles and draw your shoulder blades down and together.

Take a large step forward with your left foot, bending both knees. Keep your left knee directly over your left ankle. Point your right knee toward the floor, heel lifted. Push off with your left foot and return to the starting position. Perform 10 reps. Switch sides and repeat with your right foot.

4. Seated Incline Chest Press (chest, shoulders, and triceps)

Tip! Don't let your back sag or hunch. Keeping your abdominal muscles tight will help you maintain a straight back.

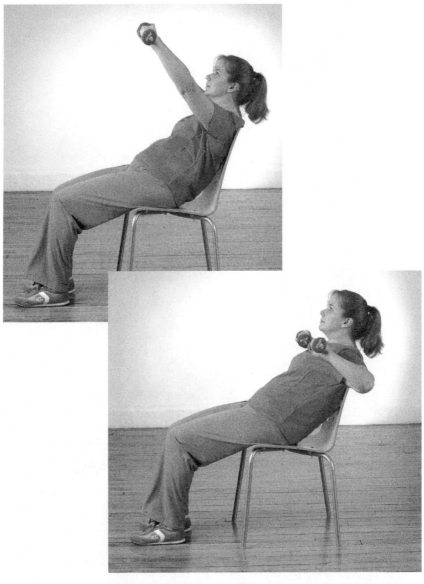

Sit on the edge of a chair with your feet flat on the floor and your knees bent directly over your ankles. Holding a weight in each hand, lean back until your upper back and shoulders rest against the back of the chair. Extend your arms in front of you to about chin height, palms facing down, wrists straight (top). Contract your abdominal muscles and pull the weights back to your sides until your elbows are bent at 90 degrees, wrists aligned with elbows (bottom). Contract your chest muscles to press the weights back up to the starting position.

5. Dead Lift (buttocks, thighs, and back)

Tip! Don't round your back as you bend forward. If this exercise is very difficult for you, increase the bend in your knees.

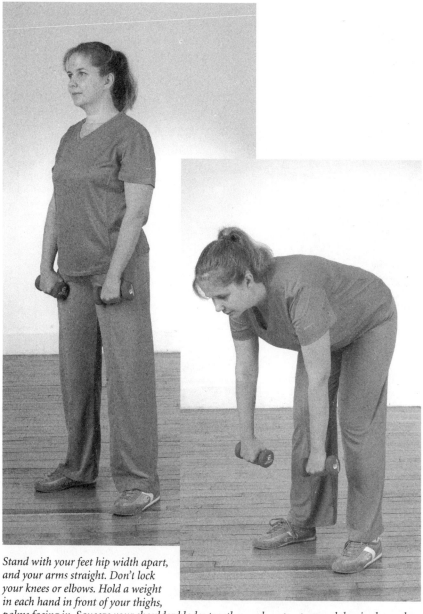

Stand with your feet hip width apart, and your arms straight. Don't lock your knees or elbows. Hold a weight in each hand in front of your thighs, palms facing in. Squeeze your shoulder blades together and contract your abdominal muscles. Keeping your knees slightly bent, bend forward from your hips, keeping the weights close to your legs. Stop when you feel a stretch in the back of your thighs. Squeeze your buttocks and, keeping your back straight, return to starting position.

6. Bent-Over Fly (upper back and shoulders)

Tip! To prevent straining your joints or chest muscles, be careful not to lift your arms higher than your shoulders or to lock your elbows.

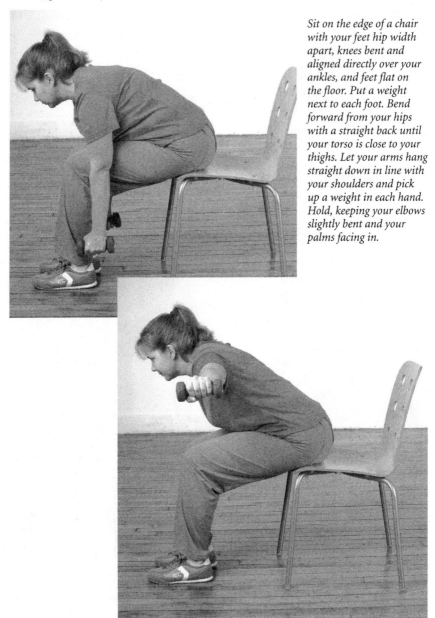

Sit on the edge of a chair with your feet hip width apart, knees bent and aligned directly over your ankles, and feet flat on the floor. Put a weight next to each foot. Bend forward from your hips with a straight back until your torso is close to your thighs. Let your arms hang straight down in line with your shoulders and pick up a weight in each hand. Hold, keeping your elbows slightly bent and your palms facing in.

Contracting your upper back muscles, lift your arms up and out to the sides until your elbows are parallel with your shoulders. Pause, then slowly lower the weights to the starting position.

7. One-Legged Bridge (buttocks, thighs, and abdominals)

Tip! When you are in the raised position, your body should be as straight as a plank from your shoulders to your raised ankle. Be careful not to twist your hips or arch your back.

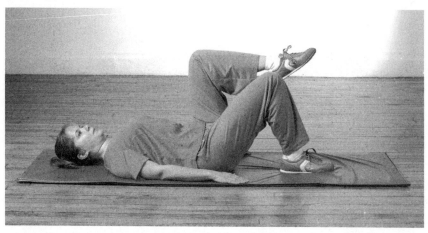

Lie on your back with your arms at your sides and your right knee bent, foot flat on the floor. Lift your left leg and bend your left knee, keeping your calf parallel to the floor.

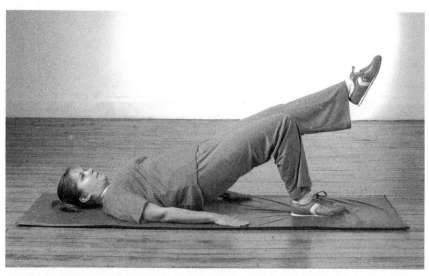

Lift your hips while simultaneously straightening your left knee, keeping your knees at the same height. Squeeze your buttocks. Return to the starting position and lower your hips to floor. Perform 10 reps. Switch sides and repeat with your right leg.

8. Crunch (abdominals)

Tip! Don't use your hands to pull up your head. Lift your upper body by tightening your abdominal muscles, not by jerking your head and neck.

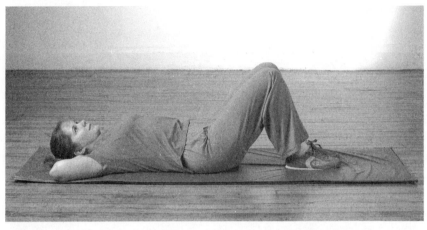

Lie on your back with your knees bent and your feet flat on the floor. Place your hands, fingers unclasped, behind your head. Contract your abdominal muscles, keeping your buttocks relaxed.

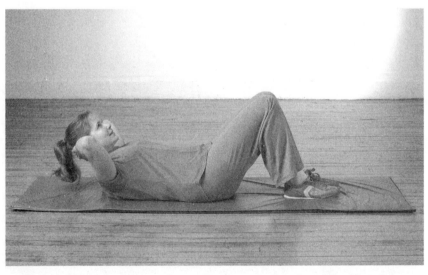

Using the strength of your abdominal muscles, curl your head, neck, and shoulders off the floor in one smooth movement. Keep your neck straight and point your chin toward the ceiling. Hold for one count, then return to the starting position.

Keep It Interesting

Once you become more physically active day by day, look for new and different ways to increase the intensity of your activities to prevent burnout.

* Take a dance class—anything from ballroom dancing to belly dancing.
* Explore hiking trails in your area.
* Sign up for a charity walk and help raise money for a good cause.
* Try new walking routes with hills that challenge you.
* Swim laps at a local pool.
* Tackle physically demanding chores, such as cleaning out the garage, washing the car, raking leaves, or painting—30 to 60 minutes of this type of work is a great calorie burner.
* Rent some workout DVDs or videos and try out different routines.
* Find a workout partner and challenge each other to work harder.
* Join a health club or local gym. Get a guest pass first to check out the classes and equipment available. You want an environment that you'll enjoy using and that's convenient and affordable.
* Train for a 5K or 10K race. A goal like this will help keep you motivated.
* Join a softball or volleyball team or play pickup basketball.
* Mix it up with different activities, such a kickboxing, spinning, tai chi, yoga, or Pilates. Plan an active vacation during which you will get to hike, cycle, kayak, surf, or swim.
* Purchase some additional home equipment, such as rubber exercise bands or a big stability ball. These exercise aids are inexpensive and bust the boredom of the same old routines. They are often sold with DVDs that demonstrate how to use them to get a great workout.
* Sneak some extra toning into your daily life. Do a set of crunches during TV commercials or squats while talking on the phone. When you're brushing your teeth, contract your butt muscles and squeeze tightly for a count of 15.

Once you get into the habit of moving more, you will discover firsthand how great it feels to exercise. By following this program consistently, you will soon experience renewed energy, a healthy glow, and a rewarding difference in the fit of your clothes and the size of your waistline.

Chapter 5

moving forward

Enjoying a healthy lifestyle is a matter of replacing bad habits with good ones, and since you've been on the alli™ diet, you've made substantial changes resulting in better health and weight loss. Congratulations! You should feel good about your accomplishments.

If you wanted to lose more than 10 or 15 pounds, you probably haven't reached your goal yet. That's fine. Just continue eating the way you have been in Phase 3 of the diet.

Be patient and you'll be sure to achieve the results you desire. And once you do meet this weight loss goal, continue to eat accordingly because *The alli™ Diet Plan* should serve as your lifestyle plan for moving forward.

Where to Go from Here

Your goal moving forward is to keep the weight off and continue to eat healthy. And your best strategy is to stick with alli™—both the capsule and the plan—because maintaining this new weight couldn't be any easier than it is with alli™. Simply continue to integrate your new way of eating and exercising into your daily life.

- Eat three nutritious reduced-calorie, low-fat meals a day containing no more than 30 percent calories from fat.
- Eat one or two low-fat snacks a day to temper your appetite.
- Be aware of portion size.
- Take a daily multivitamin at bedtime.
- Make healthy choices when eating in restaurants.
- Cook with healthy ingredients.
- Exercise regularly.
- Keep a diet journal.

The recipes and menu plans in this book are more than a delicious way to lose weight. They comprise a healthy, livable lifestyle that you can enjoy forever. This doesn't mean that keeping your weight where you want it will be easy. Maintaining your weight loss takes vigilance. But you can do it.

Settling into Your New Eating Style

After my patients lose weight I encourage them to continue their new diet and in particular to closely monitor their fat and calorie intake. Counting calories is important to maintaining a healthy weight, but watching the amount of fat you consume is simply healthy eating. A diet comprised of no more than 30 percent of daily calories from fat is best for achieving good health. Plus, when you eat a low-fat diet, you naturally eat fewer calories because a gram of fat has more than two times the calories as a gram of carbohydrate or protein.

The bottom line is that no matter how many calories you eat in a day in order to maintain your weight, you will still want to consume no more than 30 percent of your calories from fat. You may find out that you can maintain your weight on 1,600 or 1,700 calories if you're an active woman, or 2,000 calories or even more if you are a very active man. To find out the number of grams of fat you can have at any calorie level, follow the formula used on page 16.

As you settle into your new eating style, your diet journal becomes even more important because you can use it to follow your process as you experiment with different foods and with maintaining your weight.

Dealing with Small Weight Gains

As you settle into your new weight, continue to eat (and exercise) exactly as you did in Phase 3. Keep a close tab on both fat and calorie intake by continuing to use your diet journal. If you continue to lose weight but no longer want to, you can add more calories to your daily intake. Conversely, if you'd feel a bit more comfortable if you ate more, you can step up your exercise routine so you burn more calories.

Don't become a slave to the scale! Your real weight can fluctuate by a few pounds depending on a number of factors, such as water retention and hormonal balance. But if your weight continues to creep up by a few pounds, it's time to reassess your lifestyle and make some adjustments.

Review your journal to help find the cause of your weight gain. You may find you're exercising less or perhaps you've strayed from the alli™ menus and recipes. Once you determine the cause, take action to correct the problem.

You can resume taking alli™ capsules as you did in the past—one with each of your three main meals containing fat—until you get back to your weight goal. Remember, it is important to maintain a reduced-calorie, low-fat diet if you start taking alli™ again, so continue to eat as you did in Phase 3. There are probably several meal plans you have not tried yet.

Exercise. The most successful dieters maintain their weight loss not by diet alone but by committing to a daily exercise program. More than likely you are feeling significantly healthier and have more energy than when you started the the alli™ diet, so lace up your walking shoes and hit the road—every day.

Tips for Staying Fit and Thin

Living a healthy life takes discipline and practice. This applies not only to your eating habits but also to your fitness habits. To truly live a healthy lifestyle you must commit to being active every day. Try some of these tips:

- Fidget. A number of studies have shown that slim people burn around 350 calories more a day by fidgeting, tapping their toes, and wriggling while seated than those who are overweight. If you're not a natural-born fidgeter, take up a hobby such as knitting to keep your hands moving.

- Never drive when you can walk.

- Use the steps whenever possible instead of the elevator.

- When you're watching television, do something—get out your hand weights, walk in place. Better yet, try to limit the amount of time you spend watching television (particularly if you watch more than one hour per day) as studies show excessive TV watching is related linearly to obesity and weight gain as well as diabetes.

- At your kid's practice or at a game, don't just sit in the bleachers. Walk the sidelines or do a circuit of the field.

- Listen to books on tape while walking, rather than curling up with a book. Determine to walk for the length of a chapter or two.

- If you're stressed, try a walking meditation. Find a place with no traffic, like a park or beach, and walk with awareness. Quiet your mind and pay attention to the feel of your feet on the ground, the air on your skin, and the rhythm of your breathing.

- Take a walk around the block between eating dinner and dessert. You'll burn calories and the exercise might even dampen your need for the extra food.

- Rather than reaching for food or alcohol if you're angry or upset, opt for some high-intensity exercise like taking a brisk walk, jumping rope, doing jumping jacks, or sparring with an imaginary partner.

- Put on old socks and polish the kitchen or bathroom floor with your feet.

- Be a tourist in your own home town or city. Take a walking tour or just explore an unfamiliar part of the city.

- When your energy is flagging, hold off on the coffee, candy bar, or nap and get moving. Studies have shown that a brisk 10-minute walk raises energy levels for two hours, and you'll be burning calories too.

Always remember you must make a firm commitment to lifestyle changes to achieve and maintain weight loss. So continue to use your journal to record all the new and fabulous ways you have improved your life by losing weight. Read them from time to time to remind yourself of your achievements. Add to your list other goals in your life that became possible because you lost weight. Remember, few things in life are achieved without effort. Congratulate yourself on your weight loss success every time you look in the mirror. You earned it.

the alli™
diet plan
recipes

I have always been a firm believer that the combination of great taste and menu variety is the key to achieving weight loss success. So when I assembled a team of chefs, recipe developers, and nutritionists to create and test recipes for this book, I gave them a specific mission: Create great-tasting recipes that allow you to get the maximum potential from alli™ without sacrificing taste. I am happy to say that my team succeeded.

Naturally, they cut fat and calories. If they detected a change in flavor during the testing process, they put it back in. If good taste could not be achieved without staying alli™ friendly, the recipe did not make it into this book.

Next I wanted to make sure the recipes:
• Have enough variety to be enjoyed on all three phases of the alli™ diet.
• Are easy to make.

- Are not too costly.
- Are healthy, satisfying, and filling.
- Are foods that the entire family will enjoy.
- Could comfortably fit into a meal that is 30 percent calories from fat.
- The majority of dishes can be prepared and on the table in 30 minutes or less, or be prepared ahead of time so all you have to do is pop it in the oven (Check for the notation under the name of the recipe.) You'll also find a notation for dishes that freeze well.
- Don't require too much time or preparation.

The result is 200-plus recipes that will help you succeed at weight loss by eating food you love without having to eat the same dishes over and over again. My guess is many of these recipes will become family favorites.

The surprising truth is that you can slash fat and calories from almost any recipe because a lot of recipes contain too much needless fat. Consider a crab cake. Crab is low in calories and sweetly rich in taste—a 4-ounce serving contains only 116 calories and 2 grams of fat. When you form the crabmeat into a cake and sink it into a deep fryer, it absorbs oil. The result: The same 4-ounce serving jumps to 220 calories and 9 grams of fat—meaning 44 percent of its calories come from fat. In addition to absorbing fat, deep-frying actually detracts from the sweet natural flavor of the crab. Lightly sauteing is a tastier and healthier way to enjoy this delicacy.

Most people love to grill, and grilling is a natural and simple way to reduce fat. As fat melts, it drips away from the food instead of surrounding it as it does when you bake, broil, or saute.

Just make sure you pay attention to portion size. And keep in mind that just because a dish is low in fat, it is not okay to eat more than the portion specified. The key to success on the alli™ diet plan is limiting calories as well as getting a specific amount of fat grams at each meal. Eating too many calories, even if your fat intake is low, can interfere with your ability to lose weight. *The alli™ Diet Plan* recipes ensure that weight loss will never be a bore.

breakfast

specials

Sweet Potato Jacks with Apple Topping

prepare ahead • freeze

These hearty pancakes are easy to make. The homemade apple syrup adds just enough sweetness to satisfy without going overboard on calories. Use baking apples, such as McIntosh or Cortland, for the best texture.

Syrup	¼	cup packed dark brown sugar
	¼	cup orange juice
	½	teaspoon ground cinnamon
	2	medium baking apples, peeled, cored, and coarsely chopped

Pancakes	6	cups grated sweet potatoes
	1	cup all-purpose flour
	1	teaspoon baking powder
	½	teaspoon ground cinnamon
	1	teaspoon salt
	1	tablespoon honey
	1	large egg
	2	large egg whites

1 For the syrup: In a large nonstick skillet, stir together the brown sugar, orange juice, and cinnamon. Add the apples and cook over medium-high heat, stirring, for 10 minutes, or until the apples are tender and the brown sugar has melted to form a syrup. If the apples begin to dry out, add water, one tablespoon at a time, to keep them moist. Transfer to a bowl, cover, and keep warm. Wash and dry the skillet.

2 For the pancakes: In a large bowl, mix the sweet potatoes, flour, baking powder, cinnamon, salt, honey, egg, and egg whites.

3 Preheat oven to 200°F. Coat the skillet with nonstick cooking spray and place over medium heat for 3 minutes, until hot, but not smoking. For each pancake, drop about 2 tablespoons of batter into the skillet. Flatten slightly with a spatula until about 3 inches across. Cook the pancakes until golden on both sides. Repeat with the remaining batter, coating the skillet with cooking spray as needed.

Makes 12 pancakes • Serving size: 1 pancake
Per serving: 1 gram fat • 142 calories

Makes about 1½ cups syrup • Serving size: ¼ cup
Per serving: 0 grams fat • 60 calories

Banana-Nut Hotcakes

30 minutes or less

The bananas make these hotcakes so moist and flavorful that they don't need a topping. If you do add one, make sure to figure in the calories and fat.

1¼ cups all-purpose flour

1 tablespoon packed golden brown sugar

½ teaspoon baking powder

½ teaspoon baking soda

¼ teaspoon salt

1¼ cups low-fat buttermilk

¼ cup egg substitute

1 teaspoon vegetable oil

1 cup chopped ripe bananas (about 2 bananas)

2 tablespoons chopped toasted walnuts

1 In a large bowl, mix the flour, brown sugar, baking powder, baking soda, and salt.

2 In a small bowl, mix the buttermilk, egg substitute, and oil. Stir into the flour mixture. Fold in the bananas and walnuts.

3 Preheat oven to 200°F. Coat a large nonstick skillet with nonstick cooking spray and place over medium heat for 3 minutes, until hot. For each hotcake, ladle about ¼ cup of batter into the skillet. Cook until bubbles appear on top and the edges are barely dry. Turn the hotcakes and cook about 1 minute, or until the center springs back when touched. Transfer to a warm plate and keep warm in the oven. Repeat with the remaining batter, coating the skillet with cooking spray as needed.

Makes 8 hotcakes • Serving size: 2 hotcakes
Per serving: 5 grams fat • 284 calories

 To freeze, place on a waxed paper-lined cookie sheet and put in the freezer until firm. Then, double-wrap individually. Thaw completely before reheating. The hotcakes can be frozen for up to 3 months.

Pecan Waffles with Strawberry Sauce

Apricot nectar is the secret ingredient to giving these waffles a cakelike texture.

1½	cups all-purpose flour
1½	teaspoons baking powder
½	cup chopped unsalted pecans
1¼	cups apricot nectar
½	cup egg substitute
¼	cup Grade B maple syrup
2	tablespoons vegetable oil
1¼	cups Strawberry Sauce (page 300)

1 In a large bowl, mix the flour and baking powder. Stir in the pecans.

2 In a medium bowl, whisk together the apricot nectar, egg substitute, maple syrup, and oil.

3 Stir the apricot nectar mixture into the flour mixture until just combined. Do not overmix.

4 Heat a waffle iron and lightly brush the grids with oil. Pour in enough batter to cover two-thirds of the bottom grid. Bake according to the manufacturer's directions but start checking for doneness after 3 minutes. Repeat until the batter is used up; occasionally brush the grids with oil to prevent sticking.

Makes 12 regular or 6 Belgian-style waffles • Serving size: 2 regular or 1 Belgian-style waffle
Per serving: 12 grams fat • 335 calories

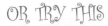
OR TRY THIS

Waffles with Strawberry Sauce

If you love waffles, you can move this breakfast treat up a phase by eliminating the pecans from the recipe. It's that simple.

Per serving: 6 grams fat • 272 calories

Almond-Pumpkin Breakfast Bread

prepare ahead • freeze

This bread-like cake is so versatile it can show up at breakfast, as a dessert, or even as a side during a special meal. Because it is easy to make and keeps well, it is offered here as a make-ahead and take-along breakfast.

- ¾ cup canned pumpkin
- ½ cup honey
- 3 tablespoons vegetable oil
- 3 tablespoons packed brown sugar
- 2 large eggs, lightly beaten
- 1 cup whole wheat flour
- ½ cup all-purpose flour
- 2 tablespoons flaxseeds
- ½ teaspoon baking powder
- ½ teaspoon ground allspice
- ½ teaspoon ground cinnamon
- ½ teaspoon ground nutmeg
- ¼ teaspoon salt
- 2 tablespoons sliced almonds

1 Preheat oven to 375°F. In a large bowl, combine the pumpkin, honey, oil, brown sugar, and eggs. Beat with an electric mixer on low speed until well blended.

2 In a small bowl, whisk together the flours, flaxseeds, baking powder, allspice, cinnamon, nutmeg, and salt. Add the flour mixture to the pumpkin mixture and blend on medium speed. Stir in the almonds.

3 Coat a 6 × 4-inch loaf pan with nonstick cooking spray. Add the batter and spread evenly. Bake at 375°F for 1 hour, or until a toothpick inserted into the center of the loaf comes out clean. Let cool in the pan on a wire rack for 10 minutes. Turn the loaf out of the pan onto the rack and let cool completely.

Makes 12 servings
Per serving: 6 grams fat • 177 calories

Blueberry Muffins
freeze

If you crave sweets for breakfast, this muffin will fill the bill without adding too many calories.

1½	cups all-purpose flour
2	teaspoons baking powder
½	teaspoon salt
1	large egg
½	cup sugar
3	tablespoons fat-free vanilla yogurt
1	tablespoon canola oil
1	teaspoon vanilla extract
½	cup light (1%) milk
2	cups blueberries, fresh or frozen

1 Preheat oven to 400°F. In a medium bowl, whisk together the flour, baking powder, and salt.

2 In a large bowl, combine the egg, sugar, yogurt, oil, and vanilla. Beat with an electric mixer on high speed for 2 minutes. Reduce the speed to low and alternately beat in the flour mixture and the milk. Beat until just combined. Stir in the blueberries.

3 Coat a 12-cup muffin pan with nonstick cooking spray. Divide the batter evenly among the muffin cups, filling them about two-thirds full. Bake at 400°F for 20 minutes, or until a toothpick inserted into the center of a muffin comes out clean. Cool on a wire rack for 5 minutes before removing the muffins from the pan.

Makes 12 muffins • Serving size: 1 muffin
Per serving: 2 grams fat • 128 calories

Cranberry Muffins
freeze

This is what to reach for when you want a high-fiber start to your day. The whole wheat flour, wheat germ, and cranberries are responsible for the high fiber content.

1⅓	cups whole wheat flour
⅓	cup wheat germ
1	tablespoon baking powder
¾	cup light (1%) milk
⅓	cup honey
¼	cup egg substitute
2	tablespoons vegetable oil
1	cup coarsely chopped cranberries

1 Preheat oven to 375°F. In a large bowl, mix the flour, wheat germ, and baking powder. In a medium bowl, mix the milk, honey, egg substitute, and oil.

2 Stir the milk mixture into the flour mixture until just combined. Do not overmix. Gently stir in the cranberries.

3 Coat a 12-muffin baking pan with nonstick cooking spray. Divide the batter among the cups, filling them about three-quarters full. Bake at 375°F for 20 to 25 minutes.

Makes 12 muffins • Serving size: 1 muffin
Per serving: 3 grams fat • 119 calories

 If you don't like eating first thing in the morning, freeze these muffins in individual wrappers and place each in a small brown bag. Grab a bag from the freezer on your way out the door in the morning. The muffin will defrost at room temperature and be ready to eat in about an hour.

Carrot-Raisin Bran Muffins

prepare ahead • freeze

Lots of nutrition and fiber—a great way to start the day.

1	cup all-purpose flour
½	cup whole wheat pastry flour
¼	cup oat bran
1½	teaspoons baking powder
1½	teaspoons ground cinnamon
½	teaspoon baking soda
¼	teaspoon salt
1	cup fat-free vanilla yogurt
½	cup packed dark brown sugar
1	large egg
2	tablespoons vegetable oil
1	teaspoon vanilla extract
½	cup finely chopped carrots
½	cup chopped raisins

1 Preheat oven to 400°F. In a large bowl, mix the flours, oat bran, baking powder, cinnamon, baking soda, and salt.

2 In a small bowl, mix the yogurt, brown sugar, egg, oil, and vanilla. Pour over the flour mixture and stir until just moistened. Stir in the carrots and raisins until evenly distributed.

3 Coat a 12-cup muffin pan with nonstick cooking spray. Divide the batter evenly among the muffin cups, filling them about two-thirds full. Bake at 400°F for 20 to 25 minutes, or until a toothpick inserted into the center of a muffin comes out clean. Cool on a wire rack for 5 minutes before removing the muffins from the pan.

Makes 12 muffins • Serving size: 1 muffin
Per serving: 3 grams fat • 150 calories

Raisin Bran Muffins with Orange Glaze

prepare ahead • freeze

The orange glaze adds amazing flavor and keeps the muffins moist.

Muffins	2	cups shredded All-Bran cereal
	¾	cup hot water
	¼	cup canola oil
	¾	cup low-fat buttermilk
	¼	cup fresh orange juice
	2	tablespoons light molasses
	2	tablespoons honey
	1	large egg
	1¼	cups all-purpose flour
	2	teaspoons baking soda
	½	teaspoon salt
	1	cup raisins
Glaze	¼	cup fresh orange juice
	¼	cup sugar

1 Preheat oven to 400°F. For the muffins: In a medium bowl, mix the cereal, water, and oil, stirring until soft.

2 In another bowl, mix the buttermilk, orange juice, molasses, honey, and egg. Add to the cereal mixture and mix well.

3 In a large bowl, mix the flour, baking soda, and salt. Add the cereal mixture and stir until just incorporated. Stir in the raisins. Do not overmix.

4 Coat a 12-cup muffin pan with nonstick cooking spray. Divide the batter evenly among the muffin cups, filling them about two-thirds full. Bake at 400°F for 15 minutes, or until a toothpick inserted into the center comes out clean. Cool on a wire rack.

5 For the glaze: Mix the orange juice and sugar in a small saucepan. Bring to a boil and stir to dissolve the sugar. Brush on top of the muffins.

Makes 12 muffins • Serving size: 1 muffin
Per serving: 6 grams fat • 208 calories

Asparagus Omelet with Summer Herbs

30 minutes or less

Divide the recipe in half to make an omelet for one or double the recipe if cooking for a crowd. Use whichever fresh herb you like; basil, dill, and tarragon are especially good choices.

  4 large egg whites
  2 large eggs
  ¼ cup fat-free milk
  2 tablespoons chopped scallions
  ¼ cup chopped fresh herb
  6 asparagus spears, trimmed, woody stalks shaved, and cut into
      1-inch pieces
  ¼ cup water
  ½ cup fat-free cottage cheese

1 In a medium bowl, whisk together the egg whites, eggs, and milk. Stir in the scallions and herb. Season with salt and pepper.

2 Place the asparagus and water in a large microwave-safe bowl. Cover with vented plastic wrap and microwave on high power for a total of 4 to 6 minutes, or until crisp-tender; stop and stir after 2 minutes. Drain and pat dry.

3 Coat a medium nonstick omelet pan or skillet with nonstick cooking spray. Set over medium heat until hot. Pour half of the egg mixture into the skillet and cook until almost set, about 5 minutes. Spoon half of the cottage cheese on top of the Eggs and scatter half of the asparagus across the surface.

4 Fold the omelet in half, cover, and cook for 2 to 3 minutes, or until the eggs are set. Transfer to a plate and keep warm while preparing the second omelet.

Makes 2 servings
Per serving: 5 grams fat • 165 calories

Ratatouille Omelet

30 minutes or less

This veggie-egg mix and a green salad make a healthy brunch.

1   teaspoon oil
1   small onion, peeled and thinly sliced
1   tablespoon minced garlic
1   small eggplant, peeled and chopped
2   small zucchini, chopped
2   tomatoes, seeded and coarsely chopped
6   large eggs
½   teaspoon dried oregano
½   cup chopped fresh basil (optional)

1 Warm the oil in a large ovenproof nonstick skillet over medium heat. Add the onion and cook for 5 minutes, or until softened. Add the garlic, eggplant, and zucchini; cook for 8 minutes, or until the vegetables are soft and lightly browned. Add the tomatoes and season with salt and pepper.

2 In a medium bowl, lightly beat the eggs with a fork. Add the oregano and season with salt and pepper. Pour over the vegetables and cook for 5 minutes, or until the bottom is starting to brown and the eggs look softly set.

3 Broil about 4 inches from the heat until the top looks puffed and golden. If desired, sprinkle with the basil.

Makes 4 servings
Per serving: 9 grams fat • 192 calories

 The easiest way to seed tomatoes is to slice them in half and, holding one half over the sink (or a bowl), simply squeeze. Remove any lingering seeds by scraping the inside of the tomato with a teaspoon.

Eggs-and-Potato Hash

30 minutes or less

Lower in fat than its traditional counterpart thanks to the absence of bacon, this delicious decidedly American breakfast dish is also perfect as a light dinner when served with a small green salad.

½ tablespoon oil

¾ pound red potatoes, peeled and cut into chunks

½ cup diced onion

1 garlic clove, peeled and chopped

¾ cup chopped tomato

4 large eggs

¼ cup chopped fresh cilantro

1 Warm the oil in a large nonstick skillet over high heat. Add the potatoes and onion; cook, stirring frequently, for 5 minutes, or until the onion starts to brown. Add the garlic and season with salt and pepper. Cover and cook for 10 minutes, or until the potatoes are just tender. If the potatoes start to stick, add a little water or chicken broth to the pan.

2 Add the tomato and cook for 3 minutes, or until just softened.

3 Use a large spoon to make 4 depressions in the mixture. Break an egg into each depression. Season the eggs with salt and pepper, cover, and cook for 3 to 4 minutes, or until the eggs are set to your liking. Sprinkle with the cilantro.

Makes 4 servings
Per serving: 7 grams fat • 172 calories

soup to

start

Hot and Cold Melon Soup

30 minutes or less • prepare ahead

If you don't care for cold soup that's also spicy hot, you can eliminate the pepper sauce. On the other hand, to make the soup spicier, use a diced jalapeño or even a serrano pepper instead of the hot sauce. Serve as a light appetizer or dessert.

10	cups chopped honeydew melon
⅓	cup fresh lime juice
½	cup fruity white wine, such as Gewürztraminer or Chenin Blanc
2	tablespoons honey
½	teaspoon hot pepper sauce

In a large bowl, mix the honeydew, lime juice, wine, honey, and pepper sauce. Working in batches, transfer to a food processor or blender and process until smooth. Cover and refrigerate for at least 2 hours, until well chilled.

Makes 8 servings
Per serving: 0 grams fat • 108 calories

Asparagus Soup

prepare ahead

The creaminess in this makeover of traditional cream of asparagus soup comes from pureed vegetables and low-fat sour cream.

2	pounds asparagus spears
1	tablespoon oil
1	cup chopped onions
1	cup chopped, well-cleaned leeks (white and tender green parts)
¼	cup all-purpose flour
8	cups fat-free chicken broth
½	cup low-fat sour cream
1	tablespoon dried tarragon

1 Trim the woody ends from the asparagus and peel off the scales with a vegetable peeler. Cut off the tips (about 1 to 1½ inches) and slice them in half lengthwise, if thick. Cut the stalks into 1-inch pieces.

2 Bring a large pot filled halfway with water to a boil over high heat. Add the asparagus tips to the water and cook for 2 minutes, or until just tender and bright green; do not overcook. Remove the tips from the water with a slotted spoon and run under cold water to stop the cooking. Pat dry.

3 Add the stalk pieces to the boiling water and cook for 2 minutes. Drain in a colander.

4 Place the oil in a large saucepan over medium heat. Add the onions and leeks and cook for 5 minutes, or until softened. Add the asparagus stalks and cook for 3 minutes.

5 Add the flour, stirring to coat the vegetables. Cook for 2 minutes. Add the broth and cook for 20 minutes, or until the asparagus is tender. Let cool for 5 minutes.

6 Working in batches, transfer the soup to a blender and puree. Return the soup to the saucepan. Whisk in the sour cream. Stir in the tarragon and the asparagus tips. Season with the salt and pepper. Bring to a simmer to heat through.

Makes 6 servings
Per serving: 5 grams fat • 125 calories

Tomato-Corn Bisque

30 minutes or less • prepare ahead • freeze

In the summer, when corn is at its freshest and sweetest, simply cut the corn off the cob. Use two or three ears, depending on their size.

1	large onion, peeled and thinly sliced
1	red sweet pepper, seeded and finely chopped
1	tablespoon oil
5	large tomatoes, peeled, seeded, and chopped, or 1 can (28 ounces) whole tomatoes, chopped
5	cups fat-free chicken broth
1	cup corn kernels, fresh or frozen
1	teaspoon dried basil
¼	cup water
2	tablespoons cornstarch
¼	cup minced fresh parsley

1 In a large saucepan, cook the onion and red pepper in the oil over medium-high heat for 5 minutes, or until soft. Stir in the tomatoes. Simmer for 5 minutes.

2 Add the broth, corn, and basil. Bring to a boil, then reduce the heat and simmer for 15 minutes.

3 In a cup, mix the water and cornstarch until smooth. Add to the soup and stir over heat until thickened. Let cool for 5 minutes.

4 Puree in batches in a food processor or blender. Season with salt and pepper. Serve sprinkled with the parsley.

Makes 6 servings
Per serving: 3.4 grams fat • 120 calories

 To make chopping canned tomatoes easier (and neater), simply open the can and, using a fork, mash the tomatoes while they are still in the can.

Buttery Squash Soup

30 minutes or less • prepare ahead • freeze

Serve this soup for lunch with half of a sandwich or as a dinner entrée. You can substitute acorn squash or pumpkin for the butternut squash.

2	tablespoons butter
1	cup finely chopped onion
½	cup finely chopped carrot
2	garlic cloves, peeled and minced
1	large butternut squash, peeled, seeded, and cubed
5	cups fat-free chicken broth
1	cup tomato puree
2	limes, cut into wedges

1 Melt the butter in a large saucepan over medium heat. Add the onion, carrot, and garlic; cook, stirring, for 5 minutes. Reduce the heat to low, cover, and cook for 5 minutes.

2 Stir in the squash, broth, and tomato puree. Bring to a simmer and cook for 30 minutes.

3 Mash the squash to a chunky puree with a potato masher or the back of a spoon. Season with salt and pepper. Squeeze the lime wedges into each serving.

Makes 8 servings
Per serving: 3 grams fat • 105 calories

French Onion Soup

prepare ahead • freeze

The onions are cooked in wine instead of butter to cut the calories in this classic dish. Serve it with a salad with a no-fat dressing of your choice for a complete meal. For a quick meal, make the soup ahead and refrigerate or freeze. All you have to do is reheat and add the bread topping.

- 4 cups thinly sliced onions
- ½ cup white wine
- 5 cups fat-free beef broth
- 1 teaspoon Worcestershire sauce
- 4 slices French bread
- 4 ounces reduced-fat Swiss cheese, shredded

1 Place the onions and wine in a large saucepan and cook over medium heat for 5 minutes, stirring frequently. Reduce the heat, partially cover the pan, and cook for 15 minutes, or until the onions are soft.

2 Add the broth and Worcestershire sauce. Bring to a boil, cover, and simmer for 10 minutes to blend the flavors.

3 Preheat oven to 400°F. Place the bread on a baking sheet and bake for 5 minutes, or until just lightly browned. Place the cheese on top of the bread and bake for 1 minute, or until the cheese melts.

4 Ladle the soup into bowls and float the bread on top.

Makes 4 servings
Per serving: 3 grams fat • 246 calories

Super-Quick Pumpkin Soup

30 minutes or less • prepare ahead • freeze

This dish is so simple, it is almost as easy as opening a can of soup. But it is so much more tasty, creamy, and satisfying! Make sure to use plain canned pumpkin—pumpkin pie mix contains sugar and spices.

1	medium onion, peeled and finely chopped
1	tablespoon vegetable oil
1½	cups canned cooked unsweetened pumpkin
2	cups fat-free chicken broth
½	teaspoon dried oregano
¼	teaspoon hot pepper sauce
¼	cup toasted unsalted pumpkin seeds

1 In a medium saucepan, cook the onion in the oil over medium heat for 10 minutes, or until soft.

2 Stir in the pumpkin and then whisk in the broth in a slow stream. Add the oregano and hot pepper sauce. Simmer for 15 minutes. Stir in the pumpkin seeds. Season with salt and pepper.

Makes 4 servings
Per serving: 4.7 grams fat • 98 calories

Ukrainian Borscht

prepare ahead

There are many variations of this bright red soup, that can be served hot or cold. This version is from the Ukraine. It traditionally contains potatoes, which are eliminated here to save calories. The cabbage adds valuable fiber.

4 cups fat-free beef broth
4 large beets, peeled and shredded
½ medium cabbage, shredded
¼ cup white vinegar
1 tablespoon sugar
2 teaspoons soy sauce
½ cup canned tomato puree
1 cup fat-free plain yogurt

1 In a large saucepan, cook the broth and beets over medium heat for 25 minutes, or until tender.

2 Add the cabbage, vinegar, sugar, and soy sauce. Cover and cook for 10 minutes, or until the cabbage begins to soften.

3 Add the tomato puree, cover, and cook for 10 minutes. Season with salt and pepper. Serve topped with the yogurt.

Makes 4 servings
Per serving: 1 gram fat • 134 calories

Chicken Soup with Soba Noodles

30 minutes or less • prepare ahead • freeze

Edamame are fresh green soybeans that are so good, many people eat them as a snack. Like other soybeans, they're high in protein.

3	ounces soba noodles
1	tablespoon olive oil
1	cup chopped onion
1	cup diced carrot
1	tablespoon minced fresh ginger
1	garlic clove, minced
4	cups fat-free chicken broth
2	tablespoons soy sauce
1	pound boneless, skinless chicken breasts, chopped
1	cup shelled edamame
1	cup light (1%) milk

1 Prepare the noodles according to the package directions. Drain and set aside.

2 Warm the oil in a large saucepan over medium heat. Add the onion and cook for 4 minutes, or until soft. Add the carrot, ginger, and garlic; cook for 1 minute. Add the broth and soy sauce; bring to a simmer.

3 Add the chicken and edamame; bring to a boil. Reduce the heat to medium-low and simmer for 10 minutes, or until the chicken is cooked. Add the noodles and milk; cook until heated through.

Makes 8 servings
Per serving: 5 grams fat • 194 calories

Boston Clam Chowder

prepare ahead

The only thing missing from this New England favorite is heavy cream.

    2   cans (6½ ounces each) minced clams
    1   bottle (8 ounces) clam juice
    1   cup chopped onion
    ½   cup chopped red sweet pepper
    1   teaspoon diced garlic
    1   cup chopped potatoes
    1   teaspoon Worcestershire sauce
    ½   teaspoon dried thyme
    3   tablespoons cornstarch
    1½ cups light (1%) milk
    1½ cups fat-free evaporated milk
    ½   cup chopped fresh parsley

1 Drain the liquid from the clams into a medium saucepan; set the clams aside. Add the bottled clam juice, onion, red pepper, and garlic to the saucepan. Cook over medium heat for 5 minutes.

2 Add the chopped potatoes, Worcestershire sauce, and thyme. Bring to a boil, cover, and simmer for 10 minutes, or until the potatoes are tender.

3 In a small bowl, dissolve the cornstarch in the light milk and stir into the saucepan. Stir in the evaporated milk. Cook, stirring, until slightly thickened and bubbly. Stir in the clams. Simmer, stirring, for 1 minute. Season with salt and black pepper and sprinkle with the parsley.

Makes 4 servings
Per serving: 2 grams fat • 290 calories

Texas Black Bean Soup

prepare ahead • freeze

Garnish with a dollop of fat-free sour cream and finely chopped onions, if desired.

1	cup chopped onion
½	cup chopped carrot
½	cup chopped celery
2	garlic cloves, peeled and minced
1	tablespoon olive oil
1	can (14.5 ounces) whole tomatoes, coarsely chopped
3	cups fat-free chicken broth
⅓	cup chopped fresh parsley
2	tablespoons tomato paste
1	tablespoon fresh lime juice
1	teaspoon ground cumin
⅛	teaspoon cayenne
3	cans (16 ounces each) black beans, rinsed and drained

1 In a large nonstick saucepan, cook the onion, carrot, celery, and garlic in the oil for 10 minutes, or until soft. Transfer the mixture to a food processor and process until smooth.

2 Return the vegetables to the saucepan. Stir in the tomatoes (with juice), broth, parsley, tomato paste, lime juice, cumin, cayenne, and two-thirds of the beans.

3 In a small bowl, mash the remaining beans with a fork and add to the saucepan. Season with salt and pepper. Bring to a boil; reduce the heat and simmer for 30 minutes, or until thickened.

Makes 8 servings
Per serving: 3 grams fat • 196 calories

Navy Bean Soup

prepare ahead • freeze

There are dozens of ways to make this well-known soup, which was a staple aboard U.S. Navy ships in the 1950s, hence its name.

¾   cup dried navy beans, soaked overnight and drained
6   cups fat-free beef broth
1   cup peeled and finely chopped parsnips
1   cup peeled, seeded, and chopped tomatoes
1   cup chopped onion
2   yellow frying peppers, finely chopped
2   tablespoons minced garlic
1   teaspoon dried thyme

1 Drain the beans and place in a large saucepan. Add the broth and bring to a boil. Reduce the heat and simmer for 25 minutes.

2 Add the parsnips, tomatoes, onion, peppers, garlic, and thyme. Cover and simmer until the beans are tender, about 20 minutes.

3 Ladle about 1 cup of the soup into a blender and process until smooth. Stir back into the pan. If the soup isn't thick enough, blend more of the mixture.

Makes 8 servings

Per serving: 0.5 gram fat • 127 calories

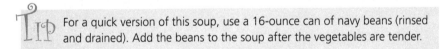

Tip   For a quick version of this soup, use a 16-ounce can of navy beans (rinsed and drained). Add the beans to the soup after the vegetables are tender.

Two-Potato Bisque

prepare ahead

Heavy cream is replaced by buttermilk and fat-free milk to pare down calories and fat.

1 large sweet potato or yam, peeled and cut into 1-inch cubes
1 large baking potato, peeled and cut into 1-inch cubes
1 cup chopped onion
2 garlic cloves, peeled and minced
1 bay leaf
1 teaspoon dried thyme
⅛ teaspoon cayenne
2 cups fat-free chicken broth
1 cup low-fat buttermilk
1 cup fat-free milk
2 tablespoons fresh lime juice

1 In a large saucepan, mix the sweet potato, baking potato, onion, garlic, bay leaf, thyme, cayenne, and broth. Bring to a boil over high heat. Reduce the heat to medium-low, cover, and simmer for 15 minutes, or until the potatoes are tender. Discard the bay leaf.

2 Working in batches, transfer the mixture to a food processor or blender and process until smooth. Return to the saucepan and stir in the buttermilk, milk, and lime juice. Season with salt and pepper. Cook over low heat until heated through; do not boil.

Makes 6 servings
Per serving: 0 grams fat • 91 calories

salads: main meal
or on the side

Classic Spinach Salad

30 minutes or less

Turkey bacon is a much leaner alternative to regular bacon and brings the fat content of this side-dish salad way down.

- 2 slices turkey bacon
- 2 teaspoons cornstarch
- ½ teaspoon grated orange zest
- 1 cup orange juice
- 1 teaspoon chopped garlic
- 8 cups spinach, torn into bite-size pieces
- 8 ounces mushrooms, wiped clean and sliced
- ¼ cup sliced scallions
- 3 oranges, peeled, halved, and sliced crosswise

1 In a small skillet, cook the bacon over medium heat until crisp. Drain on paper towels and then crumble. Wipe out the skillet with a paper towel.

2 In a small bowl, mix the cornstarch, orange zest and juice, and garlic until the cornstarch dissolves. Season with salt and pepper. Pour into the skillet and cook, stirring, over medium heat, for 2 minutes, or until the mixture thickens and boils. Continue to stir for 2 minutes longer; remove from the heat.

3 In a large bowl, mix the spinach, mushrooms, scallions, and reserved bacon. Add the hot dressing and toss. Add the oranges and toss again.

Makes 4 servings
Per serving: 2 grams fat • 145 calories

OR TRY THIS

Wilted Spinach Salad

It is a French tradition to serve this salad wilted. Bring the dressing to a boil in a large skillet, remove from the heat, and add the spinach. Turn the spinach with tongs for 1 minute, or until wilted. Transfer to a platter and arrange the mushrooms, scallions, oranges, and bacon on top.

Little Caesar Salad

30 minutes or less • prepare ahead

The incredibly creamy no-oil dressing keeps calories and fat low in this side salad. The garlic and anchovy flavors are rather strong, just as they should be, but if you'd prefer a milder flavor, use less.

Dressing	1½	teaspoons balsamic vinegar
	1	teaspoon fresh lemon juice
	1	teaspoon minced garlic
	½	teaspoon anchovy paste
	½	teaspoon Dijon mustard
	½	teaspoon Worcestershire sauce
	¼	cup fat-free cottage cheese
	¼	cup light (1%) milk
	1	tablespoon grated Parmesan cheese
Salad	1	head romaine lettuce
	1	pint cherry tomatoes, halved
	½	cup plain low-fat croutons
	1½	tablespoons grated Parmesan cheese

1 For the dressing: In a blender or food processor, combine the vinegar, lemon juice, garlic, anchovy paste, mustard, and Worcestershire sauce; process until blended.

2 Add the cottage cheese, milk, and the 1 tablespoon Parmesan. Process until the dressing is smooth and creamy.

3 For the salad: Coarsely chop the lettuce and place in a large bowl. Add the tomatoes, croutons, and dressing. Toss to combine. Serve sprinkled with the 1½ tablespoons Parmesan.

Makes 4 servings
Per serving: 4 grams fat • 174 calories

Greek Salad

30 minutes or less • prepare ahead

What goes into this main-dish salad is usually at the whim of the chef. What is constant, however, is the use of fresh vegetables and olive oil.

Dressing ½ cup balsamic vinegar

2 tablespoons chopped fresh oregano

2 tablespoons olive oil

2 teaspoons Dijon mustard

Salad 8 asparagus spears, woody ends removed, trimmed, and cut into 1-inch pieces

2 tablespoons water

4 cups mixed greens

1 can (14 ounces) hearts of palm, rinsed, drained, and cut into 1-inch pieces

1 ripe avocado, pitted, peeled, and sliced

2 cups sliced cucumbers

2 large tomatoes, cut into wedges

½ large red onion, peeled and thinly sliced

2 hard-cooked eggs, sliced

4 large pitted black olives, sliced in half

2 ounces feta cheese, crumbled

1 For the dressing: In a small bowl, whisk together the vinegar, oregano, oil, and mustard. Season with salt and pepper.

2 For the salad: Place the asparagus and water in a microwave-safe bowl. Cover with plastic wrap, vent, and microwave on high power for 2 minutes. Plunge the asparagus into a bowl of cold water, drain, and pat dry.

3 Transfer the asparagus to a large bowl. Add the greens, hearts of palm, avocado, cucumbers, tomatoes, onion, eggs, olives, and cheese. Add the dressing and toss lightly to combine.

Makes 4 servings
Per serving: 20 grams fat • 291 calories

PHASE **1 2 3**

Skinny Chef's Salad

30 minutes or less • prepare ahead

Fruit makes a nice change of pace in a side salad. Use any type of fruit you desire, such as strawberry slices, blueberries, orange or grapefruit wedges, pineapple chunks, or kiwifruit slices.

⅔ cup fat-free sour cream
¼ cup red wine vinegar
2 scallions, sliced
2 tablespoons honey mustard
1 head Boston lettuce
3 cups bite-size fruit (see note above)
2 ounces cooked turkey breast, thinly sliced
½ cup shredded low-fat cheddar cheese
½ cup alfalfa sprouts

1 In a small bowl, whisk together the sour cream, vinegar, scallions, and mustard. Season with salt and pepper.

2 Line plates with the lettuce. Arrange the fruit, turkey, cheese, and sprouts on top. Serve the dressing on the side.

Makes 4 servings

Per serving: 3 grams fat • 170 calories (using 1 cup each of strawberries, oranges, and pineapple chunks). Calories may differ based on the fruits selected.

Warm Eggplant, Tomato, and Mozzarella Salad

30 minutes or less

This perfectly matched trio is a light version of eggplant Parmesan. Turn it into a main meal by serving some protein on the side.

1   can (14 ounces) crushed tomatoes
2   teaspoons tomato paste
1   garlic clove, peeled and chopped
1   medium eggplant, cut crosswise into 8 slices
1   tablespoon oil
4   ounces part-skim mozzarella, cut into 8 slices
8   thick tomato slices
½   cup tightly packed fresh basil leaves

1   In a small saucepan, mix the crushed tomatoes, tomato paste, and garlic. Bring to a boil over medium heat and cook for 10 minutes, or until the sauce thickens slightly. Cover and keep warm.

2   Place the eggplant slices on a broiler pan and brush the tops with half of the oil. Broil about 4 inches from the heat for 4 minutes. Turn, brush with the remaining oil, and broil for 4 minutes, or until soft.

3   Transfer the eggplant to a baking sheet lined with foil. Place a slice of cheese on each eggplant piece and then add a tomato slice. Bake at 375°F for 10 minutes, or until the cheese begins to melt. Sprinkle with the basil and serve with the tomato sauce.

Makes 4 servings
Per serving: 8 grams fat • 160 calories

California Fruit Salad

30 minutes or less

Try this for a light lunch. The avocado is the source of most of the fat, but you're getting good-for-you, heart-healthy monounsaturated fat.

1	ripe avocado, halved, pitted, and peeled
2	kiwifruits, peeled and sliced
2	red or pink grapefruit, sectioned
2	cups sliced strawberries
½	cup fat-free raspberry vinaigrette
8	cups mixed salad greens

1 Slice 1 half of the avocado into 8 wedges; set aside for garnish. Cut the remaining half into cubes and place in a medium bowl. Add the sliced kiwifruit, grapefruit, and strawberries. Drizzle with ¼ cup of the dressing and toss gently to combine.

2 Put the greens in a large bowl, drizzle with the remaining ¼ cup dressing, and toss. Add the fruit mixture and toss gently to combine. Serve with the avocado wedges arranged on top.

Makes 4 servings
Per serving: 7 grams fat • 219 calories

OR TRY THIS

Chambord Compote

The fruit salad without the greens can be a dessert option. Cut the whole avocado into cubes and combine with the rest of the fruit. Mix in 1 tablespoon powdered sugar and 1 tablespoon Chambord (raspberry liqueur).

Makes 8 servings
Per serving: 4 grams fat • 113 calories

Aloha Fruit Salad with Macadamia Crunch

30 minutes or less • prepare ahead

This colorful salad is tasty any time of the day.

1	cup pineapple chunks
3	kiwifruits, peeled and cut into chunks
1	papaya, peeled and cut into chunks
1	mango, peeled and cut into chunks
1	large banana, peeled and sliced
1	cup seedless red grapes
¼	cup honey
2	tablespoons fresh lime juice
10	cups romaine lettuce
⅓	cup chopped unsalted macadamia nuts
2	tablespoons chopped crystallized ginger

1 In a large bowl, mix the pineapple, kiwifruits, papaya, mango, banana, and grapes. Mix the honey and lime juice in a cup. Drizzle over the fruit and toss gently until evenly coated. Cover and refrigerate for up to 1 hour.

2 Divide the lettuce among 8 serving plates. Top with the fruit salad and sprinkle with the nuts and ginger just before serving.

Makes 8 servings
Per serving: 5 grams fat • 186 calories

Watercress and Strawberry Salad

30 minutes or less • prepare ahead

When early summer rolls around, watercress and strawberries make a perfect match that can go with any entrée.

2 cups trimmed watercress, coarsely chopped
2 heads Belgian endive, torn into small pieces
1 cup sliced strawberries, fresh or frozen
¼ cup coarsely chopped unsalted pecans
½ cup Poppy Seed Dressing (page 340)

In a large bowl, combine the watercress, endive, strawberries, and pecans. Add the dressing and toss well.

Makes 4 servings
Per serving: 8 grams fat • 160 calories

 If fresh strawberries are unavailable or out of season in your area, use frozen strawberries and thaw as directed on the package.

Baby Greens with Avocado, Strawberries, and Walnuts

30 minutes or less

This side salad is elegant enough for a dinner party yet easy enough for a casual weekday lunch. Cut the avocado just before serving to keep it from discoloring.

2 tablespoons raspberry vinegar

1 tablespoon oil

3 tablespoons orange juice

1 tablespoon fresh lime juice

1 tablespoon chopped fresh basil

½ teaspoon dry mustard

1 ripe avocado, halved, pitted, and peeled

8 cups mixed baby salad greens

3 large tomatoes, cut into wedges

1 small red onion, peeled and thinly sliced

½ cup chopped toasted unsalted walnuts

1 pint fresh strawberries, hulled and sliced (about 2 cups)

1 In a small bowl, whisk together the vinegar, oil, juices, basil, and mustard. Season with salt and pepper.

2 Slice 1 half of the avocado into 8 wedges; set aside for garnish. Cut the remaining half into cubes.

3 Put the greens in a large bowl. Add the avocado cubes, tomato, and onion. Drizzle with the dressing, sprinkle with half of the walnuts, and toss. Add the strawberries and toss again. Sprinkle with the remaining walnuts.

4 Serve with the avocado wedges arranged on the side.

Makes 8 servings
Per serving: 10 grams fat • 140 calories

 To get the most flavor out of walnuts and other nuts, toast them. Spread the nuts on a baking sheet and bake at 350°F for 10 minutes, or until golden, but make sure to watch them carefully since they can burn quickly. Toss the nuts frequently while they bake so they toast evenly.

Grilled Chicken Caesar Salad

30 minutes or less • prepare ahead

This main-dish salad is a popular lunch item, but be careful ordering it in a restaurant. The calories and fat will be double, or possibly more.

2 recipes Little Caesar Salad (page 162)
1 pound boneless, skinless chicken breasts, trimmed of fat
2 roasted red sweet peppers, cored, seeded, and cut into strips

1 Prepare a double batch of the dressing for the Caesar salad. Place half of the dressing in a small bowl and refrigerate until needed. Place the remaining dressing in a large bowl, add the chicken, and marinate in the refrigerator for 1 hour. Bring to room temperature.

2 Lightly coat a gas or charcoal grill grate with grilling spray and heat to medium-high. Remove the chicken from the marinade. Grill the chicken, basting frequently with the marinade, for 5 to 10 minutes per side, or until no longer pink in the center when tested with a sharp knife. Slice into ½-inch strips. Discard any remaining marinade.

3 Transfer the reserved salad dressing to a blender and process for 15 seconds. Prepare the salad as directed and top with the peppers and chicken.

Makes 4 servings
Per serving: 4 grams fat • 239 calories

OR TRY THIS

Shrimp Caesar Salad

For a change, make this with shrimp instead of chicken. Use 1 pound cooked shrimp. If the shrimp are large, slice them in half lengthwise. The calories and fat are about the same.

Grilled Chicken Salad Véronique

30 minutes or less

For easier preparation, use leftover chicken and serve this main-meal salad cold. Replace the grilled onions with sliced sweet onion.

2   boneless, skinless chicken breasts cut in half and trimmed of fat

2   sweet onions, peeled and cut into 8 wedges each

½   cup Balsamic Mustard Dressing (page 332) or fat-free balsamic vinaigrette

8   cups mixed salad greens

2   cups seedless grapes

½   cup tightly packed fresh basil

1 Lightly coat a gas or charcoal grate with grilling spray and heat to medium-high. Brush the chicken and onions with 2 tablespoons of the dressing. Grill the chicken over indirect heat, turning once, for 6 to 7 minutes per side, or until no longer pink when tested with a sharp knife. Grill the onions over indirect heat for 3 to 5 minutes per side, or until soft. Cut the chicken into ½-inch slices.

2 In a large bowl, toss together the greens, grapes, basil, and the remaining dressing. Serve topped with the chicken and onions.

Makes 4 servings
Per serving: 2 grams fat • 204 calories

Roasted Chicken Salad with Raspberry Vinaigrette

30 minutes or less • prepare ahead

Here's an easy make-ahead recipe for leftover chicken or turkey.

½ cup bottled fat-free raspberry vinaigrette dressing
8 cups mixed baby salad greens
1 pound skinless and cooked chicken, cut into bite-size pieces
1 can (11 ounces) mandarin oranges, drained

In a large bowl, toss ¼ cup of the dressing with the greens until well coated. Top with the chicken and orange segments. Drizzle with the remaining ¼ cup dressing.

Makes 4 servings
Per serving: 4 grams fat • 259 calories

Grilled Shrimp with Corn-and-Tomato Salad

30 minutes or less • prepare ahead

This main-dish salad is best in summer, when you can cut the corn from the cob. It makes a wonderfully light and special supper.

- ¼ cup olive oil
- 2 cups corn kernels
- 1 pint cherry tomatoes, cut in half
- 1 small red onion, thinly sliced
- 2 tablespoons chopped fresh parsley
- 1 tablespoon chopped fresh chives
- 1 pound large shrimp, peeled and deveined
- 1 tablespoon fresh lemon juice
- 6 cups watercress

1 Warm 1 teaspoon of the oil in a large nonstick skillet over high heat. Add the corn and cook, stirring, for 2 minutes, or until softened. Transfer to a large bowl and let cool. Stir in the tomatoes, onion, parsley, chives, and 2 tablespoons of the remaining oil. Season with salt and pepper.

2 Coat a gas or charcoal grill grate with grilling spray and heat to medium-high. In a large bowl, mix the shrimp and the remaining oil. Grill the shrimp, turning once, for 3 minutes, or until pink and curled. Transfer to a clean bowl and stir in the lemon juice.

3 Line a serving platter with the watercress. Top with the shrimp and the corn mixture. Serve while the shrimp is still hot.

Makes 6 servings
Per serving: 11 grams fat • 228 calories

Warm Potato and Tuna Salad

30 minutes or less • prepare ahead

Colorful veggies dress up everyday canned tuna for this salad.

- 2 medium red potatoes, quartered
- ¼ pound green beans
- 2 cups baby spinach
- 1 can (6 ounces) tuna packed in water, drained and flaked
- 2 tablespoons bottled pesto
- 8 cherry tomatoes, cut in half

1 Bring a medium saucepan of salted water to a boil over high heat and add the potatoes. Cook for 5 minutes. Add the beans to the potatoes and cook for 3 minutes, or until the potatoes are tender when tested with a sharp knife. Drain and place in a large bowl. Add the spinach and toss with tongs until slightly wilted.

2 In a small bowl, mix the tuna and pesto. Serve the tuna over the potato mixture. Sprinkle with the tomatoes.

Makes 2 servings
Per serving: 8 grams fat • 307 calories

Field Greens with Pears and Walnuts

30 minutes or less

Pears jass up this accent for a low-fat entrée. Make sure the pears are very ripe.

2	tablespoons walnut oil
1	tablespoon apple juice
1	tablespoon balsamic vinegar
½	teaspoon Dijon mustard
6	cups mixed salad greens
2	ripe Bartlett pears, thinly sliced
¼	cup chopped unsalted walnuts
2	ounces blue cheese, crumbled

1 In a small bowl, whisk together the oil, apple juice, vinegar, and mustard. Season with salt and pepper.

2 In a large bowl, mix the greens, pears, and walnuts. Drizzle with the dressing and toss until evenly coated. Sprinkle with the cheese.

Makes 6 servings
Per serving: 11 grams fat • 154 calories

 Tip The blue cheese adds 33 calories and 3 grams of fat. You can eliminate it, if desired, to save on fat and calories.

meatless

main meals

Autumn Bean and Squash Stew

prepare ahead • freeze

As with many stews, the flavors will be enhanced if you make it in advance and allow it to stand in the refrigerator overnight. An added bonus is quick dinner the next day.

1	large onion, peeled and thinly sliced
1	garlic clove, peeled and minced
1	tablespoon chili powder
1	teaspoon dried oregano
2	teaspoons oil
2	cups peeled, seeded, and chopped tomatoes
4	cups fat-free vegetable broth
1½	cups cubed butternut squash
1	green sweet pepper, cored, seeded, and finely chopped
1	cup corn kernels
1	can (16 ounces) pinto beans, rinsed and drained

1 In a large ovenproof pot, cook the onion, garlic, chili powder, and oregano in the oil over medium heat for 5 minutes. Add the tomatoes and cook for 5 minutes.

2 Add the broth, squash, and sweet pepper; bring to a simmer.

3 Cover and bake at 375°F for 45 minutes. Stir in the corn and beans. Bake, uncovered, for 15 minutes, or until the vegetables are tender. Let cool for 5 minutes.

4 Ladle about 1 cup of the stew into a blender and process until smooth. Stir back into the pot. If the stew isn't thick enough, blend more of the mixture.

Makes 6 servings
Per serving: 5 grams fat • 245 calories

Texas-Style Stuffed Peppers

prepare ahead

Meat-loving Texans consider this a side dish, but it makes a great low-fat, high-fiber vegetarian entrée. Serve with a green salad.

4   large red sweet peppers
4   scallions, minced
1   garlic clove, peeled and minced
1   tablespoon oil
2   medium tomatoes, seeded and chopped
1   jalapeño pepper, seeded and thinly sliced
2   tablespoons minced fresh parsley
1   teaspoon dried oregano
1   teaspoon ground cumin
2   cups corn kernels
1   cup rinsed and drained canned black beans
1   can (4 ounces) tomato sauce
2   tablespoons grated Parmesan cheese

1 Cut the tops off the sweet peppers at the widest part. Remove the seeds and inner membranes, making sure not to pierce the peppers. Steam the peppers in a large steaming basket for about 3 minutes, or until slightly soft. Cool.

2 In a large skillet, cook the scallions, garlic, and oil over medium heat for 4 minutes, or until soft.

3 Add the tomatoes, jalapeño pepper, parsley, oregano, and cumin. Bring to a boil and cook, stirring frequently, for 10 minutes, or until the mixture has thickened.

4 Add the corn, partially cover, and simmer about 5 minutes. Stir in the beans and continue to simmer another 5 minutes. Cool for 5 minutes.

5 Preheat oven to 400°F. Divide the stuffing among the peppers. Stand upright in a baking dish just large enough to hold the peppers. Top with the tomato sauce and cheese. Bake for 20 minutes, or until heated through.

Makes 4 servings
Per serving: 6 grams fat • 242 calories

Grilled Vegetables with Garlic Vinaigrette

30 minutes or less

3   medium eggplants, cut into ½-inch slices
3   medium zucchini, cut into ½-inch slices
2   large red sweet peppers, cored, seeded, and cut into chunks
12 large mushrooms
2   medium russet potatoes, peeled and cut into 1-inch chunks
1   tablespoon oil
2   tablespoons Roasted Garlic Puree (page 327)
1   tablespoon balsamic vinegar
1   tablespoon grated Parmesan cheese

1 Coat a gas or charcoal grill grate with grilling spray and heat to medium-high. Brush the vegetables with the oil. Place the potatoes in an oiled hinged grilling basket and grill for approximately 5 to 8 minutes, until soft but not yet brown.

2 Add the balance of the vegetables to the basket; grill for 4 to 5 minutes per side, or until tender.

3 In a large bowl, mix the garlic puree and vinegar, and a few drop of water as needed. Add the vegetables, sprinkle with the cheese, and toss to combine.

Makes 4 servings
Per serving: 6 grams fat • 294 calories

 Try this dish roasted instead of grilled. Line a roasting pan with foil or spray it with cooking spray. Add the vegetables in one layer and drizzle them with the oil and vinegar. Bake at 350°F for about 50 minutes. Sprinkle with cheese, toss to combine.

Cheddar-Stuffed Acorn Squash

prepare ahead

Acorn squash is available in markets year-round. Its tough outer skin can be hard to cut through, so be careful—make sure you have a sharp knife and a steady surface to work on.

2	large acorn squash
1	tablespoon oil
½	cup finely chopped onion
½	cup finely chopped celery
2	garlic cloves, peeled and minced
1	cup fresh bread crumbs
¼	cup unsalted sunflower seeds
¼	cup raisins
2	tablespoons fresh lemon juice
½	teaspoon dried sage
½	teaspoon dried thyme
½	cup shredded low-fat cheddar cheese

1 Cut the squash in half lengthwise. Scoop out and discard the seeds. Coat a 13 × 9-inch baking dish with nonstick cooking spray. Add the squash, cut sides up.

2 Warm the oil in a large nonstick skillet over medium heat. Add the onion, celery, and garlic; cook for 5 minutes, or until soft.

3 Stir in bread crumbs, sunflower seeds, raisins, lemon juice, sage, and thyme; cook for 1 minute. Remove from the heat and stir in the cheese. Season with salt and pepper.

4 Heap the stuffing into the squash cavities. Bake at 350°F for 30 minutes, or until the squash is tender when tested with a sharp knife.

Makes 2 servings
Per serving: 9 grams fat • 420 calories

Moroccan Vegetable Stew

prepare ahead

This spicy dish is fun to make for a crowd. If you are making it ahead, reheat it gently.

½ teaspoon ground cinnamon
½ teaspoon ground cumin
½ teaspoon ground ginger
½ teaspoon sweet paprika
1 container (32 ounces) fat-free chicken broth
   Pinch of saffron
2 medium white potatoes, cut into wedges
4 turnips, peeled and cut into wedges
4 parsnips, peeled and cut into thick slices
4 medium carrots, shaved and cut into thick slices
2 rutabagas, peeled and cut into thick slices
2 large zucchini, cut into thick slices
2 cups couscous
1 can (16 ounces) chickpeas, rinsed and drained
½ cup raisins

1 In a cup, mix the cinnamon, cumin, ginger, and paprika. Pour the broth into the base of a steamer. Add the saffron and 1 teaspoon of the spice mixture. Bring to a simmer.

2 In a steamer basket, combine the potatoes, turnips, parsnips, carrots, and rutabagas. Cover and cook for 15 minutes, or until the vegetables are easily pierced with a knife. Add the zucchini and simmer for 5 minutes. Transfer the vegetables to a bowl.

3 Measure out 2 cups of the broth from the steamer and place in a medium saucepan. Bring to a boil, remove from the heat, and stir in the couscous. Cover and set aside for 10 minutes, or until the liquid is absorbed. Fluff with a fork.

4 Meanwhile, add the chickpeas and raisins to the broth remaining in the steamer. Add the remaining spice mixture. Bring to a simmer.

5 Spoon the couscous onto a large platter and make a well in the middle. Fill the well with the steamed vegetables. Scatter the chickpea mixture on top.

Makes 8 servings
Per serving: 2 grams fat • 408 calories

Vegetarian Chili

prepare ahead • freeze

This is good at any meal, even breakfast! And it's a great source of fiber.

2   cups finely chopped onions
2   cups finely chopped celery
2   cups finely chopped carrots
1   green sweet sweet pepper, cored, seeded, and finely chopped
4   garlic cloves, minced
2   tablespoons oil
2   tablespoons all-purpose flour
1   tablespoon chili powder
4   cups crushed tomatoes
1   cup corn kernels
2   cups fat-free vegetable or chicken broth
1   can (16 ounces) black beans, rinsed and drained

1 In a large pot, cook the onions, celery, carrots, pepper, and garlic in the oil over medium heat for 10 minutes, or until tender. Stir in the flour and chili powder.

2 Add the tomatoes, corn, and broth. Cover and simmer for 15 minutes. Add the beans and cook, uncovered, for 15 minutes, or until the vegetables are tender and the liquid has thickened.

Makes 6 servings
Per serving: 7 grams fat • 267 calories

Tomato and Zucchini Gratin with Rice

prepare ahead

Serve with a slice of crusty Italian bread, Roasted Garlic Puree (page 327), and a fresh green salad.

2	cups cooked rice
2	large tomatoes, thinly sliced
2	medium zucchini, thinly sliced
1	large red onion, peeled and thinly sliced
½	cup packed fresh basil, coarsely chopped
½	teaspoon garlic salt
¼	teaspoon ground black pepper
¼	cup grated Parmesan cheese
½	cup fat-free chicken broth
½	cup fresh bread crumbs

1 Coat a 1½-quart casserole dish with nonstick cooking spray. Spread half of the rice in the dish. Top with half of the tomatoes, zucchini, and onion. Sprinkle with half of the basil, salt, pepper, and cheese. Repeat to use the remaining rice, vegetables, basil salt, pepper, and cheese.

2 Pour the broth over the top and sprinkle with the bread crumbs. Bake at 375°F for 30 minutes, or until the vegetables are soft.

Makes 2 servings
Per serving: 5 grams fat • 380 calories

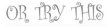

OR TRY THIS

Tomato and Zucchini Gratin

Omit the rice from this dish and you have a delicious low-fat, low-calorie side dish. At only 126 calories and 3 grams of fat per serving, it is a great way to fill out a meal without going over your fat balance.

Mac and Cheese

prepare ahead • freeze

This is a reduced-fat version of the traditional dish, good for those times when you're really hankering for comfort food. Serve with a large green salad and a zero-fat dressing.

8 ounces elbow macaroni
½ cup all-purpose flour
3 cups light (1%) milk
5 ounces reduced-fat cheddar cheese, shredded
½ cup grated Parmesan cheese
¼ teaspoon grated nutmeg
¼ teaspoon salt
¼ teaspoon ground black pepper
⅛ teaspoon cayenne pepper
3 tablespoons dry bread crumbs
¼ teaspoon sweet paprika

1 Cook the macaroni according to the package directions. Drain and return to the pot; set aside.

2 Place the flour in a medium saucepan and slowly whisk in ½ cup of the milk until smooth. Whisk in the remaining milk. Cook over medium heat, whisking often, for 10 minutes, or until the sauce thickens.

3 Remove the sauce from the heat and stir in the cheddar, Parmesan, nutmeg, salt, black pepper, and cayenne. Stir until the cheese is melted and the sauce is smooth. Pour over the macaroni in the pot and stir to coat.

4 Coat a 9 × 9-inch baking dish with nonstick cooking spray. Add the macaroni mixture. Sprinkle with bread crumbs and paprika. Bake at 375°F for 30 minutes, or until sauce is bubbling and the crumbs are lightly browned.

Makes 4 servings
Per serving: 9 grams fat • 368 calories

Spinach-Stuffed Mushrooms

30 minutes or less • prepare ahead

You can serve these one per person as a first course or as finger food for a party. Use smaller mushrooms to serve as hors d'oeuvres.

16	large mushrooms
½	cup minced onion
1	teaspoon oil
1	package (10 ounces) frozen chopped spinach, thawed and drained
1	cup 1% fat dry-curd cottage cheese
2	tablespoons crumbled blue cheese
1	tablespoon soy sauce
½	teaspoon dried tarragon
½	teaspoon dried rosemary

1 Remove the stems from the mushrooms and chop finely. Place in a large nonstick skillet and add the onion and oil. Cook over medium heat for 3 minutes, or until soft.

2 Remove from the heat and stir in the spinach, cottage cheese, blue cheese, soy sauce, tarragon, and rosemary. Season with salt and pepper to taste. Divide the filling among the mushroom caps.

3 Cover a baking sheet with foil and coat with nonstick cooking spray. Place the mushrooms on the sheet and bake at 400°F for 20 minutes, or until the mushrooms are soft.

Makes 4 servings
Per serving: 3 grams fat • 113 calories

Grilled Marinated Eggplant

30 minutes or less • prepare ahead

This dish can also be prepared under the broiler. Serve with a big green salad or Classic Spinach Salad.

½ cup soy sauce

⅓ cup dry sherry

¼ cup packed dark brown sugar

¼ cup unseasoned rice vinegar

2 tablespoons vegetable or canola oil

1 tablespoon ground ginger

2 garlic cloves, peeled and minced

2 large eggplants, cut into ½-inch slices

1 recipe tomato-pepper salsa (page 316)

1 In a small bowl, mix the soy sauce, sherry, brown sugar, vinegar, oil, ginger, and garlic.

2 Place the eggplant slices in a shallow glass or ceramic dish and pour the soy sauce mixture over them, making sure the slices are well coated. Marinate at room temperature for 1 hour.

3 Coat a gas or charcoal grill grate with grilling spray and heat to medium-high. Remove the eggplant from the marinade. Grill for 5 minutes on each side over indirect heat. Serve topped with the salsa.

Makes 4 servings
Per serving: 4 grams fat • 178 calories

Sesame Fried Tofu

30 minutes or less

Sauteing tofu gives it robust flavor and texture. Two kinds of sesame seeds add visual appeal, but you can use all white seeds if black aren't available.

1	pound firm tofu, drained
2	large egg whites, lightly beaten
¼	teaspoon salt
3	tablespoons dry bread crumbs
2	tablespoons white sesame seeds
1	tablespoon black sesame seeds
¼	teaspoon toasted sesame oil
12	scallions, cut into 1-inch pieces

1 Cut the tofu crosswise into 12 slices and drain well on several layers of paper towels. Working in batches, place the tofu in a large nonstick skillet and cook over medium-high heat for 5 minutes on each side. The tofu will brown slightly and lose some of its liquid. Transfer to a plate and cool.

2 In a shallow bowl, whisk together the egg whites and salt. On a large plate, mix the bread crumbs and sesame seeds.

3 Dip each tofu slice into the egg whites and then into the sesame seeds.

4 Warm the oil in a large nonstick skillet over medium heat. Working in batches, cook the tofu for 3 minutes per side, or until lightly browned. Transfer to a plate and keep warm. Add the scallions to the skillet and cook for 3 minutes, or until beginning to brown. Serve the tofu topped with the scallions.

Makes 4 servings
Per serving: 8 grams fat • 167 calories

Grilled Tofu Burgers

prepare ahead

A flavorful soy sauce marinade turns plain tofu into savory burgers. Be sure to use firm tofu so it holds together on the grill.

2	packages (16 ounces each) firm tofu
¼	cup soy sauce
¼	cup dry red wine
¼	cup rice vinegar
2	tablespoons toasted sesame oil
1	tablespoon oil
1	tablespoon hot chili oil
1	tablespoon chopped garlic
6	steak rolls

1 Drain the tofu and cut into six 1½-inch slices. To remove excess moisture from the tofu, line a baking sheet with several layers of paper towels, add the tofu in a single layer, and top with more paper towels. Cover with a second baking sheet and a few heavy canned items; let stand for 1 to 2 hours. Transfer the tofu to a glass or ceramic dish.

2 In a small bowl, mix the soy sauce, wine, vinegar, oils, and garlic. Pour over the tofu, cover, and marinate in the refrigerator overnight.

3 Coat a gas or charcoal grill grate with grilling spray and heat to medium-high. Remove the tofu from the marinade. Grill over indirect heat, basting frequently with the soy sauce mixture, for 12 to 15 minutes, or until lightly browned on both sides.

4 Toast the rolls on the grill for 30 seconds. Serve the tofu on the rolls.

Makes 6 servings
Per serving: 8 grams fat • 137 calories (for burger)
Per serving: 10 grams fat • 304 calories (for burger and roll)

Portobello Burgers

30 minutes or less

Portobello mushrooms offer a unique taste alternative to beef.

> 4 large portobello mushrooms
> 4 hamburger rolls
> 4 lettuce leaves
> 4 tomato slices
> ½ cup Chile Mayonnaise (page 328)

1 Coat a grill rack or broiler pan with nonstick cooking spray. Preheat the grill or broiler.

2 Coat the mushroom caps with cooking spray and season with salt and pepper. Grill or broil for 5 minutes per side, or until soft and tender.

3 Lightly toast the rolls on the grill or under the broiler. Serve the mushrooms on the rolls with the lettuce, tomatoes, and mayonnaise.

Makes 4 servings
Per serving: 5 grams fat • 194 calories

Pita Sandwiches to Go

Make low-calorie, low-fat brown bag lunches by mixing a medley of vegetables with one of the creamy low-fat salad dressings on pages 334–337. Open the top of a 6-inch whole wheat pita, tuck a lettuce leaf or other greens inside, and stuff with any of these vegetables, shredded or cut into bite-size pieces.

- Broccoli
- Celery
- Mushrooms
- Sprouts
- Zucchini
- Cabbage
- Cucumbers
- Radishes
- Red or green sweet peppers
- Carrots
- Green beans
- Scallions
- Tomatoes

Makes 1 serving
Per serving: 2 grams fat • 250 calories

Vegetarian Antipasto

30 minutes or less • prepare ahead

This dish is great party fare. You can assemble it a day ahead and add the dressing just before serving. The antipasto is best served at room temperature.

Dressing	3	tablespoons olive oil
	2	tablespoons balsamic vinegar
	2	tablespoons herb-infused vinegar, such as basil or thyme
	1½	tablespoons Italian seasoning
	¼	teaspoon sweet paprika

Antipasto	2	cups rinsed and drained canned red kidney beans
	1	cup rinsed and drained canned chickpeas
	1	large red onion, peeled and thinly sliced
	1	red sweet pepper
	1	green sweet pepper
	24	green beans
	3	large carrots, julienned
	1½	cups broccoli florets
	12	asparagus spears
	12	large mushrooms, stems removed
	1	head garlic from Roasted Garlic Puree (page 327), broken into cloves and peeled
	4	ounces part-skim mozzarella cheese, cut into cubes
	½	cup pitted black olives

1 For the dressing: In a small bowl, whisk together the oil, vinegars, and Italian seasoning. Season with salt and pepper.

2 For the antipasto: Place the kidney beans and chickpeas in a small bowl and add 2 tablespoons of the dressing. Toss to coat. Top with the onion slices. Cover and marinate at room temperature.

3 Broil the peppers, rotating until charred on all sides. Wrap the peppers in a damp dish towel and set aside for 5 minutes. Peel off the blackened skin. Cut into chunks.

4 Arrange the beans and carrots in a large steaming basket. Cover and steam for 4 to 5 minutes, or until crisp-tender. Rinse under cold water. Pat dry.

5 Arrange the broccoli florets in the steaming basket and steam for 2 to 3 minutes, or until crisp-tender. Rinse under cold water and pat dry.

6 Trim the woody ends from the asparagus and peel off the scales. Arrange in the steaming basket and steam for 3 to 5 minutes, or until crisp-tender. Rinse under cold water and pat dry.

7 When ready to serve, drain the marinade from the chickpea mixture and return the liquid to the bowl with the dressing.

8 Arrange the steamed vegetables and the mushrooms decoratively on a large platter. Remove the onion rings from the chickpeas; set aside. Scatter the chickpeas over the top. Whisk the dressing and drizzle over the vegetables.

9 Scatter the onion rings and garlic cloves over the vegetables. Top with the cheese and olives.

Makes 6 servings
Per serving: 13 grams fat • 319 calories

Mini Pizzas Two Ways

30 minutes or less • prepare ahead

Each version makes a quick lunch depending on the ingredients you have on hand. These pizzas also make great party snacks. For meal, serve with a salad on the side.

> 8 frozen mini bagels, thawed and cut in half
> Margherita Topping or Vegetable Topping

1 Line a baking sheet with foil and arrange the bagel halves, cut sides up, in a single layer. Bake at 375°F for 5 minutes.

2 Top the bagels as directed below and bake for 12 to 15 minutes, or until the cheese is melted and the pizzas are lightly browned around the edges.

Margherita Topping

> 1 cup tomato sauce
> 1 teaspoon dried Italian seasoning
> 4 ounces feta cheese, crumbled
> 1 cup chopped tomatoes
> 8 basil leaves, shredded

Spread the tomato sauce on the bagel halves and sprinkle with the Italian seasoning. Top with the cheese and tomatoes. Sprinkle with the basil.

Vegetable Topping

> 1 cup pizza sauce
> ⅔ cup soy cheese
> ¼ cup chopped red sweet pepper
> ¼ cup chopped green sweet pepper
> 8 large mushrooms, sliced
> ½ teaspoon dried oregano

Spread the pizza sauce on the bagel halves. Top with the cheese, peppers, and mushrooms. Sprinkle with the oregano.

Makes 4 servings
Per serving: 8 grams fat • 344 calories (with Margherita Topping)
Per serving: 5 grams fat • 291 calories (with Vegetable Topping)

Nachos

Just about everyone loves nachos, and there is no reason for you to give them up. This low-fat version can be lunch when you are in the mood for something sinful.

12	corn tortillas
1	can (16 ounces) pinto beans, rinsed and drained
1	red sweet pepper, cored, seeded, and minced
1	green sweet pepper, cored, seeded, and minced
4	scallions, chopped
½	cup shredded low-fat Monterey Jack cheese
1	cup Tomato-Pepper Salsa (page 316) or bottled low-fat salsa
3	jalapeño peppers, ribbed, seeded and minced
½	cup Guacamole (page 323)
½	cup fat-free sour cream

1 Preheat oven to 400°F. Cut the tortillas into quarters. Place the pieces in a single layer on a baking sheet and bake at 400°F for 5 minutes, or until crisp but not brown. Let cool for a few minutes.

2 Coarsely mash the beans. Spread the beans on the tortillas, making sure to leave a small edge for picking up the pieces. Sprinkle with the red and green peppers, scallions, and cheese. Bake for 5 minutes, or until the cheese melts.

3 Top with the salsa. Sprinkle with the jalapeños. Serve with the guacamole and sour cream on the side.

Makes 6 servings (2 tortillas per serving)
Per serving: 6 grams fat • 279 calories

succulent fish
& seafood

Caribbean Fish Stew

30 minutes or less • prepare ahead

Grouper is indigenous to the Caribbean but can often be found in many North American markets. If it's not available, substitute cod, flounder, halibut, or even crabmeat.

1	teaspoon oil
1	cup chopped onion
2	garlic cloves, peeled and minced
2	cups canned crushed tomatoes
1	cup clam juice
1	cup canned light coconut milk
1	cup water
½	teaspoon crushed saffron threads
¾	pound small red potatoes, peeled and cut into ½-inch cubes
½	pound grouper fillet, cut into cubes
½	pound red snapper fillet, cut into cubes
½	pound large shrimp, peeled and deveined
24	littleneck clams
1	fresh thyme sprig

1 Warm the oil in a large nonstick pot over medium heat. Add the onion and garlic; cook for 5 minutes, or until soft.

2 Add the tomatoes, clam juice, coconut milk, water, saffron, and potatoes. Cook for 15 minutes, or until the potatoes are just tender.

3 Add the grouper, snapper, shrimp, clams, and thyme. Cover and cook for 5 minutes, or until the clams have opened and the shrimp have turned color. Discard the thyme sprig and any unopened clams.

Makes 6 servings
Per serving: 6 grams fat • 299 calories

Mussels Marinière

This is one of the most tasty low-fat French dishes. To remove the beards (fine threads) from the mussels, pull them with your fingers or gently tug on them with pliers.

- 3 pounds mussels, scrubbed and beards removed
- 2 cups white wine
- ½ cup chopped shallots
- 2 garlic cloves, sliced
- ½ cup chopped fresh parsley

1 Discard any mussels that do not close when you tap on them. Remove the beards just before cooking.

2 In a large saucepan, mix the wine, shallots, and garlic. Bring to a boil over high heat. Add the mussels, cover, and cook, shaking the pan periodically, for 8 to 10 minutes, or until the mussels open. Discard any that do not open. Remove the mussels from the pan with a slotted spoon and divide among individual shallow bowls.

3 Cook the wine mixture for 5 minutes, to reduce slightly. Add the parsley and pour over the mussels.

Makes 4 servings
Per serving: 2 grams fat • 164 calories

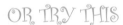
OR TRY THIS

Mussels Marinière over Pasta

You can add ½ cup of cooked pasta per person for no additional fat and a total of 264 calories.

Fisherman's Stew

30 minutes or less • prepare ahead

True fisherman's stew contains whatever happens to be the catch of the day.
This version takes advantage of low-calorie seafood.

1	tablespoon oil
2	cups chopped red onions
2	tablespoons chopped garlic
2	cups chopped tomatoes
1½	cups clam juice
1	cup fat-free chicken broth
1	cup tomato sauce
12	mussels, scrubbed and beards removed
12	clams, scrubbed
12	large shrimp, peeled and deveined
½	cup packed fresh basil, chopped
¼	cup chopped fresh oregano

1 Heat the oil in a large pot and add the onions and garlic. Cook, stirring often, for
5 minutes, or until the onions are soft. Stir in the tomatoes; cover and cook for
2 minutes. Stir in the clam juice, broth, and tomato sauce; bring to a boil. Cover,
reduce the heat, and simmer for 5 minutes. If the mixture becomes too thick, thin it
with broth or water.

2 Increase the heat to medium-high and add the mussels, clams, and shrimp. Cover
and cook, shaking the pot occasionally, until the mussels and clams open and the
shrimp is opaque, about 5 minutes. Discard any unopened mussels and clams. Add
the basil and oregano. Season with salt and pepper. Stir well.

Makes 4 servings
Per serving: 6 grams fat • 270 calories

Fish Sticks

30 minutes or less • prepare ahead

Everyone's favorite childhood dish is reborn in this version. Serve them with low-fat Tartar Sauce (page 330) or Hot-Hot Sauce (page 329). You can also form this recipe mix into little balls to serve as an appetizer or party fare.

1	pound cod or flounder fillets, cut into 2-inch pieces
2	tablespoons low-fat mayonnaise
½	teaspoon salt
¼	teaspoon ground black pepper
⅓	cup all-purpose flour
¼	cup egg substitute
1½	cups crushed baked potato chips
¼	cup grated Parmesan cheese
¼	teaspoon cayenne pepper

1 Place the fillets in a food processor and pulse to chop evenly. Transfer to a medium bowl and mix in the mayonnaise, salt, and pepper. Form the mixture into small rolls, about 4 × ½ inch.

2 Place the flour on a plate. Pour the egg substitute into a shallow bowl. In another shallow bowl, mix the potato chips, Parmesan, and cayenne.

3 Coat the fish sticks with the flour, shaking off the excess. Dip into the egg substitute and then roll in the potato chip mixture to coat completely.

4 Coat a baking sheet with nonstick cooking spray and arrange the fish sticks on the sheet, not touching. Bake at 400°F for 8 minutes. Turn and bake for 4 minutes more, or until golden brown.

Makes 12 sticks • Serving size: 3
Per serving: 8 grams fat • 261 calories

Crab Cakes with Red Pepper Sauce

30 minutes or less • prepare ahead

Even restaurants are forgoing the traditional deep-fry method of cooking crab cakes. Sauteing the patties in only a small amount of fat allows the natural sweetness of the crab to come through.

1	large egg white
1	tablespoon fresh lemon juice
2	teaspoons Worcestershire sauce
1	teaspoon Old Bay seasoning
½	teaspoon dry mustard
2	tablespoons + ½ cup fat-free mayonnaise
1	pound lump crabmeat
1	cup fresh bread crumbs
2	roasted red sweet peppers
1	tablespoon oil or butter

1 In a medium bowl, whisk together the egg white, lemon juice, Worcestershire, Old Bay, mustard, and 2 tablespoons of the mayonnaise. Stir in the crab and bread crumbs. Form into 4 patties.

2 Place the peppers in a food processor or blender and process until chopped. Add the remaining ½ cup mayonnaise and puree. Transfer to a small bowl and season with salt and pepper.

3 Warm the oil or butter in a large nonstick skillet over medium-high heat. Add the crab patties and cook for 3 minutes a side, or until golden brown. Serve with the pepper mixture.

Makes 4 servings
Per serving: 6 grams fat • 231 calories

PHASE **1**

You can make this recipe during Phase 1 by cooking the crab cakes in a nonstick skillet coated with nonstick cooking spray. The cakes will be a little drier, but you will cut the calories by 30 and cut the grams of fat in half.

Sweet and Spicy Shrimp

30 minutes or less

Chinese mustard is very hot. To cool this dish, you can substitute a creamy mustard, such as Dijon. If you use milder mustard, skip the water.

1	pound large shrimp, peeled and deveined
1½	teaspoons olive oil
2	tablespoons minced shallots
1	tablespoon minced fresh ginger
1	tablespoon minced garlic
2	cups diced tomatoes
2	teaspoons water
1	teaspoon Chinese mustard
¼	cup rice vinegar
2	tablespoons honey

1 Place the shrimp in a large bowl. Drizzle with the oil, season with salt and pepper, and toss to coat.

2 Coat a large nonstick skillet with cooking spray and place over medium-high heat for 1 minute. Add the shallots and ginger; cook for 3 minutes. Add the garlic; cook for 1 minute. Stir in the tomatoes and cook for 3 minutes, or until softened.

3 In a cup, mix the water and mustard. Add to the skillet. Stir in the vinegar and honey. Cook for 2 minutes, or until the sauce is reduced and thickened.

4 Add the shrimp. Cook for 3 minutes, or until the shrimp are opaque.

Makes 4 servings
Per serving: 3 grams fat • 180 calories

Sizzlin' Shrimp with Black-Eyed Peas

30 minutes or less • prepare ahead

This is the type of dish you'd find in tiny family-run cafes in the Caribbean.

1	tablespoon oil
½	teaspoon chili powder
⅛	teaspoon ground cinnamon
20	large shrimp, peeled and deveined
1	small red onion, peeled and finely chopped
1	red chile pepper, sliced, ribbed, seeded, and finely chopped
1	garlic clove, peeled and finely chopped
1	tablespoon honey
3	tablespoons fresh lime juice
3	tablespoons fresh lemon juice
1	can (16 ounces) black-eyed peas, rinsed and drained

1 In a medium bowl, mix the oil, chili powder, and cinnamon. Add the shrimp, stir, and let stand at room temperature for 1 hour or refrigerate for up to 4 hours.

2 In another medium bowl, mix the onion, pepper, garlic, honey, and lime and lemon juices. Stir in the black-eyed peas.

3 Place a large nonstick skillet over medium-high heat until hot. Add the shrimp and cook for 4 minutes per side, or until the shrimp have changed color. Serve with the black-eyed peas.

Makes 4 servings
Per serving: 5 grams fat • 183 calories

Shrimp Salad Sandwiches

30 minutes or less • prepare ahead

This is great for lunch when you have leftover shrimp. The dressing is a nice accent to lobster and crab as well. For extra fiber, use whole wheat pitas.

⅓   cup fat-free sour cream
3   tablespoons mango chutney
2   tablespoons fat-free mayonnaise
½   pound cooked shrimp, coarsely chopped
½   cup sliced celery
⅓   cup sliced scallions
⅓   cup currants
4   whole wheat pita breads
4   romaine lettuce leaves

1 In a medium bowl, mix the sour cream, chutney, and mayonnaise. Add the shrimp, celery, scallions, and currants; toss to mix well. Refrigerate for 15 minutes.

2 Slice about one-third from the top of each pita. Insert a lettuce leaf in each and fill with the shrimp salad.

Makes 4 servings
Per serving: 2 grams fat • 214 calories

Tuna Noodle Casserole

prepare ahead • freeze

This comfort food is lightened up with low-fat mushroom soup and just a sprinkling of high-flavor cheese.

> 1 cup macaroni
> 1 cup chopped celery
> ⅓ cup chopped onion
> 1 can (10¾ ounces) low-fat condensed cream of mushroom soup
> ¾ cup evaporated fat-free milk
> 1 can (9¼ ounces) white albacore tuna packed in water, drained
> 2 tablespoons grated low-fat Parmesan cheese

1 Cook the macaroni according to the package directions. Drain and return to the pot.

2 Coat a large saucepan with nonstick cooking spray and place over medium heat for 1 minute. Add the celery and onion; cook for 3 minutes. Stir in the soup and milk. Cook for 2 minutes, or until heated through. Stir in the tuna and macaroni.

3 Coat a 1½-quart casserole dish with cooking spray. Add the macaroni mixture and sprinkle with the cheese. Bake at 350°F for 25 to 30 minutes, or until bubbling.

Makes 4 servings
Per serving: 4 grams fat • 262 calories

Chili-Spiced Tuna with Grilled Tomato Sauce

30 minutes or less • prepare ahead

The mango in this recipe is used as a garnish, but the flavor is a nice complement to the tuna for a taste of the tropics.

Tomato Sauce	2	large ripe tomatoes (about 2 pounds), sliced ½ inch thick
	1	tablespoon oil
	¼	cup chopped fresh cilantro
	¼	cup fresh lime juice

Spice Rub	1½	teaspoons cumin seeds
	½	teaspoon coriander seeds
	1	tablespoon packed brown sugar
	1	tablespoon coarse salt
	½	teaspoon chili powder
	½	teaspoon ground cinnamon

Tuna	4	tuna steaks (about 4 ounces each), 1 inch thick
	1	teaspoon olive oil
	1	ripe mango, peeled and sliced (optional)

1 For the tomato sauce: Lightly coat gas or charcoal grill grate with grilling spray and heat to medium-high. Brush the tomato slices lightly with oil and grill over indirect heat until soft, about 3 minutes, turning frequently.

2 Mash the tomatoes in a bowl and mix in the cilantro, lime juice, and the remaining oil.

3 For the spice rub: Toast the cumin and coriander seeds in a skillet for 2 minutes, shaking the pan constantly. Transfer to a small food processor and process to a coarse powder. Add the sugar, salt, chili powder, and cinnamon. Process again. Rub tuna with the spice rub and let stand until the tuna reaches room temperature.

4 For the tuna: Lightly brush the tuna steaks with oil. Over indirect heat, grill for 3 minutes on each side for medium rare or longer to reach desired doneness.

5 Divide the tomato sauce among 4 plates. Top with the tuna. Serve with the mango.

Makes 4 servings
Per serving: 6 grams fat • 260 calories

Hot Grilled Tuna Kabobs

30 minutes or less • prepare ahead

Be careful! Wasabi paste is hot, so adjust accordingly if you are sensitive to the heat.

1	pound fresh tuna steak, cut into 1-inch cubes
½	cup oil
2	tablespoons toasted sesame oil
¼	cup soy sauce
3	tablespoons unseasoned rice vinegar
3	tablespoons peeled and minced fresh ginger
2	tablespoons minced garlic
3	scallions, chopped
¼	cup chopped fresh cilantro
6	large mushrooms, stemmed and quartered
1	large red sweet pepper, cored, seeded, and chopped into 1½-inch pieces
1	large red onion, peeled and chopped into 1½-inch pieces
1	tablespoon wasabi paste
2 to 4	tablespoons water

1 Place the tuna in a glass or ceramic dish. In a small bowl, mix the oils, soy sauce, vinegar, ginger, garlic, scallions, and cilantro. Pour over the tuna, mix, cover, and marinate in the refrigerator for 2 to 3 hours. Bring to room temperature.

2 Remove the tuna from the marinade, reserving the marinade.

3 Thread 8 skewers with tuna, mushrooms, pepper, and onion, alternating the tuna and vegetables.

4 In a cup, mix wasabi, water, and ¼ cup of the marinade; discard remaining marinade.

5 Lightly coat a gas or charcoal grill grate with grilling spray and heat to medium-high. Grill, brushing with the wasabi mixture, for 3 to 4 minutes on each side, or until the tuna is done as desired.

Makes 4 servings
Per serving: 10 grams fat • 236 calories

Cod and Tomato Stew

30 minutes or less • prepare ahead

Fresh fish and good-quality tomatoes are essential to make this easy dish a standout recipe, which is a traditional, deeply flavorful Portuguese way to enjoy the sea's freshest catch.

1¼	pound cod fillet, skin removed
2	tablespoons all-purpose flour
2	teaspoons olive oil
1	cup finely chopped onion
1	pound ripe tomatoes, coarsely chopped
2	teaspoons soy sauce
1	teaspoon chopped fresh oregano or ½ teaspoon dried oregano

1 Cut the cod into 1-inch pieces and lightly coat the pieces with the flour, shaking off the excess.

2 Warm the oil in a large nonstick skillet over high heat. Add the cod and onion; cook, turning the pieces often, until the fish turns opaque and browns.

3 Reduce heat to medium. Add the tomatoes, soy sauce, and oregano. Season with salt and pepper. Cover and simmer for 5 minutes, or until tomatoes are heated through.

Makes 4 servings
Per serving: 3 grams fat • 166 calories

Grilled Marinated Swordfish

30 minutes or less • prepare ahead

This succulent fish is perfect topped with any of the salsas on pages 314 to 319.

2	teaspoons grated lime zest
1	teaspoon grated orange zest
¼	cup fresh lime juice
⅓	cup fresh orange juice
1	small onion, peeled and chopped
1	garlic clove, peeled and minced
1	teaspoon olive oil
1	tablespoon honey
¼	teaspoon salt
½	teaspoon ground black pepper
4	swordfish fillets (4 ounces each)

1 In a bowl, mix the zests, juices, onion, and garlic. Stir in the oil, honey, salt, and pepper.

2 Place the fish in a resealable plastic bag and add the juice mixture. Turn to coat well. Marinate in the refrigerator for 1 hour. Bring to room temperature.

3 Lightly coat a gas or charcoal grill grate with grilling spray and heat to medium-high. Grill the swordfish, brushing frequently with the marinade, for 5 minutes a side, or until the fish is opaque and flakes easily when tested with a fork. Discard the remaining marinade.

Makes 4 servings
Per serving: 6 grams fat • 190 calories

Grilled Citrus-Scented Swordfish with Ginger

30 minutes or less • prepare ahead

Be sure not to include the bitter white pith of the citrus fruit when removing the zest. Wrap the fruit in plastic wrap and keep for another use.

⅔ cup soy sauce

¼ cup dry sherry

¼ cup orange juice

2 tablespoons oil

2 scallions, finely chopped

1 garlic clove, peeled and minced

2 teaspoons minced fresh ginger

1 teaspoon grated lemon zest

1 teaspoon grated orange zest

1 teaspoon grated lime zest

4 swordfish steaks (about 4 ounces each), cut 1 inch thick

1 In a shallow glass or ceramic dish, mix the soy sauce, sherry, orange juice, oil, scallions, garlic, ginger, and zests. Add the swordfish steaks, cover, and marinate for 1 to 4 hours in the refrigerator. Bring to room temperature.

2 Lightly coat a gas or charcoal grill grate with grilling spray and heat to high. Grill the swordfish steaks for 4 to 5 minutes on each side, or until cooked through. Discard the marinade.

Makes 4 servings
Per serving: 6 grams fat • 195 calories

Poached Salmon Two Ways

30 minutes or less • prepare ahead

Perfectly poached salmon is succulent in its own right, but these sauces offer a change of taste and a lot of additional flavor with just a speck of extra fat. Although nearly all the fat in these two recipes comes from the salmon itself, it is an important source of heart-healthy omega-3 fatty acids, so do make this a regular Phase 3 treat. Make the sauce the night before.

> 1 large center-cut salmon fillet (about 1 pound)
> 1 lemon, thinly sliced
> 1 bay leaf
> ½ teaspoon peppercorns
> 1 cup dry white wine
>   Water to cover
>   Dill Sauce or Balsamic Tomato Sauce

1 Cut the salmon into 4 equal pieces. Place in a deep skillet large enough to hold them in a single layer. Add the lemon, bay leaf, peppercorns, and wine. Add enough water to just cover the fish.

2 Bring to a simmer over high heat; do not boil. Reduce the heat to medium-low, cover, and simmer for 10 minutes, or until the fish flakes easily when tested with a sharp knife.

3 Remove the salmon from the liquid with a metal spatula and gently pat dry with paper towels. Serve with your choice of sauce.

Dill Sauce
> ½ cup fat-free sour cream
> ½ cup light (1%) milk
> 1 tablespoon chopped fresh dill
> ½ teaspoon sugar

1 In a small bowl, mix the sour cream and milk. Cover with plastic wrap and refrigerate until ready to use.

2 Stir in the dill and sugar. Season with salt and pepper. Refrigerate until cold.

Balsamic Tomato Sauce 1 can (14½ ounces) stewed tomatoes
1 tablespoon balsamic vinegar
1 teaspoon dried oregano

1 Place the tomatoes, vinegar, and oregano in a blender and process until smooth.

2 Transfer tomato mixture to a small saucepan, season with salt and pepper, and warm over medium heat.

Per serving: 13 grams fat • 249 calories (with Dill Sauce)
Per serving: 12 grams fat • 214 calories (with Balsamic Tomato Sauce)

 Chicken breasts can be poached in the same manner and served with the same sauces.

Pan-Seared Red Snapper with Olive Crust

30 minutes or less • prepare ahead

If red snapper isn't readily available, try sea bass, grouper, or rockfish.

¾ cup dried bread crumbs

1 tablespoon dried oregano

16 black olives, pitted and finely chopped

3 tablespoons grated Parmesan cheese

Ground black pepper

4 red snapper fillets (4 ounces each)

1 tablespoon oil

1 In a shallow bowl, mix the bread crumbs, oregano, olives, cheese, and pepper. Firmly press the fillets into the mixture to create a uniform coating on both sides. Refrigerate for about an hour to allow the crust to set.

2 Warm the oil in a large nonstick skillet over medium-high heat. Add the fillets and cook for 3 to 4 minutes on each side, or until the fish is opaque and flakes easily when tested with a fork.

Makes 4 servings
Per serving: 10 grams fat • 368 calories

Brook Trout with Tomato and Red Onion Relish

30 minutes or less

Brook trout has a clean, pristine taste much like the streams in which it lives.

2	cups cherry tomatoes, halved
1	teaspoon olive oil
1	cup chopped red onion
¼	cup balsamic vinegar
1	teaspoon molasses
1	tablespoon grated lemon zest
1	tablespoon chopped fresh parsley
1	teaspoon dried herbes de Provence
4	trout fillets (5 ounces each)

1 Line a baking sheet with foil and arrange the tomatoes, cut sides down, on the sheet. Broil the tomatoes about 4 inches from the heat for 5 minutes, or until the skins wrinkle and begin to brown. Set aside and leave the broiler on.

2 Warm the oil in a large nonstick skillet over medium-high heat. Add the onion and cook for 5 minutes, or until soft. Add the vinegar and molasses; bring to a boil. Reduce the heat to medium and simmer for 2 minutes, or until slightly reduced. Stir in the tomatoes, lemon zest, parsley, and herbes de Provence. Keep warm.

3 Lightly coat a broiler pan with nonstick cooking spray. Place the fillets on the pan and season with salt and pepper. Broil about 4 inches from the heat for 5 minutes, or until opaque and the fish flakes when tested with a fork. Serve topped with the warm tomato mixture.

Makes 4 servings
Per serving: 10 grams fat • 238 calories

Baked Halibut with Red Pepper and Parsley Crust

30 minutes or less

Halibut is a meaty, lean fish with a delicate taste. Feel free to substitute Chilean sea bass or salmon.

4 halibut fillets (about 4 ounces each)
1 red sweet pepper, cored, seeded, and finely chopped
1 cup chopped fresh parsley
1 tablespoon minced garlic
1 tablespoon olive oil
1 teaspoon Italian seasoning

1 Coat a large nonstick skillet with nonstick cooking spray. Place the pan over high heat for 1 minute. Add the halibut and cook for about 15 seconds per side, or until the pieces have a brown tinge.

2 Coat a 9 × 9-inch baking dish with cooking spray. Add the fish in a single layer and season with salt and pepper.

3 Preheat oven to 400°F. In a small bowl, mix the sweet pepper, parsley, garlic, oil, and Italian seasoning. Season with salt and pepper. Spoon over the fish and press into the flesh with the back of a spatula.

4 Bake at 400°F for 15 to 20 minutes, or until the fish flakes easily when tested with a fork.

Makes 4 servings
Per serving: 6 grams fat • 171 calories

Seared Scallops with Asparagus and Ginger

30 minutes or less

The soft, fleshy texture and delicate, sweet flavor of scallops are enjoyed by even those who are not particularly fond of fish.

1	pound asparagus spears
¾	cup fat-free chicken broth
1	tablespoon cornstarch
1	teaspoon soy sauce
12	ounces sea scallops, cut in half
1	cup sliced mushrooms, wiped clean
1	garlic clove, peeled and minced
1	teaspoon toasted sesame oil

1 Trim the woody ends from the asparagus and cut diagonally into 2-inch lengths. Bring 1 inch of water to a boil in a large saucepan over high heat. Add the asparagus, cover, and cook for 3 to 5 minutes, or until crisp-tender. Do not overcook. Drain and rinse under cold water.

2 In a bowl, mix the broth, cornstarch, and soy sauce until the cornstarch dissolves.

3 Place a large nonstick skillet over high heat until hot. Add the scallops, mushrooms, garlic, and sesame oil and cook, stirring, for 4 minutes, or until the scallops are opaque. Stir in the broth mixture and cook, stirring, until the sauce thickens and boils. Add the asparagus and season with salt and pepper. Cook for 5 minutes, or until heated through.

Makes 4 servings
Per serving: 2 grams fat • 122 calories

Seafood au Gratin

prepare ahead

This makes a light, creamy sauce rather than a thick, cheese-laden one that tends to overpower the delicate seafood.

2	tablespoons low-fat mayonnaise
2	tablespoons fat-free sour cream
2	tablespoons fresh lemon juice
1	tablespoon Dijon mustard
1	tablespoon dry vermouth
2	teaspoons oil
2	garlic cloves, peeled and chopped
1	pound peeled and deveined medium shrimp
12	ounces lump crabmeat
3	tablespoons all-purpose flour
1	can (15 ounces) evaporated fat-free milk
1	cup light (1%) milk
4	tablespoons grated Parmesan cheese
2	tablespoons dry bread crumbs
¼	teaspoon sweet paprika

1 In a large bowl, combine the mayonnaise, sour cream, lemon juice, mustard, and vermouth. Refrigerate.

2 Warm the oil in a large nonstick skillet over medium-high heat. Add the garlic; cook for 1 minute. Add the shrimp; cook, turning frequently, for 3 minutes, or until opaque. Transfer to the bowl with the mayonnaise mixture. Add the crab and stir.

3 Coat a 2-quart casserole with nonstick cooking spray. Add the shrimp mixture.

4 Place the flour in a small saucepan. Gradually whisk in the evaporated milk until smooth. Whisk in the light milk. Cook, stirring constantly, for 5 minutes, or until thickened. Whisk in 2 tablespoons of the cheese. Pour over the shrimp.

5 In a small bowl, mix the bread crumbs, paprika, and the remaining cheese. Sprinkle over the shrimp mixture. Bake at 350°F for 30 to 40 minutes.

Makes 6 servings
Per serving: 7 grams fat • 304 calories

Seafood Jambalaya

30 minutes or less • prepare ahead

Just about any kind of fish can be added to this well-known and versatile Creole dish, that features spices, okra, and a hot tang to the taste. The fat and calories in this dish are spared by eliminating high-fat sausage and other meat.

2	teaspoons oil
½	pound turkey sausage
1	cup chopped onion
½	cup chopped green sweet pepper
1	large celery rib, sliced
1	teaspoon minced garlic
4	cups fat-free chicken broth
1	can (6 ounces) tomato paste
1	teaspoon Creole spice mix
1	cup long grain white rice
1	teaspoon hot pepper sauce
½	pound okra, trimmed and coarsely chopped, or 1 package (15 ounces) frozen okra, thawed and chopped
½	pound large shrimp, peeled and deveined
½	pound scallops, cut in half
½ to 1	cup water

1 Warm 1 teaspoon of the oil in a large nonstick pot over medium heat. Add the sausage and cook, turning frequently, for 3 minutes, or until lightly browned. Cut into ½-inch slices. Set aside.

2 Add the remaining oil to the pot and stir in the onion, sweet pepper, celery, and garlic. Cook, stirring often, for 10 minutes. Stir in the broth, tomato paste, and spice mix and bring to a boil.

3 Stir in the rice and pepper sauce; bring back to a boil. Reduce the heat to medium, cover, and simmer for 15 minutes. Add the okra, shrimp, scallops, sausage, and ½ cup of the water. Cover and cook for 10 minutes, or until the rice is tender. Add more water, if needed.

Makes 6 servings
Per serving: 7 grams fat • 326 calories

Chilean Sea Bass en Papillote

30 minutes or less

This classic preparation keeps the fish moist and flavorful. It is easy to make and leaves almost nothing to clean up afterward. You can substitute halibut or any thick white fish for the sea bass.

½	teaspoon saffron threads
2	tablespoons hot water
4	Chilean sea bass fillets (each 5 ounces and 1 inch thick)
1	small tomato, diced
¼	cup diced onion
1	tablespoon olive oil
2	tablespoons white wine
1	tablespoon chopped fresh parsley
2	teaspoons chopped fresh thyme
¼	cup chopped almonds

1 Steep the saffron threads in the water for 5 minutes.

2 Cut parchment paper into four 15-inch squares. Place a fillet in the center of each square. Sprinkle with the tomato, onion, oil, wine, parsley, thyme, and saffron. Season with salt and pepper. Top with the almonds.

3 Fold the edges of each square over the fish and vegetables, crimping to seal each packet. Place the packets on a baking sheet. Bake at 375°F for 15 minutes, or until the fish is cooked and the packets start to brown.

4 Place the packets on plates. Slit each packet and fold open.

Makes 4 servings
Per serving: 11 grams fat • 222 calories

Lunch-Box Tuna Salad Sandwich

30 minutes or less • prepare ahead

A tuna salad sandwich is a lunch staple that can go off the charts for fat. Contain the fat and calories by making your own. Pile your sandwich high with crunchy fresh vegetables.

1	can (3 ounces) white albacore tuna, packed in water, drained
2	tablespoons diced celery
1	tablespoon shredded carrot
½	teaspoon celery salt
1	tablespoon fat-free mayonnaise
2	slices whole wheat bread
1	tomato slice
1	lettuce leaf
¼	cup bean sprouts

In a small bowl combine the tuna, celery, carrot, and celery salt. Fold in the mayonnaise and mix well. Serve on bread with tomato slice, lettuce leaf, and sprouts.

Makes 1 serving
Per serving: 7 grams fat • 287 calories

 You can use any bread equal to the fat and calories in the whole wheat bread: 70 calories and 1 gram fat per slice.

Tuna Burgers with Wasabi Mayonnaise

30 minutes or less

Fresh tuna is a must for a good-tasting burger, but you needn't splurge on sushi grade unless you plan on eating it raw.

½ cup reduced-calorie mayonnaise
½ tablespoon wasabi powder
2 pounds fresh tuna, coarsely chopped
1 garlic clove, chopped
1 tablespoon chopped fresh parsley
1 tablespoon chopped fresh cilantro
½ teaspoon cayenne pepper
2 tablespoons Dijon mustard
¼ cup bottled teriyaki sauce
6 hamburger rolls
Tomato slices
Onion slices

1 In a small bowl, mix the mayonnaise and wasabi. Allow to stand for 10 minutes at room temperature to develop the flavor.

2 In a medium bowl, mix the tuna, garlic, parsley, cilantro, cayenne, and 1 tablespoon of the mustard. Season with salt and pepper. Shape into 6 burgers.

3 Lightly coat a gas or charcoal grill grate with nonstick cooking spray. Heat the grill to medium-high. In a small bowl, mix the teriyaki sauce and the remaining 1 tablespoon mustard.

4 Grill the patties for 4 minutes. Turn and brush with the teriyaki mixture. Grill for 4 minutes more for medium-well-doneness.

5 Toast the rolls on the grill for 30 seconds. Serve the burgers on the rolls with the wasabi mayonnaise, tomatoes, and onions.

Makes 6 servings
Per serving: 7 grams fat • 245 calories (for burger)
Per serving: 9 grams fat • 365 calories (for burger and roll)

accent on

poultry

Chicken Fingers with Honey Mustard Sauce

prepare ahead • freeze

To freeze, bread the chicken, place in a single layer on a tray lined with parchment, and freeze until solid. Transfer to a heavy-duty plastic bag. Bake directly from the freezer, adding about 10 minutes to the oven time.

Chicken
½	cup all-purpose flour
1	cup fat-free egg substitute
1½	cups fresh bread crumbs
2	teaspoons Old Bay™ seasoning
1	teaspoon dried Italian herb seasoning
¼	teaspoon ground black pepper
1	pound boneless, skinless chicken breasts, cut into short strips, approximately 2 inches long

Sauce
¼	cup honey
2	tablespoons whole-grain mustard
2	tablespoons Dijon mustard

1 For the chicken: Place the flour in a shallow bowl. Place the egg substitute in a second shallow bowl. In a third shallow bowl, mix the bread crumbs, Old Bay, Italian seasoning, and pepper.

2 Coat the chicken strips first with the flour, then with the egg substitute, and finally with the crumb mixture. Place on a plate or a large sheet of waxed paper. Mist both sides of the chicken pieces with nonstick cooking spray. Refrigerate, uncovered, for 30 minutes to allow the breading to set. Bring to room temperature.

3 Coat a large nonstick skillet with cooking spray. Set over medium-high heat until hot. Place the chicken in the skillet in a single layer (work in batches, if necessary) and cook for 1 minute on each side, or until the crumbs are browned. Transfer the strips to a foil-lined baking sheet. Bake at 375°F for 12 to 15 minutes, or until the internal temperature of the chicken reaches 160°F and the meat is no longer pink in the center when sliced into with a sharp knife.

4 For the sauce: In a small bowl, mix the honey and mustards. Serve with the chicken.

Makes 4 servings
Per serving: 5 grams fat • 360 calories

Chicken Fajitas

Fajitas were originally made and eaten by ranch hands. This lower-fat version still delivers authentic Southwest flavors.

2	whole boneless, skinless chicken breasts, trimmed of fat
1½	teaspoons oil
1	large onion, peeled and cut into thin wedges
1	green sweet pepper, cored, seeded, and cut into strips
1	red sweet pepper, cored, seeded, and cut into thin strips
⅓	cup fat-free chicken broth
¼	cup fresh lime juice
2	tablespoons soy sauce
2	teaspoons honey
2	teaspoons cornstarch
1	teaspoon minced garlic
4	flour tortillas (8-inch diameter)
2	cups shredded lettuce
1	cup Guacamole (page 323)
1	cup Tomato-Pepper Salsa (page 316) or bottled low-fat salsa

1 Lightly coat a gas or charcoal grill grate with grilling spray and heat to medium-high. Grill the chicken, turning frequently, for 5 to 10 minutes per side, or until just cooked through. Slice crosswise into thin strips.

2 Warm the oil in a large nonstick skillet over medium heat. Add the onion and peppers. Cook, stirring, for 5 minutes, or until tender.

3 In a small bowl, mix the broth, lime juice, soy sauce, honey, cornstarch, and garlic until the cornstarch is dissolved. Add to the skillet and stir constantly for 1 to 2 minutes, or until slightly thickened. Add the chicken and stir until just warm.

4 Spoon the chicken mixture onto the tortillas. Top with the lettuce, guacamole, and salsa. Roll up the tortillas.

Makes 4 servings
Per serving: 12 grams fat • 438 calories

 Tip Authentic Mexican fajitas are served from the grill, but you can cut time by using leftover poultry or beef. Just sliver the meat and start with step 2 of the directions above.

Chicken Paprikash

prepare ahead

The quality of the paprika you use in this dish really does make a difference. Use a good Hungarian brand. Serve over plain rice.

- 1 tablespoon oil
- 4 bone-in chicken breast halves, skin removed and fat trimmed away
- 2 cups peeled and chopped onions
- 1 tablespoon sweet Hungarian paprika
- 1 cup fat-free chicken broth
- 2 teaspoons tomato paste
- ½ cup fat-free sour cream
- 1 tablespoon all-purpose flour
- ¼ cup chopped fresh parsley

1 Warm the oil in a large nonstick pot over high heat. Add the chicken and quickly sear on both sides. Transfer to a plate and season with salt and pepper.

2 Reduce the heat to medium and add the onions. Cook, stirring often, for 5 minutes, or until softened. Stir in the paprika and cook 5 minutes more. Return the chicken to the pot and stir well to coat with the onions. Cover and cook for 10 minutes.

3 Stir in the broth and tomato paste. Cover and cook for 20 minutes, or until the internal temperature of the chicken reaches 160°F and the meat is no longer pink in the center when sliced with a sharp knife. Transfer the chicken to a plate and keep warm.

4 In a small bowl, whisk together the sour cream and flour. Reduce the heat to low and whisk the sour cream mixture into the pot. Cook, stirring constantly, for 3 to 4 minutes, or until thickened and bubbling.

5 Return the chicken to the pot and cook for 2 minutes. Sprinkle with the parsley.

Makes 4 servings
Per serving: 6 grams fat • 239 calories

Grilled Margarita Chicken

30 minutes or less • prepare ahead

If you like Mexican food, you'll like the flavor of this chicken. The red pepper flakes give it the classic bite that it is not nearly as hot as a jalapeño. Add, subtract, or omit the hot peppers altogether according to your taste.

- ½ cup tequila
- ½ cup orange juice
- ¼ cup + 1 tablespoon fresh lime juice
- ¼ teaspoon red pepper flakes (optional)
- 2 boneless, skinless chicken breasts, split and trimmed of fat
- 1 avocado, peeled, pitted, and coarsely chopped
- 1 medium tomato, chopped
- 1 scallion, minced
- 1 small jalapeño pepper, ribbed, seeded, and minced

1 In a shallow glass or ceramic dish, mix the tequila, orange juice, ¼ cup of lime juice, and the pepper flakes (if using). Add the chicken, cover, and marinate overnight, turning once or twice.

2 In a small glass bowl, combine the avocado, tomato, scallion, jalapeño pepper, and the remaining 1 tablespoon of lime juice. Season with salt and pepper. Cover and refrigerate until ready to use.

3 Lightly coat a gas or charcoal grill grate with grilling spray and heat to high. Remove the chicken from the marinade. Grill, brushing frequently with the marinade, for 4 to 5 minutes on each side, or until cooked through. Discard any remaining marinade.

4 Serve each portion topped with 2 tablespoons of the avocado salsa.

Makes 4 servings
Per serving: 8 grams fat • 255 calories

Poached Chicken with Avocado Sauce

30 minutess or less

This sauce has the taste of guacamole without the excess calories and fat. Make it within a few hours of serving because avocados tend to darken and lose their flavor as time passes.

Chicken
- 1 can (14 ounces) fat-free chicken broth
- 1 bay leaf
- 1 garlic clove, peeled and crushed
- 1 small red onion, peeled and quartered
- 6 boneless, skinless chicken breast halves, trimmed of fat

Sauce
- 1 ripe avocado, pitted, peeled, and coarsely chopped
- ½ green sweet pepper, cored, seeded, and coarsely chopped
- 1 small red onion, peeled and coarsely chopped
- 2 garlic cloves, peeled and halved
- ½ cup chopped fresh cilantro
- 1 tablespoon white vinegar
- ½ cup water

1 For the chicken: In a large skillet, bring the broth, bay leaf, garlic, and onion to a simmer over medium heat. Simmer for 5 minutes. Season the chicken with salt and pepper. Add the chicken to the skillet, cover, and cook for 10 minutes, or until firm and the juices run clear when tested with a fork.

2 Transfer the chicken to a plate and keep warm. Strain the broth and reserve for another use.

3 For the sauce: In a food processor, blend the avocado, sweet pepper, onion, garlic, cilantro, vinegar, and water until smooth. Season with salt and pepper. Serve with the chicken.

Makes 6 servings
Per serving: 6 grams fat • 192 calories

Sauteed Chicken with Cider Sauce

30 minutes or less

Serve with cooked carrots or, for a one-dish meal, add a small can of drained cooked carrots with the chicken in step 4.

    1   tablespoon olive oil
    4   boneless, skinless chicken breast halves, trimmed of fat
    2   small onions, peeled and cut into wedges
    2   green apples, peeled, cored, and cut into wedges
    1   cup apple cider
    ½   cup fat-free chicken broth

1 Warm the oil in a large nonstick skillet over medium-high heat. Add the chicken and cook for 4 minutes on each side. Remove from the skillet and set aside.

2 Add the onions and apples to the pan; cook for 5 minutes, or until golden.

3 Raise the heat to high and pour in the cider. Bring to a boil and cook until slightly reduced. Add the broth, stirring to scrape any browned bits from the bottom of the skillet, and bring to a boil.

4 Reduce the heat and return the chicken to the skillet. Cover and simmer for 5 minutes, or until the chicken is cooked through. Transfer the chicken to serving plates.

5 Turn the heat to high and boil the sauce until it thickens slightly, about 3 to 4 minutes. Spoon the sauce over the chicken.

Makes 4 servings
Per serving: 5 grams fat • 251 calories

Oven-Fried Chicken

30 minutes or less

This chicken bakes as crispy and juicy as the deep-fried Southern version but with a lot less fat. Cornflakes add the crunch and a lot of flavor.

¼ cup all-purpose flour
2 large egg whites, lightly beaten
1 cup crumbled cornflakes
4 bone-in chicken breast halves, skin removed and trimmed of fat

1 Place the flour, egg whites, and cornflakes in separate shallow dishes.

2 Dip each breast into the flour to coat evenly; shake off excess flour. Dip into the egg whites to coat and then into the cornflakes. Press down firmly to make the cornflakes adhere. Refrigerate for 1 hour to help the coating set.

3 Preheat oven to 400°F. Lightly coat a shallow baking dish with nonstick cooking spray. Add the breasts in a single layer and bake at 400°F for 30 minutes, or until the chicken is crisp and the juices run clear when tested with a sharp knife.

Makes 4 servings
Per serving: 2 grams fat • 192 calories

Chicken Pot Pie

prepare ahead

Get a jump on tomorrow's dinner by assembling this colorful casserole the night before. Prepare through step 4, cover with plastic, and refrigerate. Heat up the casserole on the stovetop or in the microwave, then add the biscuits and pop it into the oven.

6	cups fat-free chicken broth
4	bone-in chicken breast halves, skin removed
2	medium carrots, thinly sliced
1	medium turnip, peeled and cubed
1	large leek, well cleaned and sliced (white and tender green parts)
2	large celery ribs, sliced
½	cup frozen peas, thawed
1	tablespoon unsalted butter
1	large shallot, peeled and minced
½	cup dry white wine
½	cup all-purpose flour
1	cup light (1%) milk
2	teaspoons herbs de Provence
⅛	teaspoon grated nutmeg
1	tube (7.5 ounces) low-fat biscuit dough

1 Place the broth in a large saucepan and bring to a boil over medium heat. Add the chicken, cover, and simmer for 30 minutes, or until cooked through. Use tongs to transfer the chicken to a plate and set aside to cool. Remove the meat from the bone, cut into 1-inch pieces, and place in a large bowl.

2 While the chicken cools, add the carrots and turnip to the saucepan; cover and cook for 10 minutes. Add the leek and celery; cover and cook for 10 minutes longer. Remove the vegetables with a slotted spoon and add them to the bowl with the chicken. Add the peas to the bowl and stir gently to mix. Reserve enough broth to measure 4 cups; save any extra for another use.

3 Add the butter to the empty saucepan and cook the shallots for 5 minutes. Add the wine and cook until about 2 tablespoons of liquid remain. Add the reserved broth and bring to a simmer.

4   Place the flour in a small bowl. Whisk in the milk until smooth. Add to the saucepan in a slow stream, whisking constantly, and cook over medium heat for 5 to 8 minutes, or until the mixture thickens and begins to bubble. Add the herbs de Provence and nutmeg. Season with salt and pepper.

5   Mix the chicken and vegetable mixture with the gravy and heat thoroughly.

6   Preheat oven to 375°F. Coat a deep 10-inch pie dish with nonstick cooking spray. Pour in the chicken, vegetables, and gravy.

7   Cover the top with pieces of the biscuit dough in a single layer, making a few slashes for steam to escape.

8   Bake at 375°F for 10 to 12 minutes, or until the filling bubbles and the crust browns.

Makes 6 servings
Per serving: 5 grams fat • 357 calories

 If the pot pie gravy is a little more than the casserole dish can accommodate, reserve the excess in case you have leftovers. To reheat, pour the reserved gravy around the bottom of the casserole, cover with foil, and reheat at 400°F for about 10 minutes, or until heated through.

Roast Chicken with Winter Vegetables

Roasting a chicken is not only a delicious and comforting way to enjoy poultry; it's a great way to have ready-made filler for fajitas, sloppy joes, and sandwiches. Keep leftovers well covered in the refrigerator to maintain moistness.

1   roasting chicken (6 pounds)
1   large lemon, quartered
2   thyme sprigs or 1 teaspoon dried thyme
1   medium sweet potato, peeled and cut into 8 pieces
2   turnips, peeled and cut into 8 pieces
2   small onions, peeled and quartered
2   large carrots, shaved and cut into 1-inch pieces
2   parsnips, peeled and cut into 1-inch pieces
1   can (14 ounces) fat-free chicken broth
1   cup dry white wine
    Salt and ground black pepper

1 Remove the giblets from the chicken cavity and reserve for another use. Remove and discard any visible fat, especially from the cavity area. Lightly coat a 13 × 9-inch baking dish or small roasting pan with nonstick cooking spray. Place the chicken in the dish.

2 Place the lemon and thyme in the cavity. Surround the chicken with the vegetables.

3 In a small bowl, mix the broth and wine. Pour over the chicken. Season with salt and pepper. Bake at 375°F for 1½ hours, or until an instant-read thermometer inserted in the thickest part of the thigh registers 190°F.

4 Transfer the chicken to a cutting board and let stand for 15 minutes. Remove and discard the skin. Slice the chicken and serve with the vegetables and broth.

Makes 8 servings • Serving size: 3 ounces of white meat
Per serving: 5 grams fat • 249 calories

 This dish is just as good the second time around. Place the leftover chicken and vegetables on a large sheet of heavy-duty foil. Fold up the sides and drizzle the chicken and vegetables with about ½ cup of broth. Wrap tightly and bake at 400°F for 15 minutes, or until heated through.

Cornish Game Hens with Apricot Stuffing

Here's a great dish for a special occasion. Be sure to remove all the skin from the hens before serving, because much of the fat is concentrated there.

2	Cornish game hens
1	cup apple juice
1	cup apricot nectar
2	teaspoons soy sauce
1	tablespoon minced fresh ginger
1½	cups uncooked wild rice
1¾	cups fat-free chicken broth
½	cup dried apricots
½	cup warm water
¼	cup chopped unsalted walnuts
1	cup minced onion
1	tablespoon oil

1 Remove the giblets. Rinse the hens with cold water and pat dry.

2 In a large bowl, mix the apple juice, apricot nectar, soy sauce, and ginger. Add the hens and turn to coat. Marinate in the refrigerator overnight. Remove the hens, reserving the marinade.

3 In a medium saucepan, mix the wild rice and 1½ cups of the broth. Bring to a boil. Cover, reduce the heat, and simmer for 40 minutes, or until all the liquid is absorbed.

4 In a small bowl, soak the apricots in the water until soft, about 30 minutes. Drain and chop; add to the wild rice. Add the walnuts.

5 In a medium saucepan, cook the onion in the oil over medium heat for 5 minutes, or until soft. Add to the wild rice along with the remaining ¼ cup broth. Mix well.

6 Fill the cavities of the Cornish hens with the stuffing, packing lightly. Place any remaining stuffing in a small casserole coated with nonstick cooking spray.

7 Place the hens on a rack in a roasting pan coated with nonstick spray. Bake at 350°F, basting occasionally with the marinade, for 1 hour or until a thermometer reads 165°F. Let stand for 20 minutes. Remove the skin and cut each hen in half.

Makes 4 servings
Per serving: 13 grams fat • 398 calories

Grilled Pineapple Chicken Sandwich

30 minutes or less

Use a fresh pineapple, if possible, as it holds up well on the grill. If desired, skip the bun and serve the chicken as a dinner entrée with Tropical Rice (page 274).

3   boneless, skinless chicken breasts, split and trimmed of fat
1   cup bottled teriyaki marinade
1   pineapple, peeled, cored, and sliced into rings, or 1 can (16 ounces) pineapple rings, drained
6   hamburger rolls
1   tablespoon Chili Mayonnaise (page 328), optional

1 Place the chicken in a shallow bowl and add the teriyaki marinade. Marinate for a minimum of 3 hours or overnight in the refrigerator. Remove the chicken, reserving the marinade.

2 Lightly coat a gas or charcoal grill grate with grilling spray and heat to medium-high. Grill the chicken for 5 minutes. Turn and brush with the marinade. Grill for 5 minutes more, or until the internal temperature of the chicken registers 160°F.

3 At the same time, grill the pineapple rings, brushing with the marinade, for 1 or 2 minutes, or until heated throughout. Discard any remaining marinade.

4 Toast the rolls on the grill for 30 seconds. Serve the chicken and pineapple rings on the rolls with the mayonnaise.

Makes 6 servings
Per serving: 4 grams fat • 230 calories (without roll)
Per serving: 6 grams fat • 350 calories (with roll)

Arizona Jerk Turkey

prepare ahead

A new twist on Jamaica's hot, hot jerk sauce, this version contains jalapeño peppers instead of scorching Scotch bonnet peppers.

4	small fresh or pickled jalapeño peppers
4	scallions, sliced
2	tablespoons red wine vinegar
1	tablespoon oil
1	tablespoon ground allspice
1	teaspoon salt
½	teaspoon ground cinnamon
⅛	teaspoon ground nutmeg
½	teaspoon ground black pepper
½	boneless, skinless turkey breast (about 1½ pounds)

1 Put the jalapeño peppers and scallions in a food processor and process until chopped. With the machine running, add the vinegar, oil, allspice, salt, cinnamon, nutmeg, and black pepper. Process until the mixture forms a paste.

2 Place the turkey flat in a shallow glass or ceramic dish and spread the jalapeño paste over the flesh. Cover and marinate in the refrigerator for 2 hours or overnight. Bring to room temperature.

3 Lightly coat a gas or charcoal grill grate with grilling spray and heat to medium-high. Grill the turkey, turning every 5 minutes, for 15 to 20 minutes, or until the juices run clear when tested with a sharp knife.

Makes 6 servings
Per serving: 3 grams fat • 157 calories

Turkey Burgers

30 minutes or less • prepare ahead

This burger stays nice and moist thanks to a secret ingredient: yogurt.

> 1   pound ground turkey breast
> 2   tablespoons minced fresh parsley
> 2   tablespoons fat-free plain yogurt
> 1   tablespoon fresh lemon juice
> 2   teaspoons soy sauce
> 4   hamburger rolls
>   Whole-grain mustard
> 1   large tomato, sliced
> 1   cup alfalfa sprouts

1 In a large bowl, mix the turkey, parsley, yogurt, lemon juice, and soy sauce. Season with salt and pepper. Shape the mixture into 4 patties. Cover and refrigerate for at least 30 minutes.

2 Lightly coat a gas or charcoal grill grate with grilling spray and heat to medium-high. Grill the burgers over indirect heat for 5 minutes on each side, or until cooked through.

3 Serve the burgers on the rolls with the mustard, tomato, and sprouts.

Makes 4 servings
Per serving: 7 grams fat • 281 calories

Turkey Sloppy Joes

30 minutes or less

Here's a great use for turkey leftovers. Serve with Creamy Coleslaw (page 286).

1	small onion, peeled and sliced
1	tablespoon water
½	cup ketchup
2	tablespoons packed light brown sugar
¼	cup Dijon mustard
2	tablespoons honey
¼	cup cider vinegar
2	tablespoons Worcestershire sauce
1	teaspoon hot pepper sauce
2	teaspoons minced garlic
12	ounces cooked turkey breast, skin removed, meat shredded
4	hamburger rolls

1 In a large nonstick skillet, cook the onion and water over medium heat for 5 minutes, or until soft but not browned. Stir in the ketchup, brown sugar, mustard, honey, vinegar, Worcestershire sauce, hot pepper sauce, and garlic. Add the turkey and cook for 3 to 4 minutes, or until heated through.

2 Serve the turkey mixture on the rolls.

Makes 4 servings
Per serving: 3 grams fat • 355 calories

This recipe is a great way to use up any leftovers, from roast pork to chicken and beef.

Hero's Hoagie

30 minutes or less • prepare ahead

What makes this sandwich special is marinating the vegetables in a vineagar dressing. This can be prepared a day ahead, wrapped tightly in plastic, and kept refrigerated.

¼	cup balsamic vinegar
1	garlic clove, peeled and minced
½	teaspoon dried oregano
¼	teaspoon dry mustard
4	thin cucumber slices
1	small tomato, sliced
4	thick red onion slices
3	green sweet pepper slices
2	black olives, pitted and sliced
1	mini baguette, 6 inches long
2	romaine lettuce leaves
2	ounces sliced turkey breast
1	ounce sliced provolone cheese
1	banana chile pepper, seeded and sliced (optional)

1 For the dressing: In a medium bowl, mix the vinegar, garlic, oregano, and mustard. Add the cucumbers, tomato, onions, sweet peppers, and olives. Set aside for 30 minutes.

2 Split the baguette lengthwise to open flat, but don't cut all the way through. Evenly layer the vegetables down half of the baguette. Top with the lettuce, turkey, cheese, and chile pepper (if using). Season with salt and pepper.

3 Lay a knife lengthwise against the ingredients, fold the sandwich closed, and cut in half.

Makes 1 serving
Per serving: 12 grams fat • 364 calories

Hoagie Dressing

Make a big batch of the hoagie dressing and add a banana chile pepper (sliced in half and seeded). It has virtually no calories. Keep refrigerated in a bottle with a sprinkle cap. Sprinkle on salads and sandwiches.

Turkey Loaf

prepare ahead

Mixing ground turkey breast with extra-lean beef cuts fat from this family favorite without changing its traditional flavor. Prepare the loaf the night before, cover with plastic wrap, and refrigerate. Just pop it in the oven and you have a no-fuss meal.

½	cup chopped onion
½	cup chopped green sweet pepper
¼	cup chopped celery
2	garlic cloves, peeled and minced
1	teaspoon Italian seasoning
½	teaspoon olive oil
1	pound extra-lean ground beef
1	pound ground turkey breast
½	cup ketchup
¼	cup dried bread crumbs
¼	cup fat-free milk
¼	cup egg substitute
2	teaspoons dried oregano
2	teaspoons Worcestershire sauce

1 In a large nonstick skillet, cook the onion, pepper, celery, garlic, and Italian seasoning in the oil over medium heat for 10 minutes, or until the vegetables are soft.

2 In a large bowl, mix the beef, turkey, ketchup, bread crumbs, milk, egg substitute, oregano, and Worcestershire sauce. Stir in the cooked vegetables. Form into a loaf.

3 Coat a 9 × 5-inch loaf pan with nonstick cooking spray. Add the meat mixture. Bake at 350°F for 1 hour, or until golden brown. Let stand for 10 minutes before slicing.

Makes 8 servings
Per serving: 11 grams fat • 234 calories

dining on
meat

Beef Stroganoff

30 minutes or less • prepare ahead

Lean top round and low-fat yogurt (instead of sour cream) transform this dish into a diet ally.

2	teaspoons olive oil
½	cup finely chopped onion
1	pound lean top round beef cubes
1	pound mushrooms, sliced
1	can (8 ounces) cooked carrots
2	teaspoons minced fresh basil or 1 teaspoon dried basil
¼	cup red wine
1	cup low-fat plain yogurt
3	cups hot cooked egg noodles

1 Warm the oil in a large nonstick skillet over medium-high heat. Add the onion and cook for 2 minutes. Add the beef and cook for 10 minutes, turning to brown evenly. Using a slotted spoon, transfer the beef and onions to a bowl.

2 Add the mushrooms to the skillet and cook for 5 minutes. Return the beef and onions to the skillet. Add the carrots and sprinkle with the basil. Stir in the wine and cook for 15 minutes, or until the beef is tender. Reduce the heat to low and gradually stir in the yogurt. Heat through but do not bring to a boil. Serve over the noodles.

Makes 4 servings
Per serving: 9 grams fat • 399 calories

Grilled Cowboy Steaks with Secret Sauce and Tomato Topping

30 minutes or less

No one will ever guess what this "secret sauce" really is!

4 ripe tomatoes, seeded and coarsely chopped
2 tablespoons balsamic vinegar
½ cup firmly packed fresh basil leaves
2 ribeye steaks (about 8 ounces each), cut 1 inch thick
2 tablespoons oyster sauce

1 In a small bowl, mix the tomatoes, vinegar, and basil.

2 Coat a gas or charcoal grill grate with grilling spray and heat to medium-high. Season the steaks with salt and pepper and grill for 4 minutes on each side or until done as desired.

3 Brush the steaks with oyster sauce and slice each steak into 4 pieces. Serve topped with the tomato mixture.

Makes 4 servings
Per serving: 17 grams fat • 320 calories

Petite Filet with Caramelized Onions

30 minutes or less

This easy and fast meal is great for onion fans. Add a green salad to round it out.

1 pound onions, peeled and sliced
½ teaspoon dried thyme
½ teaspoon dried rosemary
1 tablespoon olive oil
4 filets mignons (4 ounces each)

1 In a large nonstick skillet over medium heat, cook the onions, thyme, and rosemary in the oil, stirring often, for 15 to 20 minutes, or until the onions are soft and golden. Season with salt and pepper. Transfer to a platter and keep warm.

2 Add the filets to the skillet and cook for 3 minutes per side for medium rare, or until the desired doneness is reached. Serve smothered with the onions.

Makes 4 servings
Per serving: 12 grams fat • 260 calories

Steak Kabobs

30 minutes or less • prepare ahead

Grilled kabobs are a great way to make meat go a long way. Add as many vegetables as you want.

2	tablespoons fresh lemon juice
1	tablespoon oil
1	teaspoon dried thyme
1	teaspoon ground cumin
1	pound sirloin steak, trimmed of all visible fat and cut into 1-inch cubes
1	green sweet pepper, cored, seeded, and cut into 8 pieces
1	red sweet pepper, cored, seeded, and cut into 8 pieces
8	medium mushrooms, stems removed
2	zucchini, each cut into 8 pieces
16	cherry tomatoes, stems removed
1	large red onion, peeled and cut into 16 chunks

1 In a medium bowl, mix the lemon juice, oil, thyme, and cumin. Add the steak and toss to coat. Cover and marinate in the refrigerator for at least 2 hours or overnight.

2 Thread the steak onto 4 metal skewers, alternating the cubes with the peppers, mushrooms, zucchini, tomatoes, and onion.

3 Coat a gas or charcoal grill grate with grilling spray and heat to high. Grill the kabobs, basting frequently with the marinade, for 4 to 5 minutes per side for medium rare. Discard any remaining marinade.

Makes 4 servings
Per serving: 9 grams fat • 251 calories

London Broil Two Ways

30 minutes or less • prepare ahead

Two different marinades, one sweet and the other savory, give this lean cut of beef a distinctive taste with only a touch of fat.

    1   pound London broil, 1 inch thick
        Savory Marinade or Sweet Marinade

1 Prick the meat on both sides with a fork. Place in a shallow dish, cover with the marinade, and refrigerate overnight. Bring to room temperature before grilling.

2 Coat a gas or charcoal grill grate with grilling spray and heat to high. Remove the meat from the marinade and grill, brushing frequently with the marinade, until it reaches your desired doneness. Discard any remaining marinade.

Savory Marinade   ⅓   cup red wine vinegar
                   3   garlic cloves, peeled and minced
                   2   teaspoons olive oil
                   2   bay leaves

Mix the vinegar, garlic, oil, and bay leaves.

Sweet Marinade   1   cup chopped onion
                  ¼   cup water
                  2   tablespoons distilled white vinegar
                  2   tablespoons ketchup
                  1   teaspoon salt
                  ½   teaspoon hot pepper sauce

Mix the onion, water, vinegar, ketchup, salt, and pepper sauce.

Makes 4 servings
Per serving: 9 grams fat • 162 calories

Stuffed Bell Peppers

prepare ahead • freeze

These peppers can be frozen before or after they are cooked. This dish is so substantial, it makes a meal in itself.

4   medium green sweet peppers
1   pound extra-lean ground beef
1   cup cooked rice
1   cup corn kernels
1   teaspoon Italian seasoning
3   cups tomato sauce
3   tablespoons shredded low-fat mozzarella cheese

1 Cut the tops off the peppers at the widest part. Remove the seeds and inner membranes, making sure not to pierce the peppers.

2 In a large bowl, mix the beef, rice, corn, Italian seasoning, and ½ cup of the tomato sauce. Season with salt and pepper.

3 Divide the stuffing among the peppers. Stand the peppers upright in a saucepan just large enough to hold them. Pour the remaining 2½ cups tomato sauce over the peppers and sprinkle with the cheese. Cover and cook over medium heat for 40 minutes, or until the peppers are tender.

Makes 4 servings
Per serving: 13 grams fat • 383 calories

Chili Mac

Make sure to buy the leanest ground beef possible for this quick skillet meal. Serve it with homemade tortilla chips, if desired.

½   pound lean ground beef
½   cup chopped onion
1   garlic clove, peeled and minced
1   can (16 ounces) red kidney beans, rinsed and drained
1   can (8 ounces) tomato sauce
1   can (8 ounces) stewed tomatoes
2   cups cooked elbow macaroni
1   teaspoon chili powder
⅓   cup finely shredded low-fat sharp cheddar cheese

1 Coat a large nonstick skillet with nonstick cooking spray and warm over medium heat. Add the beef, onion, and garlic and cook, stirring frequently, until the beef browns. Drain in a sieve, pressing lightly to remove the fat.

2 Return the mixture to the skillet and add the beans, tomato sauce, tomatoes (with juice), macaroni, and chili powder. Cover and simmer for 10 minutes.

3 Sprinkle with the cheese. Cover and place over low heat just until the cheese melts.

Makes 4 servings
Per serving: 12 grams fat • 400 calories

Beef and Vegetable Stew

prepare ahead • freeze

This light stew emphasizes the vegetables rather than the beef.

1	pound lean boneless beef round
½	cup all-purpose flour
1	tablespoon oil
1	medium onion, peeled and coarsely chopped
2	garlic cloves, peeled and minced
3	cups dry red wine
2	cans (14 ounces each) fat-free beef broth
¼	cup tomato paste
1	tablespoon chopped fresh thyme or 1 teaspoon dried thyme
1	pound turnips, peeled and, if large, quartered
½	pound baby red potatoes, quartered
4	large carrots, shaved and cut into chunks
2	parsnips, shaved and cut into chunks
¾	pound mushrooms, wiped clean and quartered

1 Trim the beef of all visible fat and cut into 1-inch cubes. Place the beef in a large bowl. Sprinkle the beef with the flour, turning to coat.

2 Warm the oil in a large nonstick pot over medium-high heat. Working in batches, add the beef and cook, turning constantly, for 3 to 5 minutes, until lightly browned. Remove with a slotted spoon and place in a bowl. Pat with paper towels to remove excess fat.

3 Add the onion and garlic to the pot. Cook, stirring frequently, for 6 to 7 minutes, or until the onion is tender. Stir in the wine, beef broth, tomato paste, and thyme. Using a wooden spoon, scrape up any browned bits from the bottom of the pot. Bring to a boil. Return the beef to the pot. Partially cover and simmer for 1 hour, or until the beef is tender.

4 Add the turnips, potatoes, carrots, and parsnips and simmer for 20 minutes. Add the mushrooms and simmer for 10 minutes. Season with salt and pepper.

Makes 8 servings
Per serving: 5 grams fat • 258 calories

Drunken Pork Chops

30 minutes or less • prepare ahead

Drunken (marinated in red wine) is a traditional way to tenderize meat. The technique is believed to have originated in Italy.

> 2   cups dry red wine
> 2   bay leaves
> 2   tablespoons minced fresh rosemary
> 1   teaspoon ground coriander
> ½   teaspoon ground nutmeg
> ½   teaspoon ground cloves
> 6   bone-in loin pork chops (about 5 ounces each), trimmed, cut 1 inch thick

1 In a shallow glass or ceramic dish, mix the wine, bay leaves, rosemary, coriander, nutmeg, and cloves. Add the pork, mix, cover, and marinate overnight in the refrigerator, turning occasionally.

2 Coat a gas or charcoal grill grate with grilling spray and heat to medium-high. Remove the pork from the marinade and pat dry; discard the marinade. Season the pork with salt and pepper. Grill for 6 to 7 minutes on each side, or until cooked through.

Makes 6 servings
Per serving: 5.5 grams fat • 150 calories

Stir-Fried Pork with Apples and Figs

30 minutes or less

Figs are always a treat when you're on a diet, and in this dish a little goes a long way. For variety, chicken will complement the fruit just as well as pork.

⅔ cup fat-free chicken broth

2 tablespoons soy sauce

1 tablespoon water

2 teaspoons cornstarch

½ teaspoon sugar

Pinch of cayenne pepper

10 ounces boneless pork loin, cut into cubes

1 medium red apple, peeled, cored, and cut into cubes

6 dried figs, chopped

4 ounces snow peas

1 medium carrot, cut diagonally into thin slices

2 baby bok choy, cut into 1-inch pieces

2 scallions, sliced

1 In a small bowl, whisk together the broth, soy sauce, water, cornstarch, sugar, and cayenne until the cornstarch dissolves.

2 Coat a wok or large nonstick skillet with nonstick cooking spray and place over high heat for 1 minute. Add the pork and apple; cook, stirring, until browned on all sides. Transfer to a bowl.

3 To the pan, add the figs, snow peas, carrot, bok choy, and scallions; cook, stirring, for 5 minutes, or until the vegetables are just tender. Return pork mixture to the pan and stir in broth mixture. Bring to a boil and cook, stirring, for 5 minutes, or until thickened.

Makes 4 servings
Per serving: 2 grams fat • 172 calories

Stir-Fried Pork and Greens

30 minutes or less

The sesame oil adds a nice nutty flavor to this dish. Don't hesitate to substitute other vegetables or even add more vegetables and reduce the meat. Stir-fry is a great way to enjoy vegetables.

2	teaspoons toasted sesame oil
12	ounces boneless pork loin, cut into thin strips
3	tablespoons soy sauce
2	cups broccoli florets
6	ounces green beans, cut in half
4	scallions, cut into 1-inch pieces
2	teaspoons cornstarch
	Juice of 2 oranges
1	cup packed fresh basil, roughly torn

1 Place a wok or large nonstick skillet over medium-high heat until hot. Add the oil, pork, and 1 tablespoon of the soy sauce. Cook, stirring, for 5 minutes, or until the pork starts to brown.

2 Stir in the broccoli, beans, and half of the scallions. Cook, stirring, for 3 minutes, or until the broccoli is just tender.

3 In a cup, dissolve the cornstarch in the orange juice. Add the remaining 2 tablespoons soy sauce. Pour the mixture into the pan and stir for 1 minute, or until just thickened. Season with salt and pepper. Top with remaining scallions and basil and serve.

Makes 4 servings
Per serving: 6 grams fat • 201 calories

 Pork tenderloin is one of the leanest cuts of meat available and suitable to slicing and cooking quickly. Use it in everything from quick stir-frys to oven bakes.

Grilled Cheese and Bacon

30 minutes or less

These sandwiches are really baked, but the idea is the same. And they are just as crispy as if they were grilled in butter.

4   English muffins, split
4   Canadian bacon slices
1   cup soy cheese
1   teaspoon Dijon mustard
8   fresh basil leaves

1 Toast the muffin halves for 2 minutes, or until just starting to color. Divide the bacon and cheese among 4 of the muffin halves. Spread with the mustard. Top with the basil and the remaining muffin halves.

2 Place the sandwiches on a baking sheet and bake at 400°F for 10 minutes, or until the cheese is melted and the muffins are crisp.

Makes 4 servings
Per serving: 8.5 grams fat • 285 calories

Trade Canadian bacon for regular bacon permanently. You'll get a huge fat savings. Canadian bacon has 3 grams of fat per serving, compared with 8 grams in regular bacon.

Veal Marsala

30 minutes or less • prepare ahead

Traditional recipes can have quite a bit of butter and cream. This version retains the luscious Marsala flavor with a fraction of the fat.

⅓ cup all-purpose flour
⅓ teaspoon ground black pepper
¼ teaspoon salt
1 pound veal scallops, pounded to ⅛ inch thick
1 teaspoon oil
2 cups sliced mushrooms
1 shallot, peeled and finely chopped
1 garlic clove, peeled and minced
½ cup dry Marsala wine
⅓ cup fat-free chicken broth
2 teaspoons unsalted butter
2 tablespoons chopped fresh parsley

1 On a large plate, mix the flour, pepper, and salt. Firmly press the veal into the mixture to coat both sides and shake off any excess.

2 Heat the oil in a large nonstick skillet over medium-high heat. Working in batches if necessary, quickly cook the veal until lightly browned, about 1 minute per side. Transfer to a platter.

3 Reduce the heat to low and add the mushrooms, shallot, and garlic. Cover and cook, stirring occasionally, for 3 to 4 minutes, or until browned. (If the pan gets too dry, add a little broth.) Add the wine, increase the heat to medium-high, and cook, uncovered, for 2 to 3 minutes, or until the liquid is reduced by half. Add the broth and continue to cook until the liquid is reduced by half. Stir in the butter.

4 Return the veal to the skillet and cook for 1 to 2 minutes, or until warmed through. Serve sprinkled with the parsley.

Makes 4 servings
Per serving: 7 grams fat • 206 calories

Veal Scallops with Fennel and Grapes

30 minutes or less • prepare ahead

Veal scallops are very thin, so they cook quickly. Marinating them in an herb mixture gives nice flavor to this mild meat.

1	pound veal scallops
1	tablespoon oil
1	tablespoon minced fresh parsley
½	teaspoon dried rosemary
¼	teaspoon dried savory
½	cup fat-free chicken broth
1	fennel bulb, fronds discarded, halved lengthwise and thinly sliced
½	cup minced shallots
2	cups seedless red grapes, halved

1 Place the veal between sheets of waxed paper and gently flatten with a mallet until about ⅛ inch thick.

2 In a small bowl, mix the oil, parsley, rosemary and savory. Brush over the veal. Cover with plastic wrap and refrigerate for 3 to 4 hours.

3 Coat a large nonstick skillet with nonstick cooking spray. Over medium-high heat, saute the veal in batches for 2 minutes per side, or until slightly browned. If the veal starts to stick, add a tablespoon or two of broth. Remove to a serving dish and keep warm.

4 Add the broth, fennel, and shallots to the skillet. Cook over medium-high heat for 10 minutes, or until the broth is reduced by half and the fennel is tender. Add the grapes and cook 1 minute. Pour over the veal.

Makes 4 servings
Per serving: 7 grams fat • 255 calories

Greek Lamb Kabobs

prepare ahead

A cut from the shank of the leg will render the least fat. Make sure to trim all visible fat from the lamb before cooking. This not only reduces the meal's fat content but helps prevent flare-ups while grilling.

Lamb	¼	cup low-fat plain yogurt
	2	tablespoons chopped fresh oregano
	2	garlic cloves, minced
	2	pounds boned leg of lamb, cut into 2-inch cubes

Kabobs	2	large onions, cut into 2-inch pieces
	18	mushroom caps
	1	large red sweet pepper, cut into 1-inch pieces
	1	medium zucchini, cut crosswise into ¼-inch slices
	1	large lemon, cut crosswise into 12 slices

1 For the lamb: In a large bowl, mix the yogurt, oregano, and garlic. Add the lamb, mix well, cover, and refrigerate overnight. Bring to room temperature.

2 For the kabobs: Thread 8 skewers with the lamb, onions, mushrooms, sweet peppers, zucchini, and lemon slices, alternating the meat and vegetables. Season with salt and pepper.

3 Coat a gas or charcoal grill with grilling spray and heat to high. Grill the kabobs for 4 to 5 minutes on each side, or until done as desired.

Makes 8 servings
Per serving: 6 grams fat • 198 calories

Grilled Lamb Chops with Grilled Grapes

30 minutes or less

These grapes burst with flavor when you bite into them. Serve the chops over couscous.

4   lamb chops (5 ounces each)
4   medium clusters seedless grapes
1   teaspoon olive oil
4   fresh rosemary sprigs
4   fresh thyme sprigs

1 Lightly coat a gas or charcoal grill with grilling spray and heat to medium-high. Trim the tails and fat from the chops.

2 Rinse the grapes and thoroughly pat dry with paper towels. Using a pastry brush, brush the grapes with the oil. Tuck a sprig of rosemary and thyme into each grape cluster.

3 Put the lamb chops in the center of the grill. Place the grape clusters along the edges. Grill the chops and grapes, turning frequently (to prevent the chops from flaring up), for 15 minutes, or until the grapes develop grill marks and a few start to split and the chops are the desired doneness.

Makes 4 servings
Per serving: 12 grams fat • 326 calories

pasta,

please!

Spaghetti with Summer Tomatoes, Basil, and Garlic

30 minutes or less

The best time of year to make this dish is during the summer, when tomatoes are juicy and rich in taste and basil is plentiful.

8	ounces spaghetti
3	garlic cloves, peeled and thinly sliced
2	tablespoons olive oil
¼	cup fat-free chicken broth
	Juice of 1 lemon
12	cherry tomatoes, cut in half
¾	cup coarsely chopped fresh basil

1 Cook the spaghetti according to the package directions. Drain and return to the pot.

2 Meanwhile, in a medium nonstick saucepan, cook the garlic in the oil over medium heat for 2 minutes. Add the broth, lemon juice, and tomatoes. Season with salt and pepper. Cook over low heat for 5 minutes, or until hot. Pour over the spaghetti and toss to mix. Add the basil and toss again.

Makes 4 servings
Per serving: 8 grams fat • 290 calories

Pasta with Cherry Tomatoes and Parsley

30 minutes or less

For a weeknight dinner in a flash, it can't get any better than this. Use whatever pasta you have on hand.

8   ounces pasta

2   garlic cloves, sliced

1   teaspoon olive oil

24   cherry tomatoes, cut in half

½   cup chopped fresh parsley

2   tablespoons grated Parmesan cheese

1 Cook the pasta according to the package directions. Drain and return to the pot.

2 In a large nonstick skillet, cook the garlic in the oil over medium heat for 1 minute. Toss in the tomatoes and ¼ cup of the parsley. Cook, stirring, for 3 minutes, or until the tomatoes just begin to soften.

3 Add the hot pasta and toss. Season with salt and pepper. Sprinkle with the cheese and the remaining ¼ cup parsley.

Makes 4 servings
Per serving: 3 grams fat • 226 calories

 Tip Add a can of drained baby shrimp or crab, shredded leftover chicken or meat, or fresh or leftover vegetables to this dish. If the skillet gets too dry, stir in a few tablespoons of fat-free chicken broth.

Spaghetti with Summer Squash

30 minutes or less

Here's a nice change of pace from tomato sauce.

  8   ounces spaghetti
  2   tablespoons olive oil
  4   garlic cloves, thinly sliced
  1   cup fresh bread crumbs
  ¼   cup chopped fresh parsley
  1½ tablespoons finely chopped walnuts
  1   small yellow squash, cut into 2-inch julienne
  1   small zucchini, cut into 2-inch julienne
  1   cup shredded carrot
  1   small red sweet pepper, thinly sliced

1 Cook the spaghetti according to the package directions. Drain, return to the pot, and keep warm.

2 Warm 1 tablespoon of the oil in a large nonstick skillet over medium heat. Add the garlic and cook for 1 minute. Stir in the bread crumbs and cook for 3 minutes, or until lightly browned and crunchy. Transfer to a small bowl and stir in the parsley and walnuts. Season with salt and pepper.

3 Add the yellow squash, zucchini, carrot, and the remaining 1 tablespoon oil to the skillet. Cook for 5 minutes, or until the vegetables are crisp-tender. Add to the pot with the spaghetti.

4 Add the pepper to the skillet and cook for 2 minutes, or until just softened. Add to the spaghetti and toss to combine. Add the bread crumb mixture and toss once or twice.

Makes 4 servings
Per serving: 10 grams fat • 349 calories

Spaghetti with Fresh Mushrooms and Red Sauce

30 minutes or less

Though this recipe calls for button mushrooms, you can enhance the texture and taste by using a variety of other mushrooms, such as enoki, shiitake, cremini, or oyster. Or use coarsely chopped portobello mushrooms.

8	ounces spaghetti
½	cup chopped onion
2	garlic cloves, minced
1	tablespoon olive oil
2	pounds button mushrooms, cut into quarters
1	can (16 ounces) crushed tomatoes
1	tablespoon tomato paste
2	tablespoons chopped fresh parsley
1	tablespoon chopped fresh basil
1	teaspoon sugar
1	teaspoon dried Italian seasoning

1 Cook the spaghetti according to the package directions. Drain and return to the pot.

2 In a large nonstick skillet over medium heat, cook the onion and garlic in the oil for 3 minutes. Add the mushrooms and cook for 15 to 20 minutes, or until the mushroom liquid evaporates and the mushrooms begin to brown.

3 Stir in the tomatoes (with juice), tomato paste, parsley, basil, sugar, and Italian seasoning. Bring to a boil, reduce the heat, and simmer for 10 minutes, or until the sauce is slightly thickened. Pour over the spaghetti and toss to coat.

Makes 4 servings
Per serving: 5 grams fat • 348 calories

Orzo with Cherry Tomatoes, Capers, and Pine Nuts

30 minutes or less

Orzo is pasta that's shaped like grains of rice. It cooks quickly and is a sophisticated alternative to macaroni and other more familiar noodles.

2	teaspoons olive oil
2	cups cherry tomatoes, halved
1	garlic clove, minced
1	cup orzo
2	cups fat-free chicken broth
1	tablespoon pine nuts, finely chopped
1	tablespoon grated Parmesan cheese
2	teaspoons capers, rinsed, drained, and finely chopped
1	teaspoon dried Italian seasoning

1 Warm the oil in a large nonstick skillet over medium heat. Add the tomatoes and garlic; cook for 3 minutes, or until the tomatoes are tender. Transfer to a large bowl.

2 In the same skillet, bring the orzo and broth to a boil over medium-high heat. Reduce the heat to low, cover, and simmer for 7 minutes, or until the pasta is just tender. Remove from the heat, cover, and let stand for 3 minutes, or until almost all of the liquid is absorbed. Transfer to the bowl with the tomatoes.

3 Add the pine nuts, cheese, capers, and Italian seasoning to the bowl. Season with salt and pepper; toss to combine.

Makes 4 servings
Per serving: 5 grams fat • 216 calories

Pasta Primavera

30 minutes or less

Primavera means "spring" in Italy, and the tradition is to throw whatever is fresh in the garden into the pasta. Along the way, butter and cream worked their way into the dish, often overpowering the tender, sweet vegetable flavors. This lightened version uses fat-free milk, which cuts the richness and returns the primavera to its lighter Italian roots.

8	ounces spaghetti
1	cup julienned carrots
1	cup julienned zucchini
1	cup broccoli florets
½	cup julienned scallions
3	tablespoons oil
3	tablespoons all-purpose flour
1½	cups fat-free milk
1	teaspoon Dijon mustard
1	teaspoon dried oregano
1	cup cherry tomatoes, halved
3	tablespoons grated Romano cheese

1 Cook the spaghetti according to the package directions. Drain and keep warm.

2 Meanwhile, steam the carrots, zucchini, broccoli, and scallions until tender, about 5 minutes.

3 In a medium saucepan, warm the oil over medium heat and add the flour. Stir for 3 minutes. Whisk in the milk. Lower the heat and continue to cook, whisking constantly, until the sauce thickens and comes to a simmer. Whisk in the mustard and oregano. Remove from the heat and stir in the steamed vegetables and tomatoes. Toss with the pasta and sprinkle with the cheese prior to serving.

Makes 4 servings
Per serving: 13 grams fat • 410 calories

Pasta Carbonara

30 minutes or less

This dish is traditionally made with cream, bacon, and egg yolks. These substitutions cut the fat and calories significantly.

8	ounces spaghetti
4	ounces turkey bacon, cut into 1-inch pieces
2	tablespoons minced garlic
1	cup frozen peas, thawed
3	large egg whites
1	large egg
1	cup light (1%) milk
¼	teaspoon ground nutmeg
½	cup grated Parmesan cheese
2	tablespoons chopped fresh parsley

1 Cook the pasta according to the package directions. Drain and return to the pot.

2 Meanwhile, cook the bacon in a large nonstick skillet over medium-high heat for 5 minutes, or until crisp. Add the garlic and cook for 1 minute. Add the peas and heat through. Transfer to the pot with the pasta and toss lightly.

3 In a medium saucepan, whisk together the egg whites and egg. Whisk in the milk and nutmeg. Season with salt and pepper. Whisk gently over medium heat for 5 minutes, or until thick and creamy. Pour over the pasta and toss to combine. Sprinkle with the cheese and parsley.

Makes 4 servings
Per serving: 11 grams fat • 425 calories

Linguine with Clam Sauce

To make this dish in 30 minutes, you can substitute 2 10-ounce cans of whole baby clams and their juices for the fresh clams.

1	cup dry white wine
24	littleneck clams, scrubbed, beards removed
8	ounces linguine
2	tablespoons minced garlic
2	teaspoons oil
½	cup fat-free chicken broth
½	teaspoon dried oregano
½	cup chopped fresh parsley
3	tablespoons grated Parmesan cheese

1 Bring ½ cup of the wine to a simmer in a medium saucepan over high heat and add the clams. Cover and cook, shaking the pan frequently, until the clams open, about 5 minutes. Do not overcook. Drain and reserve the cooking liquid (if necessary, strain through a double layer of cheesecloth to remove any sand or grit). Discard any clams that have not opened. Remove the clams from their shells and set aside.

2 Cook the linguine according to the package directions. Drain, return to the pot, and set aside.

3 In a large nonstick skillet, stir the garlic and oil over medium heat for 1 minute. Add the broth, the remaining ½ cup wine, the reserved clam liquid and the oregano. Bring to a boil over high heat and cook for 15 minutes, or until the mixture reduces to about 1⅓ cups.

4 Pour the liquid over the linguine, add the clams, and toss well to mix. Sprinkle with the parsley and cheese.

Makes 4 servings
Per serving: 5 grams fat • 355 calories

Penne with Broccoli and Cheese

30 minutes or less

For something entirely different, forget the pasta and try the broccoli over baked or grilled chicken or fish. Or use the broccoli as a great side vegetable.

4	cups broccoli florets
2	tablespoons oil
1	cup fat-free chicken broth
2	ounces reduced-fat cream cheese, cubed
½	teaspoon dried thyme
½	teaspoon ground black pepper
¼	teaspoon salt
8	ounces dried penne or similar tubed pasta
2	tablespoons grated Parmesan cheese

1 In a large nonstick skillet, cook the broccoli in the oil over medium-high heat for 5 minutes, or until crisp-tender. Transfer to a plate.

2 Add the broth, cream cheese, thyme, pepper, and salt to the skillet. Whisk over heat until creamy. Return the broccoli to the pan, stir to coat, and remove from the heat.

3 Meanwhile, cook the penne according to the package directions. Drain and return the penne to the pot. Add the broccoli mixture, sprinkle with the Parmesan, and toss to combine.

Makes 4 main-dish servings or 8 side-dish servings
Per serving: 10 grams fat • 336 calories (main dish servings)

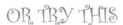

OR TRY THIS

Cheesy Broccoli

Skip the pasta and turn the recipe into a sauce or a zippy side dish for eight.

Per serving: 5 grams fat • 167 calories

Spinach Pesto with Penne and Peas

30 minutes or less

Chicken broth substitutes for much of the olive oil in standard pesto sauce to reduce the calories and fat.

1½	cups coarsely chopped fresh spinach
½	cup tightly packed fresh basil leaves
¼	cup chopped fresh parsley
3	tablespoons grated Parmesan cheese
⅓	cup fat-free chicken broth
1½	tablespoons olive oil
1	garlic clove, peeled and chopped
8	ounces penne
1	package (10 ounces) frozen baby peas, thawed

1 In a food processor, combine the spinach, basil, parsley, cheese, broth, oil, garlic, and salt and pepper to taste. Process for 3 minutes, or until the mixture is smooth and creamy.

2 Cook the penne according to the package directions. Drain and place in a large serving bowl. Stir in the peas. Add the spinach mixture and toss to coat.

Makes 4 servings
Per serving: 7 grams fat • 349 calories

 To raise the fiber count in any pasta dish, substitute whole wheat, flax, or rice pasta for standard white pasta made from semolina flour.

Spinach Risotto

30 minutes or less

Risotto, with its creamy texture, makes a satisfying main meal. Add the spinach at the last minute to retain its color and flavor. Risotto is just the thing to serve on the side with shrimp or fish.

5	cups fat-free chicken broth
1½	cups Arborio rice
1	medium onion, peeled and finely chopped
½	teaspoon paprika
1	tablespoon oil
1½	cups chopped fresh spinach
½	cup minced scallions
2	tablespoons grated Parmesan cheese

1 Bring the broth to a boil in a medium saucepan, uncovered. Reduce the heat to low.

2 In a large saucepan, cook the rice, onion, and paprika in the oil over medium heat for 3 minutes, or until the rice turns milky in color. Ladle in enough broth to just cover the rice. Simmer, stirring constantly, until the rice has absorbed all the broth.

3 Repeat, adding about 1 cup of broth at a time, until all the broth is used and the rice is tender. Do not rush the process; total cooking time should be about 25 minutes.

4 Stir in the spinach, scallions, and cheese.

Makes 4 main-dish servings or 6 side-dish servings
Per serving: 4.5 grams fat • 322 calories (main dish)
Per serving: 3 grams fat • 215 calories (side dish)

Spaghetti and Meatballs

30 minutes or less • prepare ahead • freeze

Two simple changes—substituting ground turkey for half of the usual beef and browning the onions without oil—bring down the fat in this family favorite.

½ cup diced onion
1 tablespoon minced garlic
½ pound lean ground beef (round)
½ pound ground turkey breast
⅓ cup seasoned dry bread crumbs
1 large egg white
½ teaspoon dried oregano
1 jar (26 ounces) fat-free spaghetti sauce
12 ounces spaghetti
½ cup chopped fresh parsley

1 Coat a small nonstick skillet with nonstick cooking spray and place over medium heat. Add the onion and cook for 3 to 4 minutes, or until lightly browned. Add the garlic and cook for 1 to 2 minutes.

2 In a large bowl, mix the beef and turkey. Add the onion mixture, bread crumbs, egg white, oregano, and ½ cup of the spaghetti sauce. Mix well.

3 Wet your hands with cold water and form the mixture into 12 meatballs. Roll between your palms to make them firm so they don't fall apart.

4 Put the meatballs, a few at a time, in the skillet and brown quickly. Continually turn the meatballs as they brown. Transfer to a plate lined with a paper towel to absorb any fat.

5 Place the remaining spaghetti sauce in a medium saucepan. Add the meatballs, cover, and bring to a simmer.

6 Cook the spaghetti according to the package directions. Drain and place in a large bowl. Add the sauce and meatballs; stir lightly to mix. Sprinkle with the parsley.

Makes 6 servings
Per serving: 10 grams fat • 394 calories

on the

side

Garden Peas with Fresh Mint

30 minutes or less

Getting the kids to pitch in with shelling garden-fresh peas will make them willing eaters. You can, of course, use frozen peas.

2   cups peas
1   tablespoon olive oil
2   tablespoons chopped fresh mint

Bring about 1 inch of water to a boil in a medium saucepan fitted with a steamer basket. Add the peas, cover, and steam, tossing once, for 4 minutes, or until tender. Transfer the peas to a large bowl. Stir in the oil and mint. Season with salt and pepper.

Makes 4 servings
Per serving: 4 grams fat • 86 calories

Braised Cabbage with Apples

30 minutes or less • prepare ahead

This traditional Eastern European hearty side dish kicks with fiber and flavor. You can make this in advance and reheat it before serving. It goes nicely with roast pork.

1 cup thinly sliced red onion
1 garlic clove, peeled and minced
2 teaspoons olive oil
4 cups shredded red cabbage
2 tablespoons balsamic vinegar
2 tablespoons chopped fresh oregano
1 red apple, peeled, cored, and cut into ½-inch pieces

1 In a large nonstick skillet, cook the onion and garlic in the oil over medium heat for 5 minutes, or until the onions soften.

2 Add the cabbage, vinegar, and oregano. Cover and cook, stirring occasionally, for 10 minutes. Add the apple and cook for 5 minutes, or until the cabbage is tender. Season with salt and pepper.

Makes 4 servings
Per serving: 3 grams fat • 100 calories

Grilled Portobello Mushrooms

30 minutes or less

Portobello mushrooms make a filling and tasty side dish that rounds out a meal without adding too much fat and calories. They're especially good with steaks and chops.

   2   tablespoons fat-free chicken broth
   1   tablespoon olive oil
   1   tablespoon balsamic vinegar
   3   garlic cloves, minced
   1   tablespoon chopped fresh thyme or 1 teaspoon dried thyme
   ¼   teaspoon salt
   4   large portobello mushrooms, stems removed

1 In a large shallow dish, mix the broth, oil, vinegar, garlic, thyme, and salt. Arrange the mushroom caps in a single layer in the dish, turning once to coat. Let stand at room temperature, turning occasionally, for 1 hour.

2 Coat a gas or charcoal grill grate with grilling spray and heat to medium-high. Grill the mushrooms for about 10 minutes, turning often.

Makes 4 servings
Per serving: 4 grams fat • 76 calories

Southern Red Beans and Rice

30 minutes or less

This is a variation of the traditional dish so loved in the South.

2 red sweet peppers, cored, seeded, and finely chopped
1 large onion, peeled and finely chopped
1 celery rib, finely chopped
2 garlic cloves, minced
¼ teaspoon dried thyme
1 tablespoon oil
1 can (16 ounces) red kidney beans, rinsed and drained
2 tablespoons cider vinegar
2 cups hot cooked rice
1 cup fat-free plain yogurt

1 In a large nonstick skillet, cook the peppers, onion, celery, garlic, and thyme in the oil over medium heat for 10 minutes, or until tender.

2 Add the beans and vinegar. Cook until the beans are hot, about 3 minutes. Spoon over the rice and top with the yogurt.

Makes 4 servings
Per serving: 5 grams fat • 304 calories

Boston Baked Beans

Traditional baked beans are loaded with fatty bacon. You just don't need it.

2	cups dried small white beans
4	cups water
2	bay leaves
½	teaspoon salt
2	cups chopped onions
½	cup molasses
1½	tablespoons dry mustard

1 Pick the white beans over, rinse, cover completely with cold water, and soak overnight. Drain.

2 In a large ovenproof saucepan, mix the beans, water, bay leaves, and salt. Bring to a boil over high heat. Reduce the heat to low, cover partially, and simmer for 1 hour, or until the beans have softened but are still firm. Remove and discard the bay leaves.

3 Stir the onions, molasses, and mustard into the beans. Season with salt and pepper. Cover and bake at 325°F for 4 hours, or until the beans are tender and coated with a light syrup; stir periodically and add water as needed so the beans don't dry out.

Makes 12 servings
Per serving: 0 grams fat • 167 calories

Tropical Rice

This sweet-tasting rice goes great with fish and chicken, especially if they're fresh from the grill.

¼	cup unsweetened shredded coconut
2¼	cups water
1	cup long grain white rice
1	can (8 ounces) crushed pineapple packed in juice
¼	cup fresh lime juice
1	tablespoon packed light brown sugar
1	teaspoon minced fresh ginger
½	cup chopped red sweet pepper
½	cup diagonally sliced scallions

1 Place the coconut in a small nonstick skillet and stir over medium heat for 2 to 3 minutes, or until lightly toasted. Set aside.

2 Bring the water to a boil in a medium saucepan over high heat. Stir in the rice. Reduce the heat to medium-low, cover, and cook for 20 to 25 minutes, or until the liquid is absorbed and the rice is tender.

3 Drain the pineapple over a bowl. Transfer ½ cup of the juice to a small saucepan; discard the remainder. Add the lime juice, brown sugar, and ginger; stir over medium heat until the brown sugar dissolves. Cover and simmer over low heat for 5 minutes.

4 Add the red pepper, scallions, and coconut to the saucepan. Simmer for 3 minutes.

5 Fluff the rice with a fork and place in a large bowl. Add the coconut mixture and toss to mix well. Season with salt and black pepper.

Makes 6 servings
Per serving: 2 grams fat • 171 calories

Wild Rice Salad

30 minutes or less • prepare ahead

This dish is a nice complement to poultry, lamb, and grilled kabobs.

½ cup wild rice
½ cup long grain white rice
2 oranges, peeled and sectioned
½ cup dried cranberries
½ cup sliced scallions
¼ cup water
2 tablespoons apple juice concentrate
1 tablespoon fresh lemon juice
1 tablespoon red wine vinegar
½ teaspoon dried basil
¼ teaspoon dry mustard

1 Using separate saucepans, cook the wild rice and the white rice according to the package directions. Cool and transfer both rices to a large bowl. Stir in the oranges, cranberries, and scallions.

2 In a small bowl, whisk together the water, apple juice concentrate, lemon juice, vinegar, basil, and mustard. Pour over the rice mixture and toss to coat. Season with salt and pepper.

Makes 6 servings
Per serving: 0 grams fat • 174 calories

Vegetable Risotto

30 minutes or less

Risotto is defined by its creamy texture, so be careful not to overcook it. The fat is reduced in this dish by cutting back on the cheese and eliminating added butter.

1½   cups fat-free chicken broth
1½   cups water
  2   garlic cloves, peeled and minced
  1   teaspoon herbes de Provence
  1   cup Arborio rice
 10   ounces spinach, torn into small pieces
1½   cups shredded carrots
  3   tablespoons grated Parmesan cheese

1 In a small saucepan, mix the broth, water, garlic, and herbes de Provence. Bring to a boil over medium-high heat. Reduce the heat to low.

2 Coat a large nonstick saucepan with nonstick cooking spray and place over medium heat. Add the rice and cook, stirring constantly, for 2 minutes, or until the rice is golden. Ladle 1 cup of the hot broth into the rice. Cook, stirring constantly, until the broth is almost absorbed. Add enough of the remaining broth to barely cover the rice. Cook, stirring constantly, until the broth is almost absorbed.

3 As soon as you add the last broth to the rice, stir in the spinach and carrots. Cook, stirring constantly, for 3 to 5 minutes, or until the broth is almost absorbed and the rice is tender. Stir in the cheese.

Makes 6 servings
Per serving: 1 gram fat • 149 calories

Herbes de Provence is a mixture of herbs that grow in the south of France, such as basil, lavender, rosemary, sage, and thyme. Look for it in the supermarket spice section or substitute any of the individual herbs.

Creamed Spinach

30 minutes or less

You can replace the spinach in this dish with any other greens, such as escarole or Swiss chard.

2	pounds fresh spinach
2	cups light (1%) milk
1	small shallot, peeled and chopped
2	garlic cloves, peeled and chopped
½	teaspoon dried thyme
1	teaspoon oil
1	teaspoon unsalted butter
1½	tablespoons all-purpose flour

1 Trim the spinach and rinse in cold water. Shake as much excess water from the leaves as possible. Put the spinach in a large pot, cover, and cook over medium-high heat for 3 minutes, or until just wilted. Pour into a colander. Run cold water over the spinach to cool it. Squeeze out the excess liquid and coarsely chop.

2 In a small saucepan, mix the milk, shallot, garlic, and thyme. Bring just to a boil, reduce the heat, and simmer for 20 minutes.

3 Place the oil and butter in a medium saucepan and set over medium heat to melt the butter. Add the flour and cook, stirring constantly, for 1 minute. Strain the milk into the flour mixture, stirring constantly. (Discard the solids from the milk mixture.) Cook, stirring, for 5 to 10 minutes, or until thickened. Add the chopped spinach and season with salt and pepper. Cook for 1 minute to heat through.

Makes 4 servings
Per serving: 4 grams fat • 137 calories

Tip You can make this recipe even easier by substituting frozen spinach for the fresh. Just thaw two 10-ounce packages and make sure to squeeze all of the excess water from the leaves. Start the recipe with step 2.

Garlic-Lemon Spinach

30 minutes or less

Just a little bit of olive oil and plenty of lemon prove there is no need to laden spinach with a butter sauce. The lemon accentuates the natural flavor of this savory green, which normally is overpowered by butter.

　1½　teaspoons olive oil
　　1　teaspoon minced garlic
　　1　pound fresh spinach, washed in a colander and drained
　　　　Grated zest and juice of 1 lemon

1　In a small saucepan, stir the oil and garlic over high heat for 30 seconds, or until the garlic is fragrant. Set aside.

2　Place the spinach in a large pot, cover, and cook over high heat until just wilted, about 1 to 2 minutes. (Check the spinach every 10 seconds or so and toss with tongs.) Remove from the heat and add the oil mixture. Add the lemon zest and juice; season with salt and pepper. Toss to coat.

Makes 4 servings
Per serving: 2 grams fat • 47 calories

 Substitute any leafy green vegetable for spinach in this dish: Bok choy, broccoli rabe, and even mustard greens will work nicely.

Glazed Carrots

30 minutes or less

It takes just a tad of butter to give cooked carrots a buttery flavor.

4 teaspoons water
4 teaspoons apple juice
1 tablespoon packed light brown sugar
1 teaspoon butter
¼ teaspoon ground nutmeg
¼ teaspoon salt
1 bag (16 ounces) baby carrots

1 In a medium saucepan, mix the water, apple juice, brown sugar, butter, nutmeg, and salt. Stir over medium heat until the mixture comes to a simmer.

2 Add the carrots, cover, and simmer for 15 minutes, or until the carrots are tender.

Makes 4 servings
Per serving: 1 gram fat • 64 calories

Roasting Vegetables

Roasting vegetables intensifies their color and helps their natural sugars caramelize. Good candidates include carrots, turnips, parsnips, beets, and winter squash. The key to success is high heat, uniformly sized pieces, and keeping a sharp eye on them so they don't burn.

You can roast vegetables whole, in chunks, or in small cubes. Depending on the vegetables you choose, roasting takes between 20 minutes and 1 hour. Place the vegetables in a shallow pan, mist with nonstick olive oil cooking spray, and toss to coat. Roast at 425°F, tossing the pieces occasionally, until tender and richly browned along the edges.

Rosemary Roasted New Potatoes

30 minutes or less

These potatoes are the perfect partner for lamb or chicken.

        1   tablespoon oil
        1   pound small new potatoes, cubed
        ¼   cup chopped fresh rosemary sprigs
        ¼   teaspoon salt
        ¼   teaspoon ground black pepper

1 Preheat the oven to 375°F. Pour the oil into a shallow baking dish just large enough to hold all the potatoes in a single layer. Place the dish in the oven for 2 minutes to heat the oil. Add the potatoes and stir to coat. Bake for 15 minutes.

2 Turn the potatoes and mist with nonstick cooking spray. Bake for 20 minutes.

3 Spray the potatoes again and toss with the rosemary. Bake for 5 to 10 minutes, or until the potatoes are browned on the outside and tender when tested with a sharp knife. Sprinkle with the salt and pepper.

Makes 4 servings
Per serving: 4 grams fat • 122 calories

Baked Asparagus with Gremolata

30 minutes or less

Gremolata is an Italian seasoning that combines parsley, garlic, and lemon.

- 1 pound asparagus spears, trimmed
- 1 teaspoon olive oil
- 2 tablespoons fresh bread crumbs
- 1 tablespoon grated Parmesan cheese
- 3 tablespoons chopped fresh parsley
- 1 teaspoon minced garlic
- 1 teaspoon grated lemon zest

1 Preheat oven to 375°F. In an 11 × 7-inch baking dish, toss the asparagus with the oil and arrange in an even layer. Sprinkle with the bread crumbs and Parmesan. Bake at 375°F for 15 minutes, or until the asparagus is tender.

2 To make the gremolata: In a cup, mix the parsley, garlic, and lemon zest. Sprinkle over the asparagus.

Makes 4 servings
Per serving: 2 grams fat • 44 calories

Gremolata

Mix a batch of gremolata and store it in the freezer to add zest to frozen or fresh vegetables. If you don't have fresh parsley handy, use half as much dried parsley.

Mashed Sweet Potatoes

prepare ahead

Try this at Thanksgiving in place of high-cal candied yams (you can easily double or triple the recipe). It'll become a new family favorite.

> 2   large sweet potatoes (about 1 pound each)
> ¼   cup fat-free plain yogurt
> 3   tablespoons Grade B maple syrup
> 3   tablespoons orange juice

1 Bake the potatoes at 375°F for 1 hour, or until easily pierced with a fork. Slice in half lengthwise. Scoop out the pulp, leaving a ¼-inch shell. Reserve the shells and transfer the pulp to a large bowl.

2 Mash the pulp until smooth and stir in the yogurt, maple syrup, and orange juice. Season with salt and pepper. Spoon the filling into the reserved shells. Return to the oven and bake for 10 minutes to heat through.

Makes 6 servings
Per serving: 0 grams fat • 154 calories

 To make ahead, fill the shells and refrigerate until ready to use. Pop into a 400°F oven for 30 minutes, or until piping hot.

Baked Stuffed Acorn Squash

prepare ahead

Fresh sage gives the apricot stuffing authentic Thanksgiving flavor—any time of the year.

¼ cup chopped dried apricots
¼ cup hot water
2 small acorn squash
1 teaspoon oil
½ pound mushrooms, cleaned and sliced
½ cup chopped onion
¼ cup chopped fresh parsley
2 tablespoons slivered unsalted almonds
1 teaspoon chopped fresh sage or ½ teaspoon dried sage
1 cup fresh bread crumbs

1 In a small bowl, mix the apricots and water. Set aside to soak.

2 Cut the squash in half lengthwise. Scoop out and discard the seeds. Place the squash, cut sides down, on a foil-lined baking sheet and bake at 350°F for 15 minutes. Transfer, cut sides up, to a baking dish large enough to hold the halves in a single layer.

3 Warm the oil in a large nonstick skillet over medium heat. Add the mushrooms and onion; cook for 5 minutes, or until the onion is soft. Stir in the parsley, almonds, and sage; cook for 1 minute.

4 Remove from the heat and stir in the bread crumbs and apricots (with soaking water). Season with salt and pepper.

5 Divide the mixture among the squash cavities. Mist with nonstick cooking spray. Bake for 20 minutes, or until the squash is easily pierced with a fork.

Makes 4 servings
Per serving: 4 grams fat • 198 calories

 Acorn and other winter squash have very hard skin that makes cutting difficult. To soften the rind, microwave whole squash on high power for 1 to 2 minutes; let stand for 3 minutes. Use a meat cleaver and a rubber mallet for cutting and be sure to work on a sturdy surface.

Lean and Mean Mashed Potatoes

Yukon gold potatoes have creamy, yellow-tinged flesh that looks like it's already full of butter. Adding low-fat buttermilk and fat-free sour cream to these mashed spuds completes the illusion.

2	pounds Yukon gold potatoes, cut into 1-inch cubes
1	cup low-fat buttermilk
½	cup fat-free sour cream
¼	cup chopped fresh parsley
1	tablespoon chopped fresh chives

1 Place the potatoes in a large saucepan and add cold water to cover by 1 inch. Bring to a boil over high heat. Reduce the heat to medium and cook for 15 to 20 minutes, or until the potatoes are tender when tested with a sharp knife. Drain and return to the saucepan. Off heat, mash with a potato masher until almost smooth.

2 In a small saucepan, mix the buttermilk, sour cream, parsley, and chives. Whisk over low heat for 3 minutes, or until just warm; do not boil. Pour the mixture over the potatoes and mash until thoroughly incorporated. Season with salt and pepper.

Makes 6 servings
Per serving: 1 gram fat • 189 calories

Crispy Beer Batter Onion Rings

30 minutes or less • freeze

Who says you can't have onion rings! You can even prep them ahead of time. Just do the pan frying, arrange the rings on the baking sheets, and refrigerate until you are ready to pop them into the oven.

3 large onions
1 cup all-purpose flour
1 teaspoon paprika
1 cup beer
1 tablespoon vegetable oil

1 Cut the onions crosswise into ½-inch slices and separate into rings.

2 Mix the flour and paprika in a large bowl; season with salt and pepper. Using a whisk, stir in the beer until the foam subsides.

3 Lightly coat 2 baking sheets with nonstick cooking spray. Warm the oil in a large nonstick skillet over medium-high heat.

4 Add the onion rings to the batter and toss to coat evenly. Using tongs, lift out a few onion rings at a time, allowing the excess batter to drip off. Place the onions in a single layer in the hot skillet and fry for 1 minute on each side, or until browned. Transfer the browned rings to the baking sheets. Bake at 425°F for 8 minutes, or until crisp.

Makes 6 servings
Per serving: 3 grams fat • 145 calories

Creamy Coleslaw

30 minutes or less • prepare ahead

Easy, tangy, and low in fat—what more could you ask?

2 cups shredded green or red cabbage
¼ cup chopped green sweet pepper
1 tablespoon finely chopped onion
3 tablespoons fat-free mayonnaise
3 tablespoons fat-free sour cream
1 tablespoon fresh lemon juice
2 teaspoons sugar
1½ teaspoons cider vinegar
½ teaspoon celery seeds

1 In a large bowl, mix the cabbage, pepper, and onion.

2 In a small bowl, whisk together the mayonnaise, sour cream, lemon juice, sugar, vinegar, and celery seeds. Season with salt and pepper. Pour over the cabbage and toss to coat.

Makes about 2½ cups • Serving size: ½ cup
Per serving: 0 grams fat • 34 calories

dessert
tonight

Banana Ice Cream

30 minutes or less • freeze

If you like bananas, and you like ice cream (who doesn't?), you'll love this dessert. It's as good as and as close to the real thing as you can get without adding a speck of fat.

 2 very ripe medium bananas
 ¼ cup lemon juice
 2 tablespoons fat-free vanilla yogurt
 1 teaspoon vanilla extract

1 Peel the bananas and rub the flesh with the lemon juice. Wrap each banana separately in aluminium foil and freeze for at least 2 hours.

2 Break the bananas in pieces and place in a blender or food processor. Add the yogurt and vanilla and blend until smooth.

Makes 2 servings
Per serving: 0 grams fat • 134 calories

Chocolate-Covered Strawberries

30 minutes or less • prepare ahead

This special treat satisfies your fat tooth without risking your diet. These can also be served at the end of a special meal. For the best presentation and to make dipping easier, try to buy strawberries with stems and leave the stems on.

4   ounces semisweet chocolate
24   strawberries

1 Break up the chocolate and place in a small bowl. Microwave on medium power until the chocolate is melted and thick, about 1 minute.

2 Holding each strawberry by the stem, dip it about halfway into the chocolate, allowing excess chocolate to drip off. Gently set the berries on a baking sheet lined with parchment. Refrigerate until ready to eat.

Makes 24 strawberries • Serving size: 2 strawberries
Per serving: 3 grams fat • 63 calories

Key Lime Pie

30 minutes or less • prepare ahead

The secret to keeping the fat and calories low in this dessert is to forgo the meringue or whipped cream topping—and to eat only a small slice.

1   can (14 ounces) fat-free sweetened condensed milk
2   large egg yolks
½   cup bottled Key lime juice
1   baked graham cracker crust (9 inches)

1 In a large bowl, combine the milk and egg yolks. Beat with an electric mixer on high speed for 3 minutes.

2 Preheat oven to 350°F. Slowly beat in the lime juice and continue to beat for 3 minutes. Pour into the prepared crust. Set on a baking sheet.

3 Bake at 350°F for 5 minutes. Cool and refrigerate for at least 3 hours before cutting.

Makes 8 servings
Per serving: 8 grams fat • 243 calories

 You can buy bottled Key lime juice in specialty food shops and most supermarkets that cater to Latino customers. Make sure to shake the bottle well or the pie filling will not set.

Blueberry Banana Split

30 minutes or less

Two kinds of berries turn a classic into a guiltless treat.

2 large ripe bananas
2 cups low-fat frozen vanilla yogurt
1 cup blueberries
1 cup Fresh Raspberry Sauce (page 300)
¼ cup low-fat crunchy cereal nuggets

Cut the bananas in half crosswise and then in half lengthwise. For each serving, place 2 banana pieces against the sides of a long shallow dessert dish. Top with 2 small scoops (½ cup total) of the frozen yogurt and sprinkle with the blueberries. Drizzle with the raspberry sauce and sprinkle with the nuggets.

Makes 4 servings
Per serving: 3 grams fat • 261 calories

Red, White, and Blue Parfaits

30 minutes or less • prepare ahead

You can enjoy these for breakfast, lunch, or dessert.

1 cup sliced strawberries
2 cups fat-free lemon yogurt
1 cup blueberries
1 cup low-fat granola

1 In a small bowl, mix the strawberries with ½ cup of the yogurt.

2 In a second small bowl, mix the blueberries with ½ cup of the remaining yogurt.

3 Layer the mixtures into 4 parfait glasses as follows: 2 tablespoons strawberries, 2 tablespoons blueberries, 2 tablespoons lemon yogurt, 2 tablespoons granola. Repeat layers.

Makes 4 servings
Per serving: 2 grams fat • 169 calories

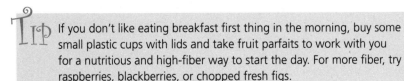

Tip If you don't like eating breakfast first thing in the morning, buy some small plastic cups with lids and take fruit parfaits to work with you for a nutritious and high-fiber way to start the day. For more fiber, try raspberries, blackberries, or chopped fresh figs.

Carrot Cake

prepare ahead

Carrot cake has a good-for-you reputation because it contains carrots, but standard recipes use so much oil that they belong on the forbidden list. Our version uses applesauce as a substitute for oil. You'll never know the difference.

1	cup all-purpose flour
1	cup whole wheat flour
2	teaspoons baking soda
2	teaspoons ground cinnamon
½	teaspoon ground nutmeg
¼	teaspoon ground cloves
6	large egg whites
1⅓	cups sugar
1	cup unsweetened applesauce
½	cup low-fat buttermilk
1½	teaspoons vanilla extract
1	can (8 ounces) crushed pineapple packed in juice
2	cups shredded carrots
½	cup chopped unsalted walnuts

1 In a medium bowl, mix the flours, baking soda, cinnamon, nutmeg, and cloves.

2 Place the egg whites in a large bowl. Beat with an electric mixer on high speed until soft peaks form. Reduce the speed and slowly beat in the sugar, followed by the applesauce, buttermilk, and vanilla.

3 Fold in the flour mixture until just combined, followed by the pineapple (with juice), carrots, and walnuts.

4 Preheat the oven to 350°F. Lightly coat a 13 × 9-inch baking dish with nonstick cooking spray. Add the batter. Bake at 350°F for 40 minutes, or until a toothpick inserted near the center comes out clean. Cool completely on a wire rack.

Makes 20 servings
Per serving: 2 grams fat • 140 calories

Baked Apples

prepare ahead

Less fat makes an old-fashioned treat still as flavorful as grandma's recipe.

4	medium baking apples such as McIntosh or Macoun
¼	cup raisins, coarsely chopped
1	tablespoon chopped toasted unsalted walnuts
2	tablespoons packed dark brown sugar
1	teaspoon ground cinnamon
¼	teaspoon ground cloves
1	tablespoon white wine
	Juice of 1 lemon
1½	teaspoons cornstarch
1	cup orange juice

1 Core the apples using a corer or paring knife and leaving a hole 1 inch wide. Coat a 9 × 9-inch baking dish with nonstick cooking spray and stand the apples in the dish.

2 In a small bowl, mix the raisins, walnuts, brown sugar, cinnamon, and cloves. Stir in the wine and lemon juice. Spoon into the cavities of the apples; if any mixture remains, spoon over the apples.

3 Place the cornstarch in a small bowl. Add the orange juice and stir until smooth. Pour around the apples. Bake at 350°F for 50 to 60 minutes, or until apples are soft when tested with a sharp knife; as the apples bake, occasionally baste them with the pan juices. Serve warm.

Makes 4 servings
Per serving: 2 grams fat • 176 calories

Spiced Apples

30 minutes or less

Serve this alone to satisfy a sweet tooth or spoon it over frozen yogurt.

4	large, firm apples (such as Macoun or Honeycrisp), peeled, cored, and thinly sliced
1	teaspoon vegetable oil
½	cup unsweetened cranberry juice
1	tablespoon packed dark brown sugar
¼	teaspoon ground cinnamon
⅛	teaspoon ground allspice
⅛	teaspoon grated nutmeg

1 In a large nonstick skillet, cook the apples in the oil over medium heat for 10 minutes, or until tender but not mushy. Transfer to a bowl and keep warm.

2 Add the cranberry juice, brown sugar, cinnamon, allspice, and nutmeg to the skillet. Cook over medium-high heat, stirring continuously, for 5 minutes, or until syrupy.

3 Return the apples to the skillet and heat for 1 minute, stirring to glaze the apples.

Makes 4 servings
Per serving: 1 gram fat • 100 calories

Tip Is it a dessert or a side dish? It can be either! These spiced apples are a wonderful complement to baked or grilled pork loin or chops.

Peachy Blueberry Crisp

prepare ahead

Don't worry about making too much of this traditional American dessert. Just reheat by zapping leftovers in the microwave—or enjoy cold. The crisp keeps well for several days.

2	pounds ripe peaches, peeled, pitted, and cut into ½-inch slices
2	cups blueberries
¼	cup sugar
⅓	cup peach nectar
1	tablespoon fresh lemon juice
2	tablespoons + ½ cup all-purpose flour
¼	cup rolled oats
2	tablespoons granulated sugar
2	tablespoons packed brown sugar
½	teaspoon ground cinnamon
3	tablespoons cold butter, cut into small pieces

1 Coat a 9 × 9-inch baking dish with nonstick cooking spray. In a large bowl, mix the peaches, blueberries, sugar, peach nectar, lemon juice, and 2 tablespoons of the flour. Transfer to the baking dish.

2 Preheat oven to 375°F. In a medium bowl, mix the oats, granulated sugar, brown sugar, cinnamon, and the remaining ½ cup flour. Cut in the butter with a pastry blender or 2 knives until the mixture resembles coarse meal. Sprinkle over the fruit.

3 Bake at 375°F for 30 to 35 minutes, or until the fruit is bubbling and the topping is lightly browned.

Makes 8 servings
Per serving: 5 grams fat • 213 calories

 To peel fresh peaches, drop them into boiling water for 20 seconds. Remove with a slotted spoon and run under cold water. The skin will come off easily with a paring knife.

Pineapple-Mango Topping with Frozen Yogurt

30 minutes or less

Try this with any fruit you like. It's best when you use fresh fruit.

1½	cups chopped pineapple
1	mango, peeled and chopped
2	tablespoons fresh lime juice
½	teaspoon coconut extract
2	cups frozen fat-free vanilla yogurt

In a blender or food processor, process the pineapple, mango, lime juice, and coconut extract until smooth. Serve over the frozen yogurt.

Makes 4 servings
Per serving: 0 grams fat • 155 calories

 Mix all of the fruit with the frozen yogurt in a food processor and blend until smooth and creamy. Serve in tall glasses for a refreshing island fruit frappe.

Mixed Fruit with Strawberry-Ginger Sauce

30 minutes or less • prepare ahead

The sauce can be made ahead, but mix it with the berries just before serving. If you don't have berries, most any other fruit will work.

4	cups sliced strawberries
¼	cup orange juice
3	tablespoons chopped crystallized ginger
½	teaspoon vanilla extract
2	cups blackberries
2	cups raspberries
2	cups blueberries

1 In a blender or food processor, combine the strawberries, orange juice, ginger, and vanilla. Process until smooth. Strain into a bowl through a fine-mesh sieve, pressing on the solids with a spatula to extract all the juice.

2 In a large bowl, toss together the blackberries, raspberries, and blueberries. Serve topped with the sauce.

Makes 6 servings
Per serving: 1 gram fat • 126 calories

Sauce alone makes 2 cups • Serving size: ⅓ cup
Per serving: 0 grams fat • 56 calories

Brown Sugar-Grilled Peaches

Save this great dessert for a summer barbecue when the grill is already fired up. Serve as is or cut the recipe in half and ladle over frozen yogurt or sorbet.

4 ripe peaches
1 tablespoon unsalted butter, melted
1 tablespoon packed dark brown sugar
½ cup Fresh Raspberry Sauce (page 300)

1 Cut the peaches in half and remove the pits. Brush the cut sides of the fruit with the butter and sprinkle with the brown sugar.

2 Coat a gas or charcoal grill grate with grilling spray and heat the grill to medium hot. Grill the peaches over indirect heat, cut sides up, for several minutes. Turn and grill until the peaches begin to soften but still hold their shape, making sure they do not burn. Serve warm or at room temperature with the raspberry sauce.

Makes 4 servings
Per serving: 3 grams fat • 91 calories

Strawberry Sauce

30 minutes or less • prepare ahead

This flavor combo makes a great topping for waffles, pancakes, and frozen low-fat desserts.

> 2 cups sliced strawberries
> ½ cup apricot nectar
> 2 tablespoons Grade B maple syrup

Combine the strawberries, apricot nectar, and maple syrup in a food processor. Process until smooth.

Makes about 2 cups • Serving size: ¼ cup
Per serving: 0 grams fat • 35 calories

Fresh Raspberry Sauce

30 minutes or less • prepare ahead • freeze

You won't believe this no-fat dessert sauce tastes so rich.

> ¼ cup raspberry vinegar
> 2 tablespoons balsamic vinegar
> 2 tablespoons water
> 2 tablespoons sugar
> 2 cups raspberries, lightly crushed

Bring the raspberry vinegar, balsamic vinegar, water, and sugar to a boil in a small saucepan over medium heat and stir until the sugar dissolves. Remove from the heat and stir in the raspberries. Serve warm or chilled.

Makes about 2½ cups • Serving size: ¼ cup
Per serving: 0 grams fat • 24 calories

snack

time

Chicken Wingettes

30 minutes or less • prepare ahead

Chicken wings are usually not a diet option because they have fatty skin and tend to be deep-fried. Removing the skin and baking the wings makes a big difference in their fat content. For a snack you can make a batch ahead and keep them refrigerated. Either pop them in the microwave to reheat or serve at room temperature.

12	chicken wing pieces, large joint
¼	cup all-purpose flour
2	large egg whites, lightly beaten
¾	cup dry bread crumbs
½	cup Hot-Hot Sauce (page 329)

1 Remove the skin from the chicken with kitchen shears.

2 Place the flour on a large plate and season with salt and pepper. Place the egg whites in a medium bowl. Place the bread crumbs on a large plate.

3 Roll the chicken in the flour and then dip into the egg whites. Let the excess whites drip off and roll the pieces in the bread crumbs to coat.

4 Coat a baking sheet with nonstick cooking spray. Place the chicken in a single layer on the sheet. Bake at 400°F for 15 minutes, turning once midway. Serve with hot sauce.

Makes 12 pieces • Serving size: 2 pieces
Per serving: 9 grams fat • 213 calories

 Tip The large joint of the wing (sometimes called a drumette) may be hard to find prepackaged in the supermarket, so make a special request to the butcher.

Artichokes and Dip

30 minutes or less

Artichokes are a low-calorie food that get a bad rap because they are usually dipped in butter. They make a great snack or appetizer because the way they are eaten—leaf by leaf—prolongs the time and enjoyment.

4	small artichokes
½	cup fat-free sour cream
½	cup fat-free mayonnaise
¼	cup finely chopped fresh parsley
1	teaspoon dried dill
1	small garlic clove, minced
2	teaspoons Dijon mustard

1 Cut the stems from the artichokes. Snap off any tough leaves near the stem and snip off the prickly tips. Cook in a large pot of boiling water for 15 minutes, or until easily pierced with a sharp knife. Drain.

2 In a small bowl, mix the sour cream, mayonnaise, parsley, dill, garlic, and mustard. Place in individual ramekins.

3 Place each artichoke upright on a serving plate with a ramekin of sauce.

Makes 4 servings
Per serving: 2 grams fat • 121 calories

Sesame Cheese Balls

30 minutes or less • prepare ahead

Eat these cheese balls as a snack or serve as low-fat party fare.

1	cup shredded low-fat sharp cheddar cheese
¼	cup low-fat cream cheese, softened
2	tablespoons fat-free ricotta cheese
1	tablespoon chopped fresh chives
1	tablespoon chopped pimiento
1	teaspoon Worcestershire sauce
2	tablespoons sesame seeds

1 In a medium bowl, mix the cheddar, cream cheese, and ricotta. Stir in the chives, pimiento, and Worcestershire sauce. Cover and refrigerate for at least 1 hour.

2 Form about 2 tablespoons of the cheese mixture into a ball and roll lightly in the sesame seeds. Continue with the rest of the mixture. Refrigerate in a sealed container until ready to use.

Makes 12 balls • Serving size: 1 ball
Per serving: 2 grams fat • 42 calories

Frozen Grapes

For a pop-in-your-mouth snack or a way to take the edge off your appetite, keep frozen grapes on hand. Choose seedless grapes that are plump, fresh looking, and securely attached to their stems. Avoid any with dry, brittle stems or those that are cracked or leaking moisture.

Wash the grapes well and pat completely dry with paper towels. Place small clusters or whole bunches on a baking sheet and set in the freezer for several hours, or until just frozen. Transfer to a plastic bag.

Serving size: 6 grapes
Per serving: 0 gram fat • 20 calories

Stuffed Celery

30 minutes or less • prepare ahead

Fat-free yogurt cheese replaces standard cream cheese in this crunchy retro snack.

½ cup Yogurt Cheese (recipe follows)
1 tablespoon crumbled blue cheese
1 teaspoon caraway seeds
8 celery ribs, cut into thirds
Paprika

In a bowl, mix the yogurt cheese, blue cheese, and caraway seeds. Fill each of the celery pieces with about 1 teaspoon of the cheese mixture. Lightly sprinkle with paprika.

Makes 8 servings
Per serving: 0 gram fat • 20 calories

Yogurt Cheese

This soft cheese is very easy to make and is a tangy stand-in for cream cheese and sour cream. To make Yogurt Cheese, line a strainer with a double layer of cheese-cloth or a coffee filter. Place the strainer over a deep bowl. Spoon two 16-ounce containers of fat-free plain yogurt into the strainer. Place the strainer with the bowl in the refrigerator and let the whey drain from the yogurt. This can take from 12 to 24 hours. The yogurt cheese will be thickened when ready. Discard the whey and transfer the cheese to a container. Cover and store in the refrigerator.

Yield: 2 cups • Serving size: 2 tablespoons
Per serving: 0 grams fat • 20 calories

Green Olive Tapenade

30 minutes or less • prepare ahead

If you love to snack on green olives, try this Mediterranean condiment. The strong, rich flavor satisfies your taste buds with just a modest amount of fat. Eat it as a spread with pita wedges.

1   teaspoon olive oil
1   shallot, finely chopped
2   plum tomatoes, chopped
1   garlic clove, minced
1   teaspoon chopped fresh oregano or ½ teaspoon dried oregano
½   cup white wine
¾   cup pitted green olives, roughly chopped
1   tablespoon grated lemon zest
2   tablespoons chopped fresh parsley

1 Warm the oil in a small nonstick skillet over medium-high heat. Add the shallot and cook for 3 minutes, or until softened. Add the tomatoes, garlic, and oregano; cook for 2 minutes, or until the tomatoes are tender. Add the wine and slowly bring to a boil. Reduce the heat to low and simmer, stirring often, for 5 minutes, or until the liquid has evaporated. (The mixture will be thick.) Transfer the mixture to a medium bowl and let cool completely.

2 Stir in the olives, lemon zest, and parsley. Cover and refrigerate for up to 2 days. Bring to room temperature before using.

Makes about 1½ cups • Serving size: 2 tablespoons
Per serving: 1 gram fat • 47 calories

Low-Fat Hummus

30 minutes or less • prepare ahead

Hummus is a Middle Eastern condiment that's also a great dip for vegetables or pita. It gets its nutty taste from tahini, which is sesame seed paste. This recipe cuts back on the tahini to cut back the fat.

- 1   can (16 ounces) chickpeas
- 2   tablespoons fresh lemon juice
- 2   tablespoons tahini
- 1   garlic clove, minced

Drain the chickpeas, reserving ¼ cup of the liquid. Place the chickpeas and liquid in a food processor. Add the lemon juice, tahini, and garlic. Process until smooth and creamy. Season with salt.

Makes about 2 cups • Serving size: 2 tablespoons
Per serving: 1 gram fat • 39 calories

Make Your Own Tortilla Chips

Low-fat tortilla chips are easy to make. All you have to do is cut commercial soft corn tacos into six wedges and set the wedges on a baking sheet that's lightly coated with nonstick cooking spray. Bake the wedges at 400°F for 5 minutes, turn them, and bake for 5 minutes more, or until brown and crispy. Six chips come in at 60 calories and 1 gram of fat.

Chili Bean Dip

30 minutes or less • prepare ahead

The high fiber in the beans makes this dip filling, so a little goes a long way.

1   can (16 ounces) pink beans
1   teaspoon chili powder
1   teaspoon onion powder
1   teaspoon chopped green jalapeño chile peppers, canned or fresh, ribs and seeds removed
¼   teaspoon cayenne pepper

1 Drain the beans and reserve the liquid.

2 Place the beans in a food processor and puree. Blend in enough bean liquid to form a smooth consistency. Add the chili powder, onion powder, chile peppers, and cayenne. Blend.

Makes about 1 cup • Serving size: ¼ cup
Per serving: 1 gram fat • 102 calories

Horseradish Dip

30 minutes or less • prepare ahead

This zippy sauce is great on a baked potato or as a dip with raw vegetables.

1 cup fat-free plain yogurt
½ cup minced scallions
2 tablespoons prepared white horseradish
2 tablespoons chopped chives

In a small bowl, mix the yogurt, scallions, horseradish, and chives.

Makes about 1½ cups • Serving size: 2 tablespoons
Per serving: 0 grams fat • 16 calories

Creamy Onion Dip

30 minutes or less • prepare ahead

This low-fat version of the party favorite gets fresh taste from cooked onions rather than dried soup mix.

2	cups finely chopped onions
1½	teaspoons olive oil
1	cup fat-free sour cream
1	teaspoon sweet paprika

In a large skillet, cook the onions in the oil over medium heat for 3 minutes, or until barely soft. Transfer to a medium bowl and stir in the sour cream and paprika. Season with salt and pepper. Cover and refrigerate until needed.

Makes about 1 ½ cups • Serving size: ¼ cup
Per serving: 2 grams fat • 72 calories

Tex-Mex Dip

30 minutes or less • prepare ahead

You don't have to suspend your diet when getting together with a crowd. Make this your take-along item.

1	can (16 ounces) fat-free refried beans
½	cup low-fat salsa
1	cup fat-free sour cream
1	cup shredded low-fat Monterey Jack cheese
2	tomatoes, chopped
½	cup Guacamole (page 323)
¼	cup sliced scallions
2	tablespoons chopped black olives
6	pita breads

1 In a medium bowl, mix the beans and salsa. Transfer to a 9-inch platter or pie plate and spread in an even layer.

2 Spread the sour cream on top of the beans. In layers, add the cheese, tomatoes, guacamole, scallions, and olives. Cover and refrigerate until ready to serve.

3 Line a baking sheet with foil and mist with nonstick cooking spray. Cut the pitas into 6 wedges each and pull the layers apart. Arrange the pita wedges on the sheet and mist with the nonstick spray. Broil about 4 inches from the heat for 2 minutes, or until the pita is just crisp. Serve with the bean mixture.

Makes 12 servings
Per serving: 4 grams fat • 190 calories

Trail Mix

30 minutes or less • prepare ahead

If you read the labels on most commercial trail mixes, you know how high in calories this health food can be. Opt to stay on the healthy food track by making your own.

2	cups low-fat granola
1	cup broken thin pretzel sticks
¼	cup sunflower seeds
¼	cup dried pineapple pieces
¼	cup dried cranberries

Spread the granola, pretzels, sunflower seeds, pineapple, and cranberries in a single layer on a nonstick baking sheet. Mist with nonstick cooking spray. Season with salt and pepper. Bake at 350°F for 15 minutes. Cool. Store in a container with a tight-fitting lid for up to 1 week.

Makes about 3 cups • Serving size: ½ cup
Per serving: 3 grams fat • 167 calories

savory salsas

and spreads

Peach-Nectarine Salsa

30 minutes or less • prepare ahead

Try this salsa on just about anything you throw onto the grill, even burgers.

- 2 peaches, peeled, pitted, and chopped
- 2 nectarines, peeled, pitted, and chopped
- ¼ cup minced red onion
- 2 tablespoons chopped fresh mint
- 2 tablespoons chopped fresh cilantro
- 2 teaspoons grated orange zest
- 2 tablespoons fresh orange juice
- 2 tablespoons fresh lime juice

Gently toss together the ingredients in a large bowl. Season with salt and pepper. Cover and refrigerate for at least 30 minutes to allow the flavors to blend.

Makes about 3 cups • Serving size: ¼ cup
Per serving: 0 grams fat • 24 calories

Blueberry Salsa

30 minutes or less • prepare ahead

...roves with age, so make it ahead. It will keep, refrigerated, for

cups fresh or frozen, thawed blueberries, coarsely chopped
¼ cup chopped tomato
½ cup minced red onion
⅓ cup chopped roasted red sweet peppers
¼ cup minced yellow sweet pepper
1 jalapeño pepper, seeded, ribbed, and minced
2 tablespoons chopped fresh basil
2 tablespoons orange juice

...medium bowl, mix the blueberries, tomato, onion, red pepper, yellow pepper, ...peño pepper, basil, and orange juice. Season with salt and pepper. Cover and ...frigerate for at least 1 hour before using.

Makes about 2 cups • Serving size: ¼ cup
Per serving: 0 grams fat • 27 calories

Curried Grape Salsa

30 minutes or less • prepare ahead

The salsa goes well with grilled meats, and it's equally good stirred into rice.

2 tablespoons chopped red sweet pepper
1 teaspoon curry powder
1 teaspoon vegetable oil
1 cup seedless red grapes, coarsely chopped
1 cup seedless green grapes, coarsely chopped
2 tablespoons prepared mango chutney
½ teaspoon finely grated fresh ginger

1 In a small skillet, stir the pepper, curry powder, and oil over medium heat for 2 minutes, or until fragrant. Transfer to a medium bowl.

2 Stir in the grapes, chutney, and ginger. Season with salt and pepper. Refrigerate for at least 1 hour to allow the flavors to blend.

Makes about 2¼ cups • Serving size: ¼ cup
Per serving: 1 gram fat • 37 calories

 Tip Raise or lower the heat in this dish by choosing a hot, medium, or mild curry powder.

Tomato-Pepper Salsa

30 minutes or less • prepare ahead

This is best in summer when the tomatoes and peppers can be picked from the vine. It can be kept in the refrigerator for up to a week.

1	large red sweet pepper, seeded and coarsely chopped
1	small red onion, peeled and quartered
1	small bunch fresh parsley
2	large tomatoes
3	tablespoons red wine vinegar
1	tablespoon fresh lemon juice
1	teaspoon ground cumin

1 Place the sweet pepper, onion, and parsley in a food processor. Pulse until finely chopped.

2 Cut the tomatoes in half crosswise and squeeze out most of the juice and seeds. Chop the tomatoes coarsely, then add to the onion mixture in the food processor. Pulse several times to make a coarse puree. Transfer to a medium bowl and stir in the vinegar and lemon juice.

3 Place the cumin in a small skillet and stir over low heat for 2 to 3 minutes, or until the cumin just starts to smoke. Stir into the salsa and season with salt and pepper. Cover and refrigerate until needed.

Makes about 2½ cups • Serving size: ¼ cup
Per serving: 0 grams fat • 22 calories

Zesty

30 minutes or

Great with pork, this salsa can be served

1	can (16 ounces) black beans, r
2	large tomatoes, seeded and finel
1	large onion, peeled and finely cho
½	cup minced fresh cilantro
3	tablespoons balsamic vinegar
1	tablespoon minced chile peppers

In a medium bowl, mix the beans, tomatoes, onion, cilantro,
Cover and let stand about 30 minutes at room temperature. C
until ready to use.

Makes about 3 cups • Serving size: ¼ cup
Per serving: 0 grams fat • 40 calories

This salsa im
several days

1¹

In a
jala
re

Pineapple Salsa

30 minutes or less • prepare ahead

You'll like this on grilled or poached chicken, fish, and even roast pork.

1	can (20 ounces) pineapple chunks packed in juice, drained
1	cucumber, peeled, seeded, and chopped
½	green sweet pepper, cored, seeded, and chopped
1	small red onion, peeled and chopped
¼	cup finely chopped fresh cilantro
1	tablespoon minced fresh ginger
3	tablespoons fresh lime juice
1 to 3	teaspoons packed light brown sugar

In a medium bowl, mix the pineapple, cucumber, pepper, onion, cilantro, ginger, and lime juice. Stir in 1 teaspoon of the brown sugar and taste for sweetness. Add more, if desired.

Makes about 2 cups • *Serving size: ¼ cup*
Per serving: 0 grams fat • **37 calories**

Banana Chutney

30 minutes or less • prepare ahead

You'll get the best flavor from this chutney if you make it the night before. Let it stand for 30 minutes at room temperature and then refrigerate. It will keep for 2 or 3 days.

1	large ripe banana, chopped
½	cup chopped red or green sweet pepper
¼	cup chopped onion
1½	tablespoons packed light brown sugar
1	tablespoon grated lime zest
3	tablespoons fresh lime juice
1	teaspoon olive oil
	Salt and ground black pepper

In a medium bowl, mix the banana, sweet pepper, onion, brown sugar, lime zest and juice, and oil. Season with salt and pepper. Allow the flavors to blend at room temperature for 30 minutes before serving.

Makes about 1 ½ cups • Serving size: ¼ cup
Per serving: 1 gram fat • 48 calories.

Peach Chutney

prepare ahead

The flavor of this chutney is a great complement to grilled or baked chicken breasts. The peaches should be very ripe.

¼ cup honey
¼ cup white vinegar
¼ cup minced onion
¼ cup minced golden raisins
1 tablespoon minced fresh ginger
¼ teaspoon ground cumin
4 ripe peaches, peeled, pitted, and coarsely chopped

1 In a medium saucepan, mix the honey, vinegar, onion, raisins, ginger, and cumin. Simmer for 10 minutes.

2 Add the peaches and simmer for 30 minutes, or until thick. Cool. Store in a tightly covered container in the refrigerator. Serve warm or cold.

Makes about 2 cups • Serving size: ¼ cup
Per serving: 0 grams fat • 69 calories

Tomato Chutney

30 minutes or less • prepare ahead

Serve this mildly spicy accompaniment with any type of meat or poultry. It's big on flavor but light in calories.

4	large tomatoes, seeded and finely chopped
½	cup minced onion
½	cup minced celery
1	tablespoon apple juice
1	bay leaf
1	apple, peeled, cored, and chopped
¼	cup cider vinegar
½	teaspoon ground cinnamon
¼	teaspoon ground allspice

1 In a medium saucepan, mix the tomatoes, onion, celery, apple juice, and bay leaf. Simmer over medium heat for 5 minutes.

2 Add the apple, vinegar, cinnamon, and allspice. Partially cover and simmer, stirring frequently, for 40 minutes, or until thick. Cool. Discard the bay leaf.

3 Refrigerate in a tightly sealed container until ready to use.

Makes about 2 cups • Serving size: 2 tablespoons
Per serving: 0 grams fat • 16 calories

Guacamole

30 minutes or less

Tomatillos, Mexican "green tomatoes," replace half of the avocados to bring down the fat and calorie content of this popular condiment. Have the other ingredients ready to go before you peel the avocados to prevent the fruit from discoloring when exposed to air.

  2   small ripe avocados, halved, pitted, and peeled
  4   tomatillos, peeled, rinsed, and chopped
  1   medium tomato, seeded and chopped
 ½   cup chopped onion
  2   jalapeño peppers, ribbed, seeded, and finely chopped
  1   tablespoon fresh lime juice
  1   garlic clove, minced
 ¼   teaspoon salt
 ⅛   teaspoon cayenne pepper

In a medium glass or ceramic bowl, mash the avocados with a fork. Add the tomatillos, tomato, onion, jalapeño peppers, lime juice, garlic, salt, and cayenne; mix well. Cover and refrigerate until ready to use, up to 2 days.

Makes about 2½ cups • Serving size: ¼ cup
Per serving: 5.5 grams fat • 70 calories

Cranberry-Walnut Spread

prepare ahead

Enjoy this on turkey sandwiches piled high with crunchy vegetables on whole grain bread.

1   can (15 ounces) whole-berry cranberry sauce
4   ounces reduced-fat cream cheese, at room temperature
2   tablespoons chopped unsalted walnuts

1 Place the cranberry sauce in a strainer set over a medium bowl. Press on the sauce with the back of a spoon until most of the juice is extracted. Discard the juice and transfer the sauce to a blender or food processor.

2 Add the cream cheese and blend until smooth.

3 Pour into a small bowl and stir in the walnuts. Refrigerate until needed.

Makes about 1 cup • Serving size: 1 tablespoon
Per serving: 2 grams fat • 62 calories

Bean and Red Pepper Spread

30 minutes or less • prepare ahead

This spread is very versatile. It tastes great stuffed into celery.

1   cup rinsed and drained canned Great Northern beans
3   tablespoons finely chopped red sweet pepper
2   scallions, finely chopped

Place the beans in a medium bowl and mash with a potato masher. Stir in the pepper and scallions. Cover and store in the refrigerator for up to 1 week.

Makes about 1¼ cups • Serving size: 1 tablespoon
Per serving: 0 grams fat • 16 calories

Thousand Island Dressing

30 minutes or less • prepare ahead

What an effortless way to perk up the flavor of plain mayo. Use on most any kind of sandwich or burger where you want an extra bit of zing.

½ cup fat-free mayonnaise
¼ cup minced shallots
¼ cup chili sauce
1 tablespoon sweet pickle relish

In a small bowl, mix the mayonnaise, shallots, chili sauce, and relish. Chill before serving.

Makes about 1 cup • Serving size: 2 tablespoons
Per serving: 0 grams fat • 30 calories

Roasted Garlic Puree

It's hard to imagine eating garlic by the clove until you've tasted it baked to a soft and smooth consistency. Its pungency gives way to a sweet and succulent taste, making it a great substitute for butter. You can also toss it into vegetables, pasta dishes, and salad dressings. Or you can eat it just so, if you desire.

The puree keeps for up to 2 weeks in the refrigerator, so make a big batch.

6 large whole garlic heads
2 tablespoons oil
   Dried thyme

1 With a sharp knife, slice off the top of each head of garlic to expose the inner cloves. Remove any loose skin, but remove as little as possible.

2 Place the garlic heads on a large square of foil. Drizzle 1 tablespoon of the oil over top and sprinkle lightly with the thyme. Wrap tightly and place on a baking sheet. Bake at 350°F for 50 to 60 minutes, or until the garlic is soft when pierced with a fork. Allow the cloves to cool.

3 Squeeze the garlic cloves out of their skin and mash them with a fork. Place the puree in a small glass container and pour the remaining 1 tablespoon oil on top. Cover and refrigerate the puree; use as needed.

Makes about 1 cup • Serving size: 1 tablespoon
Per serving: 1.7 grams fat • 35 calories

Chile Mayonnaise

30 minutes or less • prepare ahead

This mayo is a great topping for chicken, fish, and burgers. If you prefer it hot, increase the number of chiles or simply include the seeds from the peppers.

> 1 cup reduced-calorie mayonnaise
> 1 can (4 ounces) chile peppers, seeded, drained, and finely chopped

Combine the mayonnaise and chiles.

Makes 1¼ cups • Serving size: 1 tablespoon
Per serving: 5 grams fat • 53 calories

Hot-Hot Sauce

30 minutes or less • prepare ahead

The habanero is among the world's hottest peppers, in the same family with the Scotch bonnet used traditionally in Jamaican cooking. Need we say more? Remember to wash your hands immediately after working with the peppers.

2	habanero peppers, seeded and chopped
½	green sweet pepper, cored, seeded, and chopped
1	small onion, peeled and quartered
2	scallions, chopped
3	garlic cloves, peeled
½	cup packed fresh cilantro or parsley
½	teaspoon dried oregano
¼	cup olive oil
¼	cup water
3	tablespoons balsamic vinegar
	Salt and ground black pepper

1 In a food processor, combine the peppers, onion, scallions, garlic, cilantro, and oregano. Process until uniformly chopped.

2 With the processor running, pour in the oil, water, and vinegar; process until smooth. Season with salt and pepper.

Makes about 1 cup • Serving size: 1 tablespoon
Per serving: 3 grams fat • 37 calories

To tame the fire, use the much milder Anaheim chile in place of the incendiary habanero.

Tartar Sauce

30 minutes or less • prepare ahead

Use as a spread for grilled chicken sandwiches or as a dipping sauce for Fish Sticks (page 198). Either way, use sparingly.

¾ cup low-fat mayonnaise
3 tablespoons minced dill pickle
2 tablespoons minced fresh parsley
1 tablespoon fresh lemon juice
2 teaspoons chopped capers

In a small bowl, mix the mayonnaise, pickle, parsley, lemon juice, and capers.

Makes about 1 cup • Serving size: 1 tablespoon
Per serving: 2 grams fat • 16 calories

no-guilt
salad dressings

Balsamic Mustard Dressing

30 minutes or less • prepare ahead

At less than 10 calories and zero fat per serving, this dressing is good to have on hand.

⅔ cup balsamic vinegar
2 tablespoons Dijon mustard
½ teaspoon seasoned salt
½ teaspoon sugar

In a small bowl, whisk together the vinegar, mustard, salt, and sugar.

Makes about ¾ cup • Serving size: 2 tablespoons
Per serving: 0 grams fat • 9 calories

Raspberry Walnut Dressing

30 minutes or less • prepare ahead

This dressing is refreshing on salad greens or drizzled over a mixed fruit salad.

  6   tablespoons orange juice
  ¼   cup raspberry vinegar
  2   tablespoons olive oil
  2   tablespoons chopped unsalted walnuts
  1   teaspoon grated lime zest
  2   tablespoons fresh lime juice
  1   tablespoon chopped fresh basil
  ½   teaspoon dry mustard

In a small bowl, whisk together the orange juice, vinegar, oil, walnuts, lime zest and juice, basil, and mustard. Season with salt and pepper.

Makes about 1 cup • Serving size: 2 tablespoons
Per serving: 5 grams fat • 50 calories

Basil-Cream Dressing

30 minutes or less • prepare ahead

Nice over a chef's salad. Bring to room temperature and shake well before pouring. Transfer to a jar and refrigerate until needed.

1   cup low-fat cottage cheese
1   cup fat-free plain yogurt
3   tablespoons grated Parmesan cheese
2   tablespoons fresh lemon juice
1   tablespoon honey
2   teaspoons Dijon mustard
2   teaspoons minced shallot
1   teaspoon dried basil

Place the cottage cheese in a food processor and process until smooth. Transfer to a medium bowl. Whisk in the yogurt, cheese, lemon juice, honey, mustard, shallot, and basil. Season with salt and pepper.

Makes about 2 cups • Serving size: 2 tablespoons
Per serving: 1 gram fat • 30 calories

Creamy Dijon Dressing

30 minutes or less • prepare ahead

Sour cream is what makes this standard dressing creamy and rich. Here fat-free yogurt stands in as the substitute, and the result is just as luscious.

¾	cup fat-free plain yogurt
½	cup fat-free chicken broth
2	tablespoons Dijon mustard
1½	teaspoons sugar
2	teaspoons dried tarragon
2	garlic cloves, peeled and minced
½	teaspoon salt

In a medium bowl, whisk together the yogurt, broth, mustard, sugar, tarragon, garlic, and salt. Let stand at room temperature for 30 minutes to blend the flavors. Transfer to a jar and store in the refrigerator until needed.

Makes about 1 ½ cups • Serving size: 2 tablespoons
Per serving: 0 grams fat • 18 calories

Creamy Italian Dressing

30 minutes or less • prepare ahead

Make sure to use low-fat Parmesan—it makes a big fat difference.

½ cup fat-free plain yogurt
½ cup fat-free sour cream
¼ cup grated low-fat Parmesan cheese
1 tablespoon fresh lemon juice
1 teaspoon minced garlic

In a small bowl, whisk together the yogurt, sour cream, cheese, lemon juice, and garlic. Let stand at room temperature for 30 minutes to blend the flavors. Transfer to a jar and store in the refrigerator until needed.

Makes about 1 ¼ cups • Serving size: 2 tablespoons
Per serving: 0.6 grams fat • 18 calories

Creamy Raspberry Dressing

prepare ahead

This dressing is refreshing on salad greens or drizzled over a mixed fruit salad.

- 1 cup fat-free plain yogurt
- 1 bag (10 ounces) frozen unsweetened raspberries thawed and drained
- ¼ teaspoon grated lime zest
- ¼ teaspoon grated orange zest
- 1 tablespoon honey
- ¼ teaspoon dried basil

1 Line a strainer with cheesecloth. Add the yogurt and drain over a bowl for 30 minutes. Transfer to a medium bowl.

2 In a food processor, blend the raspberries, zests, honey, and basil until smooth. Add to the yogurt and mix well.

Makes about 1½ cups • Serving size: 2 tablespoons
Per serving: 0 grams fat • 28 calories

Honey-Lime Dressing

30 minutes or less • prepare ahead

Use this for a salad, but it is also nice drizzled over melon or steamed asparagus, broccoli, or green beans.

½ teaspoon grated lime zest
½ cup fresh lime juice
½ cup egg substitute
2 tablespoons honey
2 tablespoons white wine vinegar
1 teaspoon dry mustard
½ cup oil

1 In a blender or food processor, process the lime zest and juice, egg substitute, honey, vinegar, and mustard until smooth.

2 With the machine running, slowly add the oil. Season with salt and pepper.

Makes about 1¾ cups • Serving size: 1 tablespoon
Per serving: 4 grams fat • 44 calories

 This dressing will keep in a sealed container in the refrigerator 1 week.

Oriental Ginger Dressing

30 minutes or less • prepare ahead

You can even use this thick and creamy dressing as a dip.

1	teaspoon arrowroot powder
3	tablespoons seasoned rice vinegar
¼	cup fat-free chicken broth
¼	cup pineapple juice
2	tablespoons honey
1	tablespoon soy sauce
1	tablespoon toasted sesame oil
1	teaspoon grated fresh ginger
1	teaspoon minced garlic

In a small saucepan, dissolve the arrowroot in the vinegar. Whisk in the broth, pineapple juice, honey, soy sauce, oil, ginger, and garlic. Cook over medium heat, whisking, for 5 minutes, or until slightly thickened. Cool, transfer to a jar, and store in the refrigerator until needed.

Makes about 1 cup • Serving size: 2 tablespoons
Per serving: 2 grams fat • 39 calories

 Arrowroot is a thickening agent traditionally used in Asian cooking.

Poppy Seed Dressing

30 minutes or less • prepare ahead

Poppy seeds, with their slightly nutty taste and aroma, have been popular as a condiment since as early as the 1st century. This dressing is especially good with any salad that contains fruit.

¼ cup sugar
6 tablespoons orange juice
3 tablespoons raspberry vinegar
2 tablespoons minced shallot
1 tablespoon oil
1 teaspoon honey
½ teaspoon dry mustard
2 teaspoons poppy seeds
¼ teaspoon salt
¼ teaspoon ground black pepper

In a small bowl, whisk together the sugar, orange juice, vinegar, shallot, oil, honey, and mustard until the sugar dissolves. Whisk in the poppy seeds, salt, and pepper.

Makes about 1 cup • Serving size: 2 tablespoons
Per serving: 2 grams fat • 54 calories

Garlic Vinaigrette

30 minutes or less • prepare ahead

Vinaigrette is somewhat of a misnomer because classically made versions are oil based. This version cuts the fat and calories in half. Make it a staple of your maintenance program—there is no reason to go back to the full-fat variety.

1   garlic head, separated into cloves and peeled
½   cup water
½   cup red wine vinegar
1   teaspoon honey
¼   cup extra-virgin olive oil

1 Place the garlic and water in a small saucepan. Bring to a boil, reduce the heat to medium-low, and simmer for 15 minutes, or until the garlic is tender and the liquid is reduced to about 2 tablespoons. Pour into a small sieve set over a bowl.

2 With a wooden spoon, mash the garlic through the sieve and into the bowl. Whisk in the vinegar, honey, and oil. Season with salt and pepper.

Makes about 1 cup • Serving size: 2 tablespoons
Per serving: 7 grams fat • 71 calories

Orange Vinaigrette

30 minutes or less • prepare ahead

The orange flavor adds zip to field greens or a medley of fruit.

¾   cup orange juice
2   tablespoons champagne vinegar
1   teaspoon olive oil

In a small bowl, whisk together the orange juice, vinegar, and oil. Season with salt and pepper.

Makes about 1 cup • Serving size: 2 tablespoons
Per serving: 1 gram fat • 16 calories

recipes by phase

Aloha Fruit Salad with Macadamia Crunch

Arizona Jerk Turkey

Artichokes and Dip

Asparagus Omelet with Summer Herbs

Autumn Bean and Squash Stew

Baked Apples

Baked Asparagus with Gremolata

Balsamic Mustard Dressing

Banana Chutney

Banana Ice Cream

Banana-Nut Hotcakes

Basil-Cream Dressing

Bean and Red Pepper Spread

Beef and Vegetable Stew

Blueberry Muffins

Blueberry Salsa

Boston Baked Beans

Boston Clam Chowder

Buttery Squash Soup

Carrot Cake

Carrot-Raisin Bran Muffins

Chicken Fingers

Chicken Pot Pie

Chili Bean Dip

Chocolate-Covered Strawberries

Classic Spinach Salad

Cod and Tomato Stew

Cranberry Muffins

Creamy Coleslaw

Creamy Dijon Dressing

Creamy Italian Dressing

Creamy Raspberry Dressing

Curried Grape Salsa

Drunken Pork Chops

French Onion Soup

Fresh Raspberry Sauce

Frozen Grapes

Garlic-Lemon Spinach

Glazed Carrots

Green Olive Tapenade

Gremolata

Grilled Chicken Caesar Salad

Grilled Chicken Salad Véronique

Grilled Citrus-Scented Swordfish with Ginger

Grilled Cowboy Steaks with Secret Sauce and Tomato Topping

Grilled Lamb Chops with Grilled Grapes

Grilled Marinated Eggplant

Grilled Pineapple Chicken Sandwich

Grilled Vegetables with Garlic Vinaigrette

Hoagie Dressing

Horseradish Dip

Hot and Cold Melon Soup

Hot Grilled Tuna Kebabs

Lean and Mean Mashed Potatoes

Little Caesar Salad

Low-Fat Hummus

Make Your Own Tortilla Chips

Mashed Sweet Potatoes

Mixed Fruit with Strawberry-Ginger Sauce

Moroccan Vegetable Stew

Mussels Marinière

Mussels Marinière over Pasta

Navy Bean Soup

Orange Vinaigrette

Orzo with Cherry Tomatoes, Capers, and Pine Nuts

Oven-Fried Chicken

Pasta with Cherry Tomatoes and Parsley

Peach Chutney

Peach-Nectarine Salsa

Pineapple Salsa

Pineapple-Mango Topping with Frozen Yogurt

Pita Sandwiches to Go

Portobello Burgers

Red, White, and Blue Parfaits

Roast Chicken with Winter Vegetables

Roasted Chicken Salad with Raspberry Vinaigrette

Roasted Garlic Puree

Seared Scallops with Asparagus and Ginger

Shrimp Caesar Salad

Shrimp Salad Sandwiches

Sizzlin' Shrimp with Black-Eyed Peas

Skinny Chef's Salad

Southern Red Beans and Rice

Spiced Apples

Spinach Risotto

Spinach-Stuffed Mushrooms

Stir-Fried Pork with Apples and Figs

Strawberry Sauce

Stuffed Celery

Sweet and Spicy Shrimp

Sweet Potato Jacks with Cinnamon-Apple Topping

Texas Black Bean Soup

Thousand Island Dressing

Tomato and Zucchini Gratin

Tomato and Zucchini Gratin with Rice

Tomato Chutney

Tomato-Corn Bisque

Tomato-Pepper Salsa

Tuna Burgers with Wasabi Mayonnaise

Tuna Noodle Casserole

Turkey Sloppy Joes

Two-Potato Bisque

Ukrainian Borscht

Veal Scallops with Fennel and Grapes

Vegetable Risotto

Warm Potato and Tuna Salad

Wild Rice Salad

Wilted Spinach Salad

Yogurt Cheese

Zesty Bean Salsa

Include all Phase 1 Recipes in addition to the ones below.

Asparagus Soup

Baked Halibut with Red Pepper and Parsley Crust

Baked Stuffed Acorn Squash

Beef Stroganoff

Braised Cabbage with Apples

Brown Sugar-Grilled Peaches

California Fruit Salad

Caribbean Fish Stew

Chambord Compote

Cheesy Broccoli

Chicken Fingers with Honey Mustard Sauce

Chicken Paprikash

Chicken Soup with Soba Noodles

Chili-Spiced Tuna with Grilled Tomato Sauce

Crab Cakes with Red Pepper Sauce

Cranberry-Walnut Spread

Creamed Spinach

Creamy Onion Dip

Crispy Beer Batter Onion Rings

Eggs-and-Potato Hash

Fish Sticks

Fisherman's Stew

Garden Peas with Fresh Mint

Greek Lamb Kabobs

Grilled Cheese and Bacon

Grilled Margarita Chicken

Grilled Marinated Swordfish

Grilled Portobello Mushrooms

Grilled Tofu Burgers

Linguine with Clam Sauce

Lunch-Box Tuna Salad Sandwich

Mac and Cheese

Nachos

Oriental Ginger Dressing

Poached Chicken with Avocado Sauce

Poppy Seed Dressing

Raisin Bran Muffins with Orange Glaze

Rosemary Roasted New Potatoes

Sauteed Chicken with Cider Sauce

Seafood au Gratin

Seafood Jambalaya

Sesame Cheese Balls

Spaghetti with Fresh Mushrooms and Red Sauce

Spaghetti with Summer Tomatoes, Basil, and Garlic

Spinach Pesto with Penne and Peas

Stir-Fried Pork and Greens

Super Quick Pumpkin Soup

Tartar Sauce

Texas-Style Stuffed Peppers

Trail Mix

Tropical Rice

Turkey Burgers

Veal Marsala

Vegetarian Chili

Waffles with Strawberry Sauce

Warm Eggplant, Tomato, and Mozzarella Salad

Warm Potato and Tuna Salad

Include all Phase 1 and 2 Recipes in addition to the ones below.

Almond Pumpkin Breakfast Bread

Baby Greens with Avocado,
Strawberries, and Walnuts

Blueberry Banana Split

Brook Trout with Tomato and
Red Onion Relish

Cheddar-Stuffed Acorn Squash

Chicken Fajitas

Chicken Wingettes

Chilean Sea Bass en Papillote

Chili Mac

Chile Mayonnaise

Cornish Game Hens with
Apricot Stuffing

Field Greens with Pears and Walnuts

Garlic Vinaigrette

Greek Salad

Grilled Shrimp with Corn-and-
Tomato Salad

Guacamole

Hero's Hoagie

Honey-Lime Dressing

Hot-Hot Sauce

Key Lime Pie

London Broil Two Ways

Mini Pizzas Two Ways

Pan-Seared Red Snapper with
Olive Crust

Pasta Carbonara

Pasta Primavera

Peachy Blueberry Crisp

Pecan Waffles with Strawberry Sauce

Penne with Broccoli and Cheese

Petite Filet with Caramelized Onions

Poached Salmon Two Ways

Raspberry-Walnut Dressing

Ratatouille Omelet

Sesame Fried Tofu

Spaghetti and Meatballs

Spaghetti with Summer Squash

Steak Kebabs

Stuffed Bell Peppers

Tex-Mex Dip

Turkey Loaf

Vegetarian Antipasto

Watercress and Strawberry Salad

index